Focus on Exercise and Health Research

Focus on Exercise and Health Research

Thomas B. Selkirk
Editor

Nova Biomedical Books
New York

Copyright © 2006 by Nova Science Publishers, Inc.

All rights reserved. No part of this book may be reproduced, stored in a retrieval system or transmitted in any form or by any means: electronic, electrostatic, magnetic, tape, mechanical photocopying, recording or otherwise without the written permission of the Publisher.

For permission to use material from this book please contact us:
Telephone 631-231-7269; Fax 631-231-8175
Web Site: http://www.novapublishers.com

NOTICE TO THE READER

The Publisher has taken reasonable care in the preparation of this book, but makes no expressed or implied warranty of any kind and assumes no responsibility for any errors or omissions. No liability is assumed for incidental or consequential damages in connection with or arising out of information contained in this book. The Publisher shall not be liable for any special, consequential, or exemplary damages resulting, in whole or in part, from the readers' use of, or reliance upon, this material.

This publication is designed to provide accurate and authoritative information with regard to the subject matter covered herein. It is sold with the clear understanding that the Publisher is not engaged in rendering legal or any other professional services. If legal or any other expert assistance is required, the services of a competent person should be sought. FROM A DECLARATION OF PARTICIPANTS JOINTLY ADOPTED BY A COMMITTEE OF THE AMERICAN BAR ASSOCIATION AND A COMMITTEE OF PUBLISHERS.

Library of Congress Cataloging-in-Publication Data
    Available upon request

ISBN 1-59454-349-6

Published by Nova Science Publishers, Inc. ✛ New York

Contents

Preface		vii
Chapter I	Aerobic Physical Exercise Improves Membrane Fluidity of Erythrocytes in Hypertensive and Normotensive Subjects - An Electron Paramagnetic Resonance Study *Kazushi Tsuda*	1
Chapter II	Exercise and Cognition: Theoretical and Empirical Evidence for an Interaction Effect from an Integrated Cognitive Psychology/ Neuroscientific Perspective *Terry McMorris*	17
Chapter III	Exercise-Induced Oxidative Stress and Lipid Peroxidation: The Exercise Paradox *David Alexander Leaf and Michael Kleinman*	61
Chapter IV	Postprandial Lipid Metabolism and Exercise: Recent Findings and Future Directions *Christina Koutsari*	93
Chapter V	Hypothalamo-Pituitary-Adrenal Axis Adaptation to Repeated and Prolonged Exercise-Induced Cortisol Secretion in Endurance Training: Physiology is the First Target *Duclos Martine*	131
Chapter VI	The Efficacy of Psyching-Up on Strength Performance *David Tod and Michael McGuigan*	163
Chapter VII	Exercise-Induced Cardiovascular Adjustments by Muscle Receptors Stimulation *Antonio Crisafulli and Alberto Concu*	181

Chapter VIII	Thermoregulatory Responses of Athletes with a Spinal Cord Injury to Prolonged Wheelchair Exercise in Cool and Warm Conditions *M. J. Price and I. G. Campbell*	**203**
Chapter IX	Exercise Pathophysiology in Patients with Juvenile Dermatomyositis *Tim Takken, Elisabeth F. Elst and Janjaap van der Net*	**221**
Chapter X	Being From "Away" … Focus on Exercise, Nutrition, and Health Research among Immigrant Older Adults *Shanthi Jacob Johnson*	**239**
Chapter XI	Pregnancy and Exercise: Should Healthy Pregnant Women Actively Train? *Jouko Pirhonen, Elisabeth Rettedal, Tom Hartgill and Pelle Lindqvist*	**251**
Index		**269**

Preface

In the last 50 years significant numbers of men and women take little exercise in the course of their occupation. The computer keyboard, the rise of private transport, the world by television, household "labor saving" devices mean that with the minimal of physical effort people work and play. The benefits of doing regular exercise include a reduced risk of: heart disease, stroke, bowel cancer, breast cancer, osteoporosis, and obesity. In addition, many people feel better in themselves during and after exercise. Regular exercise is also thought to help ease stress, anxiety, and mild depression. This book presents new and important research from around the world dealing with various aspects and impacts of exercise as related to health.

The present study was undertaken to investigate the effects of aerobic physical exercise on membrane functions in hypertensive and normotensive subjects as described in chapter I. Physical exercise within the intensity of anaerobic threshold level was performed twice a week for 6 months to both untreated mild essential hypertensive patients and age-matched normotensive subjects. The membrane fluidity of erythrocytes was examined by means of an electron paramagnetic resonance (EPR) and spin-labeling method before and after the trial period in both groups. After the physical exercise, the blood pressure significantly decreased in the hypertensive group (mean blood pressure: before exercise 111 ± 2 mm Hg, n=8, after exercise 104 ± 1 mm Hg, n=8, $P<0.05$). In the normotensive group, the blood pressure tended to decrease. The order parameter (S) and peak height ratio (h_0/h_{-1}) in the EPR spectra of erythrocytes were significantly reduced after the exercise in both groups (S, hypertensives 0.717 ± 0.004 vs 0.691 ± 0.008, n=8, $P<0.05$, normotensives 0.716 ± 0.005 vs 0.698 ± 0.003, n=8, $P<0.05$, h_0/h_{-1}, hypertensives 5.38 ± 0.06 vs 4.89 ± 0.06, n=8, $P<0.01$, normotensives 5.36 ± 0.06 vs 4.95 ± 0.04, n=8, $P<0.01$), which showed that the exercise increased the membrane fluidity of erythrocytes. In addition, the lower the membrane fluidity of erythrocytes before exercise, the greater the exercise-induced increase in the fluidity (S, $r=-0.72$, n=16, $P<0.05$, h_0/h_{-1}, $r=-0.53$, n=16, $P<0.05$). There was no direct correlation between blood pressure reduction and the exercise-induced increase in the membrane fluidity of erythrocytes. However, the decrease in the peak height ratio (percent changes in h_0/h_{-1}) in the EPR spectra by the exercise was significantly correlated with the changes in fasting plasma insulin level ($r=0.51$, n=16, $P<0.05$). The results of the present study showed that the aerobic physical exercise significantly increased the erythrocyte membrane fluidity in both mild hypertensive and normotensive subjects. The exercise-induced increase in the fluidity might, at least in part, be linked to the changes in plasma insulin levels. Furthermore, the data suggest that the physical exercise might ameliorate membrane functions, which could contribute, at least in part, to the beneficial effects of exercise in both hypertensive and normotensive subjects.

Chapter II examines the empirical and theoretical evidence for an exercise-arousal-cognition interaction effect. Most researchers have claimed that exercise will affect cognition in an inverted-U fashion, in line with the effect of emotionally induced arousal on cognitive performance. Early research has failed to provide much support for such a claim. Results were somewhat equivocal but there is some evidence for a linear improvement in performance for complex tasks during incremental exercise to exhaustion. More recent research has provided some support for the argument that when exercise reaches an intensity that results in a significant increase in plasma concentrations of the catecholamines epinephrine and norepinephrine, there is also significant improvement in cognition. Results are not unequivocal, however. Observation of research, with animals, shows that Central Nervous System concentrations of norepinephrine, dopamine and 5-hydroxytryptomine increase during exercise. As these are brain neurotransmitters it is possible that this increase results in improved cognition during exercise. The equivocal nature of the empirical evidence for such an effect, however, suggests that other factors are involved. An integrated cognitive/neuroscientific model is proposed which shows an interaction between the increased availability of the neurotransmitters in the brain during exercise and the individual's perception of the nature of exercise as a stressor.

The pathogenesis of coronary artery disease (CAD), the leading cause of morbidity and mortality in the United States, is characterized by an underlying inflammatory response that generates free radicals and associated oxidative stress. Although participation in aerobic physical exercise is recommended to reduce CAD risk, a single bout of acute physical exercise generates free radicals and causes oxidative stress that can be measured as increased levels of lipid peroxides. In accordance with the role of oxidative stress in the pathogenesis of CAD we have found that exercise-induced oxidative stress (measured as lipid peroxides) is greater among high risk patients than healthy individuals without CAD. These findings suggest the following paradox; if aerobic exercise causes potentially deleterious oxidative stress, should physical exercise be recommended as a public health measure? Chapter III's findings in high risk populations and studies in healthy subjects by other investigators show physical exercise training reduces oxidative stress. Hence the paradox is solved. Participation in regular physical exercise reduces exercise-induced oxidative stress. This effect should lower the risk for CAD and other disease conditions related to oxidative stress by reducing cumulative burden of oxidative stress accrued during a lifetime of activities of daily living. The mechanism(s) by which aerobic physical exercise causes this effect are numerous and include both exogenous factors such as diet as well as endogenous anti-oxidant systems that may be up-regulated in response to exercise-induced oxidative stress. Further studies are warranted to evaluate the 'anti-oxidant' role of role of physical exercise in reducing CAD risk, and identify the mechanism(s) by which exercise exerts this effect.

In the past two decades, there has been a wealth of evidence for a link between postprandial triacylglycerol (TAG) metabolism and atherosclerosis. Postprandial lipemia predominantly represents the presence in plasma of large TAG-rich lipoproteins (TRL) produced from the intestine (chylomicrons), but also reflects the accumulation of TRL particles of hepatic origin (very low density lipoproteins; VLDL). The precise mechanisms by which postprandial TAG metabolism affect the pathogenesis and progression of coronary heart disease (CHD) have not been elucidated yet but it seems that a constellation of potentially atherogenic lipoprotein changes is involved, including increases in plasma TRL particles and their remnants, decreases in HDL-cholesterol and formation of small dense LDL particles. Chapter IV will present an overview of the current knowledge on postprandial lipid and lipoprotein metabolism, its regulation and link between its impairment and CHD. Exercise performed 12-16 h before a high- or normal-fat mixed meal ameliorates fasting and postprandial TAG concentrations. Important determinants of exercise-induced decreases in postprandial lipemia appear to be exercise timing and the total energy expended during exercise. The reduction in postprandial lipemia is transient, independent of qualitative differences in substrate utilisation during exercise and greater than that attributable to the energy deficit incurred. Although significant progress has been made on the effects of exercise on postprandial lipid metabolism, there are still many questions to be answered. Future directions of research in this important field of human metabolism will be discussed. Exercise represents a potent physiological stimulus upon the hypothalamo-pituitary adrenal (HPA) axis. Glucocorticoids (GC) exert many beneficial actions in exercising humans, increasing availability of metabolic substrates for the need of energy of muscles, maintaining normal vascular integrity and responsiveness and protecting the organism from an overreaction of the immune system in the face of exercise-induced muscle damage. On the other hand, when an acute bout of endurance-exercise is stopped, the hormonal profile is expected to converge towards anabolic processes. However, the authors have previously demonstrated that after a 2-h run, plasma cortisol levels remain significantly increased during almost two hours after the end of the exercise. When training for a marathon race, subjects run an average of 120-180 km/week. This implies daily sessions of prolonged and/or intense running and consequently prolonged phases of endogenous hypercortisolism (*i.e.* during exercise and during post-immediate exercise recovery). Given the antagonistic action of glucocorticoids on muscle anabolic processes as well as their immunosuppressive effects, this has led us to hypothesize that endurance-trained men might develop adaptive mechanisms in order to protect muscle and other GC sensitive tissues against this increased post-exercise cortisol secretion. Indeed, the response to GC is regulated not only by the concentration of GC but also by the availability of cortisol and the sensitivity to GC of the target tissues. Changes in availability and /or sensitivity to GC may explain the discrepancy between repeated and prolonged exercise-induced HPA axis activation and the lack of metabolic consequences of such increased cortisol secretion.

The data on the effects of endurance training on extra-cellular and intra-cellular cortisol availability are discussed. The results provide supports for the adaptation of the HPA axis to repeated and prolonged exercise-induced increases in cortisol secretion. It is an exciting challenge to understand the differences between the effects of repeated exercise-induced cortisol secretion in well-adapted athletes and the deleterious effects (metabolic, endocrine, cardiovascular) of the subtle hypercortisolism reported in some pathology (visceral obesity, metabolic syndrome, depression) representing, on the other hand, models of disadaptation to subtle hypercortisolism. Limitation of the current litterature and possible direction for future research are discussed in chapter V.

Many people believe that mental preparation influences exercise behaviour and athletic performance. Researchers have examined the effect that a range of cognitive behavioural techniques have on the display of motor skills, and it has been concluded that these interventions may positively influence exercise behaviour and enhance sporting performance. Psyching-up is one type of intervention that has received empirical attention with respect to muscular force production and refers to self-directed cognitive strategies used immediately prior to or during skill execution that are designed to enhance physical performance. Chapter VI reviews the literature examining the influence of psyching-up on maximal strength, local muscular endurance, and power. The existing research provides evidence that psyching-up may help untrained or neophyte participants improve their maximal strength and local muscular endurance during simple or isolated dynamic contractions. Preliminary evidence also suggests that psyching-up may enhance performance on movements requiring power although more research is needed. Generally, equivocal results have emerged from the few studies in which well-trained samples have been used. Also, the experimental tasks have been restricted to movements such as the handgrip, leg extension, bench press, sit-up, press-up, pull-up, and standing broad jump. Currently, it is unclear why psyching-up may assist novice performers undertaking simple dynamic movements because no explanation has any overwhelming support. To further the understanding of the psyching-up and muscular force production relationship, researchers need to use a wider range of participants, employ complex movements, include multiple control conditions, describe samples on several characteristics, and interpret the meaningfulness of their findings. Although there is insufficient evidence to indicate that well-trained athletes might profit from psyching-up prior to or during competition, such interventions may be of benefit for novice participants in health and fitness settings.

During exercise cardiovascular apparatus operates some adjustments which aim at meeting the metabolic needs of exercising muscle. Both mechanical (skeletal-muscle and respiratory pumps) and nervous (centrally and peripherally originating) mechanisms contribute to regulate blood pressure and flow to the metabolic demand. Concerning the nervous component of this regulation, there are several inputs of both central/cortical and peripheral/intravascular origin that converge to the brain-stem neurons controlling cardiovascular activity and regulate the hemodynamic responses to exercise on the basis of the motor strategy. Furthermore, evidences support the concept that also nervous signals of extravascular origin, i.e. arising from muscle mechano- and/or metabo- receptors, activate the same control areas on the basis of the muscle mechanical and metabolic involvement. Chapter VII focuses on inputs arising from exercising muscles which modulate cardiovascular system in order to connect blood pressure and flow with the actual muscle mechanical status (muscle length and strain, and tissue deformation due to muscle movements) and metabolic condition (concentration of catabolites in the extra-cellular compartment produced by muscle activity). It was reported that the stimulation of type I afferent nervous fibers from muscle receptors increases blood pressure through a mechanism of peripheral origin. Among sub-groups of type I afferents, indirect findings suggest that type Ib from Golgi tendon organs may contribute to the muscle-induced cardiovascular reflex. On the contrary, it appears that group Ia from muscle spindle primary ending and group II afferents are not involved in this reflex. Opposite, it seems ascertained that type III and IV afferent nervous fibers can be activated by exercise-induced mechanical and chemical changes in the extracellular environment into they are scattered. It is believed that type III afferents act mainly as "mechanoreceptors", as they respond to muscle stretch and compression occurring during muscle contraction, while type IV fibres act as "metaboreceptors", since they are stimulated by end-products of muscle metabolism. The activity of both type III and IV afferents can reflexely increase heart rate and systemic vascular resistance which, in turn, lead blood pressure to raise. Moreover, there are several growing evidences that also myocardial contractility, stroke volume and cardiac pre-load can be modulated by the activity of these reflexes of muscular origin. These findings suggest that signals arising from exercising muscle act to regulate cardiovascular adjustments during exercise so that blood flow can be set to meet the muscle metabolic request.

Chapter VIII examined the thermoregulatory responses of athletes with a spinal cord injury (T3/4-L1) at rest, during exercise and recovery in cool (21.5 ±1.3°C; 54.2 ±6.3% relative humidity) and warm conditions (31.3 ±0.4°C; 42.3 ±6.3% relative humidity). Subjects exercised on a wheelchair ergometer at 60% of peak oxygen uptake ($\dot{V}O_2$ peak) for 60 minutes in both conditions. Aural and skin temperatures were continually monitored. Aural temperature increased from rest by 0.6 ±0.3°C (P<0.05) during exercise in cool conditions with relatively steady state aural temperature values from 20 minutes of exercise. During exercise in warm conditions aural temperature increased continually to 1.2 ±0.5°C above resting levels (P<0.05). Differences between conditions were observed from 10 minutes of exercise (P<0.05). Skin temperatures demonstrated differences between conditions from rest in the environmental chamber until the end of recovery (P<0.05). Sensate upper body skin sites demonstrated a balance between heat gain and heat loss in both conditions. Insensate lower body skin temperatures increased by greater amounts, particularly during warm conditions, suggesting an imbalance in thermoregulation and indicating the lower body to be a potent site for heat storage. Whole body heat storage was much greater at the end of exercise in warm (5.44 ±1.8 J.g-1) when compared to cool conditions (0.99 ±1.58 J.g-1; P<0.05). Fluid consumption and changes in plasma volume and body mass were similar during exercise in both trials. During the initial 5 minutes recovery, heart rate was greater during warm conditions. The results of this study suggest that trained athletes with a spinal cord injury are able to tolerate prolonged wheelchair exercise in the conditions studied, although greater physiological strain was evident during exercise and the initial stages of recovery in warm when compared to cool conditions. The influence of regional heat storage, voluntary fluid intake and sweat rates in relation to limitations to exercise are discussed.

Juvenile Dermatomyositis (JDM) is one of the idiopathic inflammatory myopathies in childhood. In this disease the immune system targets the microvasculature of the skeletal muscle and skin, leading to myopathy and a typical skin rash. During episodes of active disease patients experience a significant reduction in exercise tolerance which is not only related to loss in muscle mass. In chapter IX the authors propose a model consisting of 5 pathways that could explain the reduced exercise tolerance in children with JDM. The five pathways are 1) the increased concentration of intramuscular cytokines, 2) the systemic inflammation process 3) the inflammation of the capillaries in the muscle 4) the result of hypo-activity and 5) the effect of steroid treatment on body mass gain and protein breakdown.

In recent decades, both human life expectancy and general health among older adults have improved in industrialized nations as described in chapter X. This trend is largely attributed to technological advancements and improved health practices that have been facilitated by research on biological and environmental determinants of health. While research can be a valuable tool in health promotion efforts, there are some segments of the population for which health concerns have not been adequately addressed, such as immigrants. Immigrants differ from non-immigrants and from other immigrant groups on many dimensions that have been associated with health outcomes, including cultural, socioeconomic, and linguistic characteristics. Immigrants also represent an increasing proportion of the population in Western nations, thus potentially influencing overall health data and necessitating their inclusion in modern health research. Health practices and outcomes among older immigrant adults are particularly important because health issues are likely to be more salient in old age, but this group is especially likely to be underrepresented in research. Health data among older immigrants is explored, highlighting trends in lifestyle choices, prevalence of health problems and service utilization. Methodological concerns that influence current data are discussed as well as recommendations to increase cultural sensitivity in future research endeavors with this population subset.

The aim of this chapter XI is to examine the evidence in the literature with regard to the safety of exercise in pregnancy. A literature search revealed fourteen randomised controlled trials which were systematically reviewed. The outcome measures looked at were both short and long term consequences of training in healthy pregnant women. The methodology of all included studies was qualitatively evaluated, though few were graded as good. The majority were small and had variable compliance from the volunteers. There was a lack of standardisation of the training schedules: the frequency ranged from 3 - 5 times per week, training intensities varied from age related maximal heart rates of 50 - 75% and exercise periods ranged from 20 – 60 minutes in length. Overall however, the exercise could be classified as moderate. The literature revealed neither the fetus nor the mother derived harm from moderate exercise in pregnancy. Pregnant women who exercised in the above manner delivered normal healthy infants. With increasing intensity of exercise it appears the children are born with a lower percentage of body fat and thereby a lower birth weight, though still within normal range. This form of training does not appear to increase the incidence of preterm birth or caesarean section. The low number of studies and small patient numbers make it difficult to draw any conclusions with regard to teratogenic effects of hyperthermia. The exclusion of women who developed obstetric complications means it is not possible to draw any conclusions as regards exercise and the risk of placental abruption or bleeding. Moderate exercise seems to have positive effects on pregnancy by way of improved physical well being. Moderate exercise also appears to increase psychological well being – the women feel better. Children born to mothers who exercised regularly showed no significant difference to those born to sedentary mothers in either a positive or a negative way. There was no apparent positive or negative effect on the infant at birth. From currently available data it appears that regular exercise of moderate intensity is both safe and commendable in pregnancy. Further research in this area is required to assess whether physical activity can increase the risks of obstetric complications or cause significant effects from hyperthermia, particularly where exercise intensity is greater than as described here.

In: Focus on Exercise and Health Research
Editor: Thomas B. Selkirk, pp. 1-16

Chapter I

Aerobic Physical Exercise Improves Membrane Fluidity of Erythrocytes in Hypertensive and Normotensive Subjects -An Electron Paramagnetic Resonance Study

Kazushi Tsuda[*]

Division of Cardiology, Department of Medicine,
Wakayama Medical University, Wakayama 641-8509, Japan

Summary

The present study was undertaken to investigate the effects of aerobic physical exercise on membrane functions in hypertensive and normotensive subjects. Physical exercise within the intensity of anaerobic threshold level was performed twice a week for 6 months to both untreated mild essential hypertensive patients and age-matched normotensive subjects. The membrane fluidity of erythrocytes was examined by means of an electron paramagnetic resonance (EPR) and spin-labeling method before and after the trial period in both groups. After the physical exercise, the blood pressure significantly decreased in the hypertensive group (mean blood pressure: before exercise 111±2 mm Hg, n=8, after exercise 104±1 mm Hg, n=8, $P<0.05$). In the normotensive group, the blood pressure tended to decrease. The order parameter (S) and peak height ratio (h_0/h_{-1}) in the EPR spectra of erythrocytes were significantly reduced after the exercise in both groups (S, hypertensives 0.717±0.004 vs 0.691±0.008, n=8, $P<0.05$, normotensives 0.716±0.005 vs 0.698±0.003, n=8, $P<0.05$, h_0/h_{-1}, hypertensives 5.38±0.06 vs 4.89±0.06, n=8, $P<0.01$, normotensives 5.36±0.06 vs 4.95±0.04, n=8, $P<0.01$), which showed that the exercise increased the membrane fluidity of erythrocytes.

---

[*] M.D. Division of Cardiology, Department of Medicine; Wakayama Medical University; Kimiidera 811-1, Wakayama 641-8509; Japan; Tel: 81-73-447-2300 (Ext. 5167) Fax: 81-73-441-0713

In addition, the lower the membrane fluidity of erythrocytes before exercise, the greater the exercise-induced increase in the fluidity (S, r=-0.72, n=16, P<0.05, ho/h-1, r=-0.53, n=16, P<0.05). There was no direct correlation between blood pressure reduction and the exercise-induced increase in the membrane fluidity of erythrocytes. However, the decrease in the peak height ratio (percent changes in ho/h-1) in the EPR spectra by the exercise was significantly correlated with the changes in fasting plasma insulin level (r=0.51, n=16, P<0.05). The results of the present study showed that the aerobic physical exercise significantly increased the erythrocyte membrane fluidity in both mild hypertensive and normotensive subjects. The exercise-induced increase in the fluidity might, at least in part, be linked to the changes in plasma insulin levels. Furthermore, the data suggest that the physical exercise might ameliorate membrane functions, which could contribute, at least in part, to the beneficial effects of exercise in both hypertensive and normotensive subjects.

Key Words: Aerobic physical exercise, membrane fluidity, erythrocytes, electron paramagnetic resonance, spin labeling, insulin, hypertension, normotension

Introduction

Many studies have shown that regular physical exercise is beneficial for both the prevention and treatment of hypertension, and can reduce cardiovascular disease morbidity and mortality [1-6]. Cade et al. [5] demonstrated that an exercise program based on walking for three months induced a significant reduction in blood pressure in subjects with mild or moderate essential hypertension. Van Hoof et al. [6] reported that using the 24-hour noninvasive ambulatory blood pressure monitoring the daytime blood pressure was significantly decreased after a 4-month physical training period. The physical exercise is, therefore, recommended as the non-pharmacological treatment for mild or borderline hypertension [7]. It has been proposed that cell membrane abnomalies may be an aetiological factor in hypertension [8-12]. They include not only functional abnormalities such as transmembrane cation fluxes [8, 9], but also structural or physical changes of the cell membranes [10-12]. Recently, an electron paramagnetic resonance (EPR) and spin labeling method has been developed to evaluate the membrane fluidity and perturbations of the membrane function by external agents [13-15]. The membrane fluidity is a physico-chemical feature of biomembranes, and has an important role in modulating cell functions such as rheological behavior and membrane microviscosity [16]. Using the EPR method our previous studies showed that the membrane fluidity of erythro-cytes was lower in both spontaneously hypertensive rats (SHR) and patients with established essential hypertension [17-19]. In a study presented recently, we demonstrated that membrane fluidity of erythrocytes in hypertension was restored in the exercise-group, but not in the non-exercise group [20]. However, the precise mechanisms underlying the effect of physical exercise on membrane fluidity and whether exercise might be beneficial for the membrane function in normotensive subjects are still unclear. In the present study, in order to identify the cellular mechanisms of aerobic physical exercise, we investigated the relationship between membrane fluidity of erythrocytes and humoral factors before and after the trial period of exercise in hypertensive and normotensive subjects by using the EPR method.

Subjects and Methods

Subjects

Eight Japanese men (age 46.2±1.4, n=8, mean±SEM) with mild essential hypertension and eight normotensive men (age 43.4±2.2, n=8) were included in the study.

All hypertensive subjects had no medication, and had no other diseases such as hematological or hepatic disorders. The physical and laboratory examinations excluded secondary hypertension, coronary heart disease, congestive heart failure, cerebral complications, renal insufficiency, diabetes mellitus and other metabolic disorders. Consent was obtained from all participants after they were explained about the nature and objective of the study. No important differences of physical activities among the investigated subjects were reported. All subjects were requested to maintain their usual casual lifestyles during the study. Before the trial period of exercise, we performed the measurements of fitness, physical examination, and checked the routine laboratory findings of blood, electro-cardiography, X-ray of chest and abdomen, and echocardiography of the heart in all participants.

Exercise Intensity

In order to determine the individual exercise intensity in the exercise group, the initial treadmill exercise test (Stress Test System ML-5000 and MAT-2000, Fukuda Denshi Co., Ltd., Tokyo Japan) with a respiratory gas-exchange monitoring (Metabosystem IS-5000, Fukuda Denshi Co., Ltd., Tokyo, Japan) was performed before the study, and the anaerobic threshold (AT) level was obtained in each subject according to the method described by Wasserman et al. [21]. In the preliminary study, we examined VO_2 values at both the AT level and the peak exercise level in hypertensive subjects (18.3±0.8 and 34.4±1.7 ml/min/kg, respectively, mean±SEM, n=14). The workload at the heart rate of the initial AT level was used as the exercise intensity in each subject.

Exercise Protocols

The physical exercise consisted of the mild program (10 minute warming-up, 15 minute jogging at the heart rate of the AT level, 5 minute walking and 30 minute calisthenics). The exercise was performed twice a week for 6 months in our laboratory. The participants were supervised by the medical stuff during the exercise. In the preliminary study, we ascertained the effects of the same intensity of exercise on cardiac diastolic function in hypertensive subjects by using the echocardiography. The time of IIA-mitral valve opening in the echocardiography (IIA-MVO) was significantly decreased after the exercise (72.2±3.2 vs

59.9±4.2 msec, n=13, P<0.05), which might indicate that the exercise was effective and improved cardiac diastolic function in hypertensive subjects.

The daytime blood pressure at rest was measured indirectly with a cuff and a mercury sphygmomanometer in a sitting position before and after the trial period. The blood pressure measurement was done three times in each subject after 30 min rest while fasting, and the means of the values were reported.

Measurement of Membrane Fluidity of Erythrocytes

Blood sampling was also performed before and after the trial period in all subjects. Blood sampling was done by venipuncture after a minimum of 30 minute rest while fasting. After plasma and buffy coat were carefully removed by centrifugation at 155 g for 10 minutes at 4° C, washed erythrocytes were resuspended in the isotonic buffer (140 mmol/L NaCl, 20 mmol/L Tris-HCl, pH 7.4) at a hematocrit of 50 %. One hundred microliter of the solution containing fatty acid spin label agents (5-nitroxide stearate; 5-NS and 16-nitroxide stearate; 16-NS, 5×10^{-5} mol/L) was added to 200 ml erythrocyte suspension, and the mixed solution was then incubated for 2 hours at 37° C with gentle shaking.

The EPR measurements were performed using an EPR spectrometer (Model JEOL JES-FE2XG, Nihon Denshi, Tokyo, Japan) with a microwave unit (Model JEOL ES-SCXA, Nihon Denshi). The microwave power was 5 mW, and the modulation frequency was 100 KHz with a modulation amplitude of 2.0 gauss (G). The temperature of the measurement was controlled at 30° C. The receiver scan width was 3280±50 G with a sweep time of 8 minutes, and the receiver gain was 4×10^3 -7.9×10^3 with a response time of 1.0 second. The fatty acid spin label agents are believed to be anchored at the lipid-aqueous interface of the cell membranes by their carboxyl ends, whereas the nitroxide group moves rapidly through a restrict angle around the point of attachment [13-15, 22, 23]. Therefore, the EPR spectra of the fatty acid spin label agents are used to detect an alteration in the freedom of motion in biological membranes and to provide an indication of membrane fluidity, which is inversely correlated with membrane microviscosity. For indices of the membrane fluidity, we have evaluated the values of outer and inner hyperfine splitting $2T'\parallel$ and $2T'\perp$ in G, respectively) in the EPR spectra for 5-NS and calculated the order parameter (S) from $2T'\parallel$ and $2T'\perp$ [22, 23]

In the EPR spectra for 16-NS, we employed the peak height ratio (ho/h-1) value for an index of the membrane fluidity [22, 23] (Fig. 1). The order parameters (S) may represent the fluidity of the outer layer of the plasma membranes, whereas the peak height ratio (ho/h-1) may express the fluidity of the inner membrane compartment [15]. The intra-assay coefficient variation of the order parameter (S) and the peak height ratio (ho/h-1) was less than 0.50 %. In the preliminary study, we also examined the inter-assay variation of the membrane fluidity of erythrocytes in hypertensive subjects within a week. The alterative degree was -0.25±0.23 % of basal value (n=7). The lesser values of the order parameter (S) and the peak height ratio (ho/h-1) are associated with the greater freedom of motion of the spin labels in the biomembrane bilayers, indicating increased membrane fluidity [17-19, 22, 23].

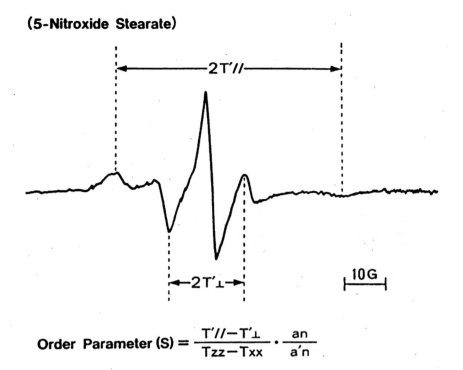

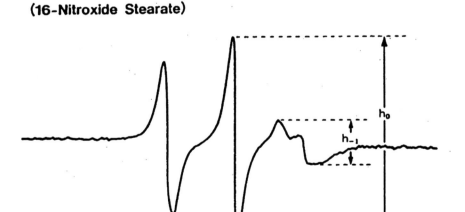

Figure 1. Typical electron paramagnetic resonance (EPR) spectra of erythrocytes for the fatty acid spin-label agents (5-nitroxide stearate: 5-NS, upper, and 16-nitroxide stearate: 16-NS, bottom); S: order parameter, 2T'll: outer hyperfine splitting, 2T'⊥ : inner hyperfine splitting, Tzz and Txx: hyperfine constants, an/a'n: isotropic coupling constant, ho/h-1: peak height ratio

Hematologic and Humoral Parameters

The blood erythrocyte count, hematocrit and hemoglobin level were measured before and after the trial period of physical exercise. The plasma renin activity (radioimmunoassay), plasma norepinephrine (high performance liquid chromatography with an electrochemical detector) and fasting plasma insulin (radio-immunoassay) as well as serum sodium, potassium, chloride, free calcium (Ca^{2+}), creatinine, cholesterol, high density lipoprotein-cholesterol, triglyceride and fasting plasma glucose were also measured. The blood sampling for the measurement of these parameters was done at the same time of the erythrocyte sampling for the EPR investigation.

Materials for EPR Measurements

The spin label agents, 5-NS and 16-NS, were purchased from Aldrich Co., Ltd. (Milwaukee, Wisconsin, USA). All other drugs were standard laboratory reagents of analytical grade.

Statistical Analysis

Values are expressed as mean±SEM. Baseline parameters before and after the exercise period were compared using Student's paired t-test. Differences between the hypertensive and normotensive subjects were analyzed with Student's unpaired t-test. Linear regression analyses were performed between exercise-induced changes in memberane fluidity and basal values of membrane fluidity of erythrocytes or changes in plasma insulin levels. A p value less than 0.05 was accepted as the level of significance.

Results

Effects of Physical Exercise on Blood Pressure in Patients with Mild Essential Hypertension and Normotensive Subjects

After the 6 month exercise period, the daytime systolic, diastolic and mean blood pressure at rest significantly decreased in the hypertensive patients (Table 1). The blood pressure in normotensive subjects tended to decrease, although the reduction in blood pressure was not significant (Table 1). The heart rate and the body mass index were not significantly changed before and after the physical exercise in both the hypertensive and normotensive groups (Table 1).

Table 1 Effects of Physical Exercise on Body Mass Index, Heart Rate and Blood Pressure in Mild Essential Hypertensive Patients and Normotensive Subjects

	Hypertensives (n=8)		Normotensives (n=8)	
	Before Exercise	After Exercise	Before Exercise	After Exercise
BMI (kg/m^2)	25.2±0.8	24.7±0.6	24.0±0.6	23.6±0.5
Heart Rate (beats/min)	69±3	68±2	75±4	73±4
Systolic Blood Pressure (mm Hg)	144±4 b	134±2 a, b	133±2	126±2
Mean Blood Pressure (mm Hg)	111±2 b	104±1 a, b	99±2	94±2
Diastolic Blood Pressure (mm Hg)	95±2 b	89±1 a, b	82±2	78±3

Values are means±SEM.   BMI: body mass index

a P<0.05 between before and after the period of physical exercise, b P<0.05 between hypertensives and normotensives

Effects of Physical Exercise on Membrane Fluidity of Erythrocytes in Hypertensive and Normotensive Subjects

Fig. 2 demonstrates the membrane fluidity of erythrocytes before and after the trial period in hypertensive and normotensive individuals. Before the exercise program, the order parameter (S) and the peak height ratio (ho/h-1) of the EPR spectra were slightly increased in hypertensive subjects compared with normotensive subjects, but the differences were not significant. The values of the order parameter (S) (Fig. 2a) and the peak height ratio (ho/h-1) (Fig. 2b) were significantly reduced after the physical exercise period in both hypertensive and normotensive groups (S value: HT 0.717±0.004 vs 0.691±0.008, n=8, P<0.05, NT 0.716±0.005 vs 0.698±0.003, n=8, P<0.05, ho/h-1 value: HT 5.38±0.06 vs 4.89±0.06, n=8, P<0.01, NT 5.36±0.06 vs 4.95±0.04, n=8, P<0.01). The finding indicated that the physical exercise might increase the membrane fluidity of erythrocytes in both hypertensive and normotensive groups. In addition, it was clearly demonstrated that the lower the membrane fluidity of erythrocyte (the higher the values of S and ho/h-1) before exercise, the greater the exercise-induced changes in the fluidity (%Δ S and %Δ ho/h-1) (r=-0.72, n=16, P<0.01 and r=-0.53, n=16, P<0.05, respectively) (Fig. 3). There was, however, no direct correlation between blood pressure reduction and the changes in the membrane fluidity of erythrocytes by the exercise.

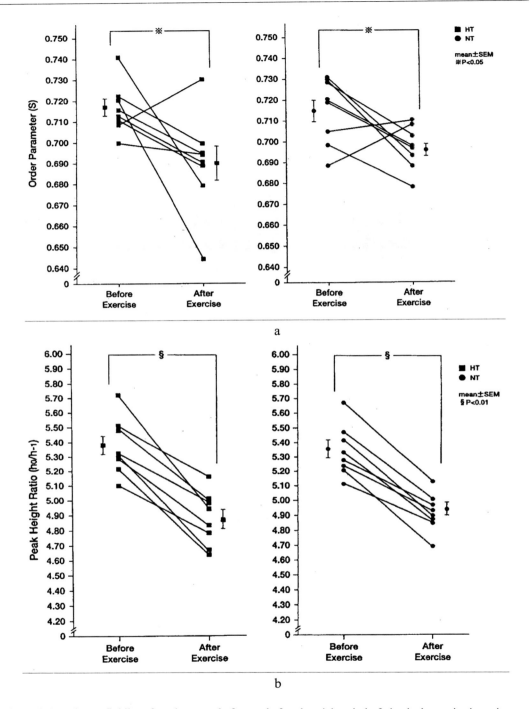

Figure 2. Membrane fluidity of erythrocytes before and after the trial period of physical exercise in patients with mild essential hypertension and normotensive subjects
a: Changes in the value of order parameter (S)
b: Changes in the value of peak height ratio (ho/h-1)
The greater the values of S and ho/h-1, the lower the membrane fluidity of erythrocytes. Bars indicate means±SEM.

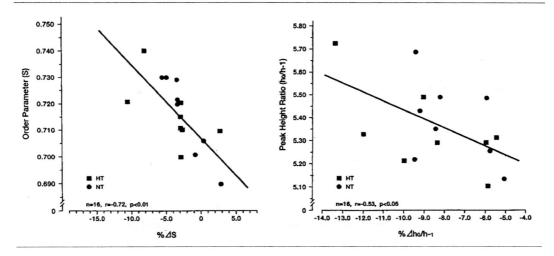

Figure 3. Relationship between membrane fluidity of erythrocytes before exercise (order parameter:S and peak height ratio:ho/h-1) and the exercise-induced changes in the fluidity (%Δ S and %Δ ho/h-1) in patients with mild essential hypertension and normotensive subjects

Hematologic and Humoral Parameters and Membrane Fluidity of Erythrocytes

As shown in Table 2, there were no significant changes by the exercise in blood erythrocyte counts, hemoglobin, hematocrit, serum sodium and potassium, serum creatinine, serum total cholesterol and high density lipoprotein-cholesterol, serum triglyceride and fasting plasma glucose in both hypertensive and normotensive subjects. The serum free Ca^{2+} was also not changed by the exercise. Plasma renin activity was significantly reduced in hypertensive group (Table 2). Plasma norepinephrine and fasting plasma insulin were slightly decreased after the trial period of exercise (Table 2).

Table 2 Hematologic and Humoral Parameters Before and After the Trial Period of Physical Exercise

	Hypertensives (n=8)		Normotensives (n=8)	
	Before Exercise	After Exercise	Before Exercise	After Exercise
Erythrocyte Counts (10^4 cells/μL)	520±11	502±12	510±8	500±6
Hemoglobin (g/dL)	15.6±0.2	15.6±0.3	15.5±0.2	15.0±0.1
Hematocrit (%)	48.0±1.0	47.8±1.0	47.0±0.5	46.3±0.2
Serum Sodium (mmol/L)	142.3±0.4	142.7±0.4	141.6±0.6	143.1±0.4
Serum Potassium (mmol/L)	4.2±0.1	4.2±0.1	4.2±0.1	4.1±0.1
Serum Chloride (mmol/L)	103.5±0.4	104.1±0.8	102.0±0.4	104.6±0.4
Serum Creatinine (mg/dL)	1.0±0.1	1.0±0.1	1.0±0.01	1.0±0.1
Total Cholesterol (mg/dL)	210±11	210±10	195±7	193±3
High Density Lipoprotein Cholesterol (mg/dL)	51±2	48±1	49±2	47±2
Triglyceride (mg/dL)	110±17	110±11	109±16	103±12
Fasting Plasma Glucose (mmol/L)	6.2±0.2	6.1±0.3	5.7±0.2	5.7±0.2
Serum Free Calcium (mmol/L)	1.26±0.03	1.28±0.01	1.32±0.02	1.28±0.01
Plasma Renin Activity (ng/mL/hr)	1.4±0.4	0.7±0.2 [a]	1.3±0.3	0.6±0.2
Plasma Norepinephrine (pg/mL)	273±43	218±24	280±59	238±45
Fasting Plasma Insulin (μU/mL)	9.6±1.6	8.2±1.5	6.4±1.0	6.2±1.0

Values are means±SEM.

a $P<0.05$ between before and after the period of physical exercise

Fig. 4 shows the relationship between the changes in fasting plasma insulin and the changes in the membrane fluidity of erythrocytes by exercise. A significant correlation was observed between the exercise-induced changes in plasma insulin level

(Δ plasma insulin) and the changes in the peak height ratio

(%Δ ho/h-1) for 16-NS of the EPR spectra ($r=0.51$, $n=16$, $P<0.05$).

No significant correlation was noted between Δ plasma insulin and %Δ S. The changes in plasma renin activity and norepinephrine concentration were not correlated with the changes in the membrane fluidity of erythrocytes.

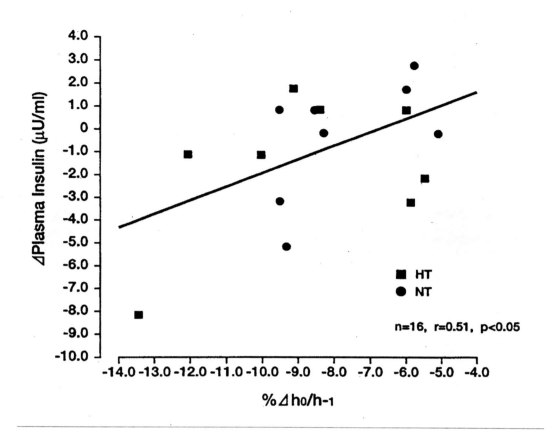

Figure 4. Relationship between the exercise-induced changes in membrane fluidity of erythrocytes (%Δ ho/h-1) and the changes in plasma insulin concentration (Δ plasma insulin) in patients with mild essential hypertension and normotensive subjects

Discussion

Many studies have suggested fairly well that regular exercise is beneficial for the prevention and treatment of hypertension and can lower both systolic and diastolic blood pressure in subjects with mild essential hypertension [1-6]. Although the American College of Sports Medicine proposes that adequate endurance exercise training consists of a program at an intensity of 50 % to 85 % of maximum oxygen consumption (VO_2max), less intense exercise (VO_2max of 40 % to 70 %) may similarly lower blood pressure [24].

The physical exercise may also attenuate other cardiovascular risk factors such as dyslipidemia and insulin resistance [25-27]. The present study demonstrated that aerobic physical exercise at the heart rate of the AT level for 6 months significantly lowered the blood pressure in subjects with borderline or mild essential hypertension. However, the cellular functions associated with these changes are not fully understood. We therefore examined alterations in the membrane fluidity of erythrocytes before and after the physical exercise in borderline hypertensive and normotensive subjects by means of the EPR method.

The order parameter (S) and the peak height ratio (ho/h-1) of the EPR spectra obtained from erythrocyte membranes significantly reduced after the trial period of physical exercise in both hypertensive and normotensive groups. The result indicated that the exercise increased the membrane fluidity of erythrocytes and ameliorated the membrane microviscosity. In the present study, there was no direct correlation between the exercise-induced blood pressure reduction and the increase in the membrane fluidity of erythrocytes. The finding might confirm the idea that alterations in the membrane fluidity of erythrocytes was not a consequence of blood pressure changes by the physical exercise.

Our previous studies already showed that erythrocyte membrane fluidity was decreased in SHR and in patients with established essential hypertension compared with normotensive controls, and suggested that cell membranes might be stiffer and less fluid in primary hypertension [17-19]. In the present study, the basal values of the order parameter (S) and the peak height ratio (ho/h-1) were not significantly different between hypertensive and normotensive subjects. It would be possible that the membrane abnormalities in borderline hypertensive subjects might not be pronounced as those of established hypertensive subjects. One more explanation is that some of the normotensive subjects in this study will have a risk of developing hypertension, because the mean blood pressure of the normotensive subjects was at the prehypertensive stage of the Seventh Report of the Joint National Committee on Prevention, Detection, Evaluation, and Treatment of Hight Blood Pressure (JNC VII) [28].

It has been proposed that the cell membrane fluidity could be affected by various factors [16]. Naftilan et al. reported that changes in lipid composition of the cell membranes in hypertensive subjects modulated the platelet membrane fluidity [29]. On the other hand, the fluidity may be regulated by endogenous humoral substances. Sauerheber et al. [30] observed that extracellular Ca^{2+} reduced the membrane fluidity of erythrocytes. We also observed that increase in the intracellular Ca^{2+} strongly reduced the membrane fluidity of erythrocytes [17]. Recent studies have suggested that hyperinsulinemia may have a role in the pathophysiology of hypertension and other cardiovascular diseases [31-37]. It was reported that human erythrocytes contained highly specific insulin receptors on the membranes [38]. With regard to the relationship between insulin and membrane functions, it was demonstrated that hyperinsulinemia was associated with the lower membrane fluidity of erythrocytes in essential hypertension [39]. Furthermore, insulin in an in vitro study significantly decreased the membrane fluidity of erythrocyte, which was partially mediated by the increase in the intracellular Ca^{2+} concentration [39]. Dutta-Roy et al. observed that insulin significantly reduced the microviscosity of human erythrocytes and consequently increased the deformability of the cells [40]. In the present study, although the reduction in plasma insulin was not significant, the exercise-induced changes in the peak height ratio (ho/h-1) of the EPR spectra were significantly correlated with the changes in fasting plasma insulin levels. The result showed that an increase in the fluidity, particularly of the inner membrane component, might partially be related to the changes in the plasma insulin concentration by the exercise. Bogardus et al. [26] examined the effects of physical training on carbohydrate metabolism in patients with non-insulin dependent diabetes mellitus, and reported that exercise improved insulin sensitivity, which was accompanied by progressive lowering of plasma insulin responses to glucose challenge. Yamanouchi et al. [27] also showed that physical exercise of daily walking improved the insulin sensitivity in patients with non-insulin dependent diabetes mellitus. Although the precise mechanisms underlying the effects of insulin on the cell functions are still uncertain, it would be possible that insulin could be a determinant factor of the membrane fluidity of erythrocytes.

One additional possible explanation is that the exercise-induced changes in the membrane fluidity might be due to the decrease in plasma endogenous digitalislike factor (EDLF) [41-44].

Koga et al. [44] measured plasma EDLF content before and after physical exercise, and reported that EDLF of the exercised hypertensive individuals was significantly reduced after 10 week mild exercise. Goto et al. [45] observed that the EDLF in human urine possessed the capacity to inhibit Na^+, K^+-ATPase activity in intact human erythrocytes. Moreover, they reported that this compound significantly increased the intracellular free Ca^{2+} concentration [45], probably through the Na^+-Ca^{2+} exchange mechanisms [46] or a direct effect upon Ca^{2+} influx into the cells [47]. Because the intracellular Ca^{2+} has an important role in the regulation of membrane fluidity [30], the decrease in plasma EDLF might produce an increase in the membrane fluidity of erythrocytes.

The physiological significance of the exercise-induced increase in the membrane fluidity is still uncertain. It is well known that membrane fluidity may be inversely correlated with membrane microviscosity and rigidity. Erythrocyte membrane functions are critically important for rapid and homogenous perfusion of oxygen in the microcirculation [40]. The lowering of the microviscosity and consequently the increased deformability may play an important role in erythrocyte diffusion in the microcirculation. It would be possible that physical exercise might ameliorate the microcirculation by decreasing erythrocyte membrane microviscosity, which could participate in the prevention of micro- and macroangiopathy and cardiovascular complications. Additional studies are necessary to assess more thoroughly the exercise-induced changes in membrane functions and their contribution to the beneficial effects of the exercise.

In summary, the results of the present study showed that aerobic physical exercise increased the membrane fluidity of erythrocytes in both hypertensive and normotensive subjects. The exercise-induced increase in the membrane fluidity might not be a consequence of blood pressure reduction, but, at least in part, linked to the changes in plasma insulin levels. Furthermore, it is strongly suggested that the improvement of membrane microviscosity of erythrocytes might contribute, at least in part, to the beneficial effects of the exercise in both hypertensive and normotensive subjects.

References

[1] Arakawa K. Hypertension and exercise. *Clin Exp Hypertens*. 1993;A15:1171-1179.
[2] Fagard RH. The role of exercise in blood pressure control: supportive evidence. *J Hypertension*. 1995;13:1223-1227.
[3] Powell KE, Thompson PD, Caspersen CJ, Kendrick JS. Physical activity and the incidence of coronary heart disease. *Annu Rev Public Health*. 1987;8:253-287.

[4] Blair SN, Kohl III HW, Paffenbarger RS, Clark DG, Cooper KH, Gibbons LW. Physical fitness and all-cause mortality. A prospective study of healthy men and women. *JAMA*. 1989;262:2395-2401.

[5] Cade R, Mars D, Wagemaker H, Zauner C, Packer D, Privette M, Cade M, Peterson J, Hood-Lewis D. Effects of aerobic exercise training on patients with systemic arterial hypertension. *Am J Med*. 1984;77:785-790.

[6] Van Hoof R, Hespel P, Fagard R, Lijnen P, Staessen J, Amery A. Effects of endurance training on blood pressure at rest, during exercise and during 24 hours in sedentary men. *Am J Cardiol*. 1989;63:945-949.

[7] 1992 Joint National Committee. The fifth Report of the Joint National Committee on Detection, Evaluation, and Treatment of High Blood Pressure (JNC-V). *Arch Intern Med*. 1993;153:154-183.

[8] Canessa M, Adragna N, Solomon HS, Connolly TM, Tosteson DC. Increased sodium-lithium countertransport in red cells of patients with essential hypertension. *N Engl J Med*. 1980;302:772-776.

[9] De Mendonca M, Garay RP, Ben-Ishay D, Meyer P. Abnormal erythrocyte cation transport in primary hypertension: clinical and experimental studies. *Hypertension*. 1981;(suppl I):I-179-I-183.

[10] Montenay-Garestier T, Aragon I, Devynck MA, Meyer P, Helene C. Evidence for structural changes in membranes of spontaneously hypertensive rats: a fluorescence polarization study. *Biochem Biophys Res Commun*. 1981;160:660-665.

[11] Orlov SN, Gulak PV, Litvinov IS, Postnov YV. Evidence of altered structure of erythrocyte membrane in spontaneously hypertensive rats. *Clin Sci*. 1982;63:43-46.

[12] Tsuda K, Minatogawa Y, Nishio I, Masuyama Y. Increased osmotic fragility of erythrocytes in essential hypertension. *Clin Exp Hypertens*. 1984;A6:2235-2247.

[13] Gaffney BJ. Spin-label measurements in membranes. *Methods Enzymol*. 1974;32:161-198.

[14] Tanaka KI, Ohnishi S. Heterogeneity in the fluidity of intact erythrocyte membrane and its homogenization upon hemolysis. *Biochim Biophys Acta*. 1976;426:218-231.

[15] Sato B, Nishikida K, Samuels LT, Tyler FH. Electron spin resonance studies of erythrocytes from patients with Duchenne dystrophy. *J Clin Invest*. 1978;61:251-259.

[16] Cooper RA. Abnormalities of cell-membrane fluidity in the pathogenesis of disease. *N Engl J Med*. 1977;297:371-377.

[17] Tsuda K, Iwahashi H, Minatogawa Y, Nishio I, Kido R, Masuyama Y. Electron spin resonance studies of erythrocytes from spontaneously hypertensive rats and humans with essential hypertension. *Hypertension*. 1987;9(Suppl III):III-19-III-24.

[18] Tsuda K, Kinoshita Y, Kimura K, Nishio I, Masuyama Y. Electron paramagnetic resonance investigation on modulatory effect of 17beta-estradiol on membrane fluidity of erythrocytes in postmenopausal women. *Arterioscler. Thromb. Vasc. Biol*. 2001;21:1306-1312.

[19] Tsuda K, Kimura K, Nishio I, Masuyama Y. Nitric oxide improves membrane fluidity of erythrocytes in essential hypertension: an electron paramagnetic resonance investigation. *Biochem Biophys Res Commun*. 2000;275:946-954.

[20] Tsuda K, Yoshikawa A, Kimura K, Nishio I. Effects of mild aerobic physical exercise on membrane fluidity of erythrocytes in essential hypertension. *Clin. Exp Pharmacol. Physiol.* 2003;30:382-386.

[21] Wasserman K, Whipp BJ, Koyal SN, Beaver WL. Anaerobic threshold and respiratory gas exchange during exercise. *J Appl Physiol.* 1973;35:236-243.

[22] Simon I. Differences in membrane unsaturated fatty acids and electron spin resonance in different types of myeloid leukemia cells. *Biochim Biphys Acta.* 1979;556:408-422.

[23] Gaffney BJ, Drachman DB, Lin DC, Tennekoon G. Spin-label studies of erythrocytes in myotonic dystrophy: no increase in membrane fluidity. *Neurology.* 1980;30:277-285.

[24] American College of Sports Medicine. Physical activity, physical fitness and hypertension. *Med Sci Sports Exercise.* 1993;25:i-x.

[25] Barnard RJ, Wen SJ. Exercise and diet in the prevention and control of the metabolic syndrome. *Sports Med.* 1994;18:218-228.

[26] Bogardus C, Ravussin E, Robbins DC, Wolfe RR, Horton ES, Sims EAH. Effects of physical training and diet therapy on carbohydrate metabolism in patients with glucose intolerance and non-insulin-dependent diabetes mellitus. *Diabetes.* 1984;33:311-318.

[27] Yamanouchi K, Shinozaki T, Chikada K, Nishikawa T, Ito K, Shimizu S, Ozawa N, Suzuki Y, Maeno H, Kato K, Oshida Y, Sato Y. Daily walking combined with diet therapy is a useful means for obese NIDDM patients not only to reduce body weight but also to improve insulin sensitivity. *Diabetes Care.* 1995;18:775-778.

[28] Chobanian AV, Bakris GL, Black HR, Cushman WC, Green LA, Izzo JL Jr., Jones DW, Materson BJ, Oparil S, Wright JT Jr., Roccella EJ, the National High Blood Pressure Education Program Coordinating Committee. Seventh report of the joint national committee on prevention, detection, evaluation, and treatment of high blood pressure. *Hypertension.* 2003;42:1206-1252.

[29] Naftilan AJ, Dzau VJ, Loscalzo J. Preliminary observations on abnormalities of membrane structure and function in essential hypertension. *Hypertension.* 1986;8(suppl II):II-174-II-179.

[30] Sauerheber RD, Lewis UJ, Esgate JA, Gordon LM. Effect of calcium, insulin and growth hormone on membrane fluidity: a spin label study of rat adipocytes and human erythrocyte ghosts. *Biochim Biophys Acta.* 1980;597:292-304.

[31] Ferrannini E, Buzzigoli G, Bonadonna R, Giorico AM, Oleggini M, Graziadei L, Pedrinelli R, Brandl L, Bevilacqua S. Insulin resistance in essential hypertension. *N Engl J Med.* 1987;317:350-357.

[32] Sowers JR, Sowers PS, Peuler JD. Role of insulin resistance and hyperinsulinemia in development of hypertension and atherosclerosis. *J Lab Clin Med.* 1994;123:647-652.

[33] Morris AD, Petrie JR, Connell JMC. Insulin and hypertension. *J Hypertension.* 1994;12:633-642.

[34] Byyny RL, LoVerde M, Lloyd S, Mitchell W, Draznin B. Cytosolic calcium and insulin resistance in elderly patients with essential hypertension. *Am J Hypertens.* 1992;5:459-464.

[35] Ohno Y, Suzuki H, Yamakawa H, Makamura M, Otsuka K, Saruta T. Impaired insulin sensitivity in young, lean normotensive offspring of essential hypertensives: possible role of disturbed calcium metabolism. *J Hypertension.* 1993;11:421-426.

[36] Shimosawa T, Ando K, Ono A, Takahashi K, Isshiki M, Kanda M, Ogata E, Fujita T. Insulin inhibits norepinephrine overflow from peripheral sympathetic nerve endings. *Biochem Biophys Res Commun*. 1992;188:330-335.

[37] Moreau P, Lamarche L, Laflamme AK, Calderone A, Yamaguchi N, de Champlain J. Chronic hyperinsulinaemia and hypertension: the role of the sympathetic nervous system. *J Hypertension*. 1995;13:333-340.

[38] Gambhir KK, Archer JA, Bradley CJ. Characteristics of human erythrocyte insulin receptors. *Diabetes*. 1978;27:701-708.

[39] Tsuda K, Kinoshita Y, Nishio I, Masuyama Y. Role of insulin in the regulation of membrane fluidity of erythrocytes in essential hypertension: an electron paramagnetic resonance investigation. *Am. J. Hypertens*. 2000;13:376-382.

[40] Dutta-Roy AK, Ray TK, Sinha AK. Control of erythrocyte membrane microviscosity by insulin. *Biochim Biophys Acta*. 1985;816:187-190.

[41] Hamlyn JM, Ringel R, Schaeffer J, Levinson PD, Hamilton BP, Kowarski AA, Blaustein MP. A circulating inhibitor of $(Na^{+}+K^{+})$ATPase associated with essential hypertension. *Nature*. 1982;300:650-652.

[42] Sagnella GA, Jones JC, Shore AC, Markandu ND, MacGregor GA. Evidence for increased levels of a circulating ouabain-like factor in essential hypertension. *Hypertension*. 1986;8:433-437.

[43] Narse K, Narse M, Tanabe A, Yoshimoto T, Watanabe Y, Kurimoto F, Horiba N, Tamura M, Inagami T, Demura H. Does plasma immunoreactive ouabain originate from the adrenal gland? *Hypertension*. 1994;23(suppl I):I-102-I-105.

[44] Koga M, Ideishi M, Matsusaki M, Tashiro E, Kinoshita A, Ikeda M, Tanaka H, Shindo M, Arakawa K. Mild exercise decreases plasma endogenous digitalislike substance in hypertensive individuals. *Hypertension*. 1992;19(suppl II):II-231-II-236.

[45] Goto A, Yamada K, Ishii M, Ishiguro T, Eguchi C, Sugimoto T. Urinary sodium pump inhibitor raises cytosolic free calcium concentration in rat aorta. *Hypertension*. 1989;13:916-921.

[46] Blaustein MP, Hamlyn JM. Sodium transport inhibition, cell calcium, and hypertension. The natriuretic hormone/Na^{+}-Ca^{2+} exchange/hypertension hypothesis. *Am J Med*. 1984;77(4A):45-59.

[47] Anner BM. The receptor function of the Na^{+}, K^{+}-activated adenosine triphosphatase system. *Biochem J*. 1985;227:1-11.

Chapter II

Exercise and Cognition: Theoretical and Empirical Evidence for an Interaction Effect from an Integrated Cognitive Psychology/ Neuroscientific Perspective

Terry McMorris
Centre for Sports Science and Medicine, University College Chichester, UK

Abstract

In this chapter we examine the empirical and theoretical evidence for an exercise-arousal-cognition interaction effect. Most researchers have claimed that exercise will affect cognition in an inverted-U fashion, in line with the effect of emotionally induced arousal on cognitive performance. Early research has failed to provide much support for such a claim. Results were somewhat equivocal but there is some evidence for a linear improvement in performance for complex tasks during incremental exercise to exhaustion. More recent research has provided some support for the argument that when exercise reaches an intensity that results in a significant increase in plasma concentrations of the catecholamines epinephrine and norepinephrine, there is also significant improvement in cognition. Results are not unequivocal, however. Observation of research, with animals, shows that Central Nervous System concentrations of norepinephrine, dopamine and 5-hydroxytryptomine increase during exercise. As these are brain neurotransmitters it is possible that this increase results in improved cognition during exercise. The equivocal nature of the empirical evidence for such an effect, however, suggests that other factors are involved. An integrated cognitive/neuroscientific model is proposed which shows an interaction between the increased availability of the neurotransmitters in the brain during exercise and the individual's perception of the nature of exercise as a stressor.

Introduction

The effect of exercise on cognitive functioning has been studied for almost 40 years. That such an effect actually exists tends to be taken for granted. However, examination of the empirical evidence does not unequivocally support this assertion. In this chapter, we examine the empirical evidence in some detail, placing particular emphasis on how weak experimental designs may be resulting in a failure to demonstrate unequivocal support for an exercise-cognition interaction effect. It is my contention that problems with research designs have come about due to the fact that few researchers have taken into account the effect of exercise induced biochemical changes, in the periphery, on neurochemical activity in the Central Nervous System (CNS). Moreover, I argue that those studies that have examined the problem from a neuroscientific perspective have been guilty of taking a simplistic approach to the peripheral-central biochemical interaction.

In the final section of the chapter, I present an integrated cognitive psychology/neuroscientific theoretical model to explain how this interaction may occur. In order to support the reasoning behind the presentation of this model it is necessary, firstly, to examine the development, over the last 40 years, of the theoretical rationale for an exercise-arousal-cognition interaction and to show how research results have slowly led to the refinement of this rationale.

Early Development of a Theoretical Rationale: A Cognitive Psychology Approach

The early studies examining the effect of exercise on cognitive performance took an atheoretical stance (e. g. Gutin & Di Gennaro, 1968a; McAdam & Wang, 1967; Meyers, Zimmerli, Farr & Baschnagel, 1969). Indeed, some of the early research used exercise protocols that appear to have been arrived at somewhat arbitrarily. Gutin and Di Gennaro (1968a) had subjects undertake 1 min of step ups, using the Harvard Step Test protocol. Meyers et al. (1969) used a similar step up protocol but had subjects work for 5 mins. McAdam and Wang's (1967) subjects carried out a run-jog-walk protocol for 10 mins. According to the authors, this was "designed to work up a mild sweat, but not to fatigue".

These authors did not state why they thought that exercise would affect cognition. They may have perceived exercise as being a stressor, having a similar effect on cognition as other stressors such as noise or temperature. It may also have been that they saw the similarities between the physiological changes that occur during exercise and those that occur when arousal level rises due to emotions. During exercise there are increases in heart rate, respiratory rate, blood pressure and sweating (Åstrand & Rodahl, 2002). Such increases can, also, be seen when arousal level rises due to emotions (Cooper, 1973; Davidson, MacGregor, Stuhr, Dixon & MacLean, 2000). It should be stated, however, that while *all* of these changes occur when people exercise they do not necessarily all occur when emotions are high. Indeed different people will exhibit different somatic responses to emotions (Lacey & Lacey, 1970).

McMorris and Keen (1994) suggested caution in equating exercise induced arousal with emotionally induced arousal. They argued that when physiological changes are the result of exercise they

"are induced and mediated by the activated musculature and are responding to exercise load, i.e., attempting to maintain homeostasis. Somatic arousal rising from emotions, however, is induced by the brain and destroys homeostasis."

McMorris and Keen (1994) accepted that exercise is a stressor and, therefore, would affect arousal, but they questioned the claims of authors, like Davey (1973), that heavy exercise would equate with high levels of arousal. They argued that, if during maximal exercise, the individual is in a state of homeostasis it may not be possible to equate this with the highly emotionally aroused person, who is no longer in a state of homeostasis.

Despite their reservations about the exact nature of exercise induced arousal, McMorris and Keen (1994) endorsed the claims of Davey (1973) with regard to presenting a rationale for the exercise-arousal-cognition effect. Davey (1973) argued that as exercise intensity increased so did arousal. On that basis he claimed that exercise would affect cognitive performance in an inverted-U fashion, based on Yerkes and Dodson's (1908) theory. According to Yerkes and Dodson, when arousal is low, performance will be poor. As arousal rises it will reach an optimal level, the top of the inverted-U. If arousal continues to rise, however, performance will begin to deteriorate until it eventually returns to a level equal to that shown during low levels. Davey argued that exercise of moderate intensity would induce optimal performance while heavy exercise would inhibit performance.

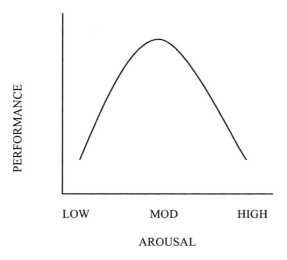

Figure 1. Graphical depiction of Yerkes and Dodson's (1908) inverted-U hypothesis

Later researchers (e.g. Allard, Brawley, Deakin & Elliott, 1989; Fleury, Bard & Carrière, 1981; Isaacs & Pohlman, 1991) have drawn on Easterbrook's (1959) development of Yerkes and Dodson's (1908) theory as the basis of the theoretical underpinning for their research. According to Easterbrook's cue utilisation theory, when arousal level is low the individual has too broad an attentional focus and attends to both relevant and irrelevant information and thus performance is poor. As arousal rises, however, attention reaches an optimal level, when only task relevant cues are processed. This corresponds to the top of the curve in Yerkes and Dodson's theory. If arousal continues to rise, however, attention will narrow and even relevant cues will be missed, hence a deterioration in performance. Easterbrook's theory has the advantage over Yerkes and Dodson's in that it provides an explanation as to how arousal affects performance.

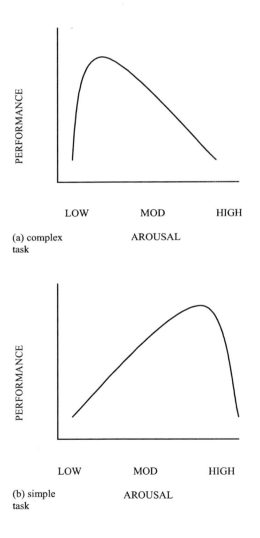

Figure 2. Graphical depiction of the effect of task difficulty on the inverted-U effect (from McMorris, T. 2004. *Acquisition and performance of sports skills*, Chichester, Wiley. Printed with permission).

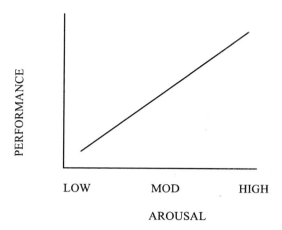

a) well learned task

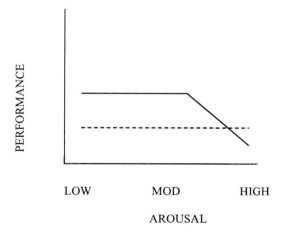

b) novel task

Figure 3. Graphical description of drive theory (from McMorris, T. 2004. *Acquisition and performance of sports skills*, Chichester, Wiley. Printed with permission).

Yerkes and Dodson (1908) believed that the type of task would affect the arousal-performance relationship. Oxendine (1984) supported this claim and stated that, if a task was complex, moderate levels of arousal would result in optimal performance and high levels would cause a deterioration. If, however, the task was simple it would require high levels of arousal for optimal performance to be exhibited. Fleury, Bard, Jobin and Carrière, (1981) argued that simple tasks would not be affected at all, even by high levels of arousal. Landers (1980) stated that familiar tasks would be less likely to be adversely affected by high levels of arousal than unfamiliar tasks.

These arguments are not dissimilar to drive theory (Hull, 1943; Spence, 1958). According to drive theory, increases in arousal will result in an improvement in performance *if habit strength is high*. If habit strength is low, increases in arousal will either have no effect or will result in a breakdown in performance. Hull and Spence asserted that the equation is further complicated by the incentive value of completing the task. They stated that there will be an interaction between arousal, habit strength and incentive value. This interaction could be explained by the formula,

$$P = D \times H \times I$$

where P is performance, D is drive or arousal, H is habit strength and I is incentive value. Although drive theory may provide better explanations than inverted-U theories for the empirical data so far engendered by research, very few authors have used it as either a rationale for their studies or a tool to explain their results.

Although most of the early research took either Yerkes and Dodson's (1908) or Easterbrook's (1959) theories of arousal as their rationale, this was not the case for the group from the Université de Poitiers (e. g. Delignières, Brisswalter & Legros, 1994; Brisswalter, Arcelin, Audiffren & Delignières, 1997; Arcelin, Delignières & Brisswalter, 1998; Collardeau, Brisswalter & Audiffren, 2001) or those from our own laboratory (e. g. McMorris & Keen, 1994; McMorris & Graydon 1996a; 1996b; 1997a; 1997b). These authors used Kahneman's (1973) theory of allocatable resources to support their hypotheses that exercise would affect cognition. Kahneman's theory is based on the assumption that we have a limited amount of CNS resources. He believes that these resources are not fixed but that they increase as arousal rises. If the amount of allocatable resources in the CNS increase as arousal rises, one would expect performance to improve when compared to that at low levels of arousal. The greater the resources the more efficient the performance. If arousal continues to increase, however, it is thought that there comes a point when the increased number of available resources becomes redundant (Humphreys & Revelle, 1984). Moreover, Landers (1980) argued that large increases would lead to what he termed "random firing of nerve cells" in the CNS. This would of course result in an inhibition in performance. In other words, an inverted-U effect is hypothesized. Kahneman, however, did not perceive that the situation was that simple. He stated that there were two major factors, one being arousal with a resultant increase in resources, and the second being the allocation of those resources. Allocation of the resources was the role of what he called "cognitive effort", often referred to simply as "effort". Kahneman believes that, even at low levels arousal, if cognitive effort allocates resources to the task in hand, performance can be as good as that when arousal is optimal.

Research Support for the Cognitive Psychology Rationale

As we saw above, the designs of early research were very limited. However, Tomporowski and Ellis (1986) published a landmark study which was to alter the sophistication of research designs quite radically. Tomporowski and Ellis stated that it was not possible to draw definite conclusions from the research because of poor experimental designs. They particularly drew attention to the weak exercise protocols which I outlined earlier (e. g. Gutin & Di Gennaro, 1968a; Meyers et al., 1969; McAdam & Wang, 1967).

As Tomporowski and Ellis (1986) stated, such designs do not take into account individual differences between subjects, therefore it is possible that subjects were working at different exercise intensities relative to their own fitness. For example, Davey (1973) had all subjects work at 420 kg/m of work over 15 secs; 840 kg/m over 30 secs; 2800 kg/m over 2 mins; 4200 kg/m over 5 mins; and 7000 kg/m over 10 mins, regardless of their own level of fitness. Individuals' maximum workloads differ therefore, although these workloads are identical, they are at different percentage of each individual's maximum. Hence the stress is not identical.

Although Tomporowski and Ellis (1986) were generally correct in their criticisms of research designs, there were some studies that had used incremental exercise to exhaustion as the criterion for maximal exercise intensity (e. g. Bard & Fleury, 1978; Fleury, Bard & Carrière, 1981; Fleury, Bard, Jobin & Carrière, 1981: Gutin & Di Gennaro, 1968b; McGlynn, Laughlin & Bender, 1977). By definition this is individual. Some studies, however, used sub-maximal protocols, which did not take into account individual differences (e. g. Davey, 1972; 1973; Flynn, 1972; McGlynn, Laughlin & Bender, 1977; McGlynn, Laughlin & Rowe, 1979).

Research since the Tomporowski and Ellis (1986) review has generally taken account of individual differences (see McMorris & Graydon, 2000; Tomporowski, 2003, for reviews). The criteria for what constitutes moderate intensity exercise, however, has differed greatly. Allard et al. (1989) determined moderate exercise as being represented by cycling on a cycle ergometer at 30% and 60% of the subjects' physical work capacity, as determined by the PWC 170 test (see Åstrand & Rodahl, 1977, for a description of this test). Isaacs and Pohlman (1991) tested subjects at 40% and 70% of maximum volume of oxygen uptake (Max VO$_2$), while Fleury and Bard (1990) deemed 60% Max VO$_2$ to be representative of moderate intensity exercise. McMorris (1975) tested subjects at 75% of their maximum power output ($\dot{W}_{max}$) while McMorris and Keen (1994) used 70% $\dot{W}_{max}$ as their criterion for moderate exercise. To further complicate matters, Fleury and Bard tested subjects' cognitive performance *after* completion of the exercise protocol, while the other authors tested *during* exercise. If subjects are tested after the completion of the exercise there is no guarantee that they are in the same physiological state as when exercising (Reilly & Smith, 1986).

The situation regarding heavy exercise is even more complicated. Several authors worked subjects to exhaustion and *then* administered the cognitive tests (e. g. Côté, Salmela & Papathanasopoulu, 1990; Fleury & Bard, 1990; Salmela & Ndoye, 1986). These authors claimed to be testing subjects at fatigue. There is no doubt that their protocols did require subjects to reach fatigue, as defined by Edwards (1983). Edwards stated that fatigue was demonstrated when the person could not maintain a given workload. The problem, however, arises when one takes into account the fact that fit subjects can recover quickly from even fatiguing exercise. There is, therefore, no guarantee that the subject's physiological state was the same during cognitive testing as it was while exercising.

In order to try to overcome this problem, other authors (e. g. Isaacs & Pohlman, 1990; McMorris and Keen, 1994; McMorris, 1995) carried out the cognitive tests while the subjects were still exercising. Isaacs and Pohlman tested subjects while working at 100% Max VO_2, while McMorris and Keen, and McMorris tested their subjects while working at 100% $\dot{W}_{max}$. $\dot{W}_{max}$ is by definition maximal exercise, because any rise in resistance or speed results in fatigue. Max VO_2, however, does not represent maximal work, because the individual can continue working at the same intensity after Max VO_2 has been reached, due to an increase in the contribution of the anaerobic glycolytic metabolic pathway (Maughan, Gleeson & Greenhaff, 2003). More importantly, however, it should be noted that even working at $\dot{W}_{max}$ means that the subject is still in a state of homeostasis, unlike the individual who is fatigued.

The fact that different criteria were used to determine exercise intensity and that some cognitive testing took place after exercise while others took place during exercise, does mean that the actual exercise intensities would, in fact, be different from one another. This would be true for moderate intensity exercise as well as heavy and fatiguing exercise. Nevertheless, the criteria are sufficiently similar to make examination of the results of the effect of exercise on cognitive performance a worthwhile venture.

Moderate and Long Duration Exercise

So far we have only reviewed the effect of incremental exercise of short to moderate lengths. A number of authors have examined the effect of steady state, sub-maximal, long duration exercise on cognition. As with incremental exercise different protocols have been used. Time varies from 13 min (Féry, Ferry, Vom Hofe & Rieu, 1997) to 90 mins (Marriott, Reilly & Miles, 1993). The majority have worked subjects for $\geq$ 20 min. Exercise intensities have also varied a great deal. The majority have taken into account individual differences and had subjects exercise at a percentage of their MaxVO_2 (e. g. Tomporowski, Ellis & Stephens, 1987; Paas & Adam, 1991; Hogervorst, Riedel, Jeukendrup & Jolies, 1996; Féry et al., 1997). Nevertheless, some can be criticised for simply setting a heart rate that fails to take into account individual differences (Marriott et al., 1993; Tsorbatzoudis, Barboukis, Danis & Grouios, 1998).

Types of Cognitive Task

It should also be noted that different types of cognitive task have been used in the research. Several theorists have claimed that the nature of the task will have a bearing on how it is affected by arousal (Douchamps, 1988; Humphreys & Revelle, 1984; Landers, 1980; Oxendine, 1984; Sanders, 1983). The tasks used have generally been classical laboratory research tasks.:- simple reaction time (McMorris & Keen, 1994; McMorris, 1995; Brisswalter et al., 1997), choice reaction time (Chmura, Nazar & Kaciuba-Uścilko, 1994; Côté et al., 1992; Delignières et al., 1994; Levitt & Gutin, 1971; Meyers et al., 1969; Reynolds, 1976; Salmela & Ndoye, 1986; Travlos & Marisi, 1995; Williams, Pottinger & Shapcott, 1985), coincidence anticipation (Bard & Fleury, 1978; Fleury & Bard, 1990; Fleury, Bard &

Carrière, 1981; Isaacs & Pohlman, 1990), visual search/signal detection (Allard et al., 1989; Bard & Fleury, 1978; Fleury & Bard, 1990; Fleury, Bard, Jobin & Carrière, 1981), and short term memory (Davey, 1972; 1973; Sjöberg, 1980). Several authors have examined the effect of exercise on solving simple arithmetical problems (Beh, 1989; Flynn, 1972; Gutin & Di Gennaro, 19698a; 1968b; Lawless, 1988; McAdam & Wang, 1967; Zervas, 1990). While McGlynn, Laughlin and Bender (1977) and McGlynn, Laughlin and Rowe (1979) had subjects carry out a comparative judgement task, in which they had to match lines for length.

McMorris and Graydon (1996a; 1996b; 1997a; 1997b), Marriott et al. (193) and Tenenbaum, Yuval, Elbaz, Bar-Eli and Weinberg (1993) examined subjects on tachistoscopically presented decision-making tests. McMorris and Graydon, and Marriott et al. examined soccer and Tenenbaum et al. looked at team handball. McMorris and Graydon decided to use this type of task as they wished to examine subjects in an activity in which they were experienced, thereby limiting problems with learning effects. Such problems have affected research results. The amounts of habituation trials given to subjects have varied greatly in the research. It has not always been possible for researchers to randomise order of presentation of exercise intensities. For pragmatic reasons, it is easiest to examine subjects during one incremental test rather than use a counterbalanced design. This of course means that the higher intensities are always being examined last. McMorris and Graydon resolved this problem by designing tests that were shown to be reliable in multiple test/re-test situations. Marriott et al. used a control situation.

Research Results

We begin this section by examining the research results concerned with the effect of incremental exercise on the cognitive performance of a variety of different mental tasks. Results concerning simple reaction time have been mixed. McMorris and Keen (1994), and McMorris (1995) found simple reaction time to be unaffected by moderate exercise but inhibited by maximal exercise. Brisswalter et al. (1997) found fit subjects to be unaffected by exercise of any intensity while unfit subjects demonstrated an inverted-U effect. These results do not support the claims of Oxendine (1984), who argued that simple tasks would be facilitated by high levels of arousal. Nor are they in agreement with Fleury, Bard, Jobin and Carrière (1981), who stated that simple tasks would be unaffected by exercise. These results may be explained by drive theory. Although the task is simple, it is unfamiliar to the subjects, therefore habit strength is low. According to drive theory, when habit strength is low, high levels of arousal will either result in a breakdown in performance, as in the McMorris studies, or have no effect, as for the fit subjects in the Brisswalter et al. study. It does not account for the unfit subjects in that study, however.

Table 1. Research results concerning the effect of incremental exercise on simple reaction time

Author(s)	Exercise protocol	Results
McMorris & Keen, 1994	rest, 70%, 100% $\dot{W}_{max}$	inhibition at $\dot{W}_{max}$
McMorris, 1995	rest, 70%, 100% $\dot{W}_{max}$	inhibition at $\dot{W}_{max}$
Brisswalter et al., 1997	rest, 20%, 40%, 60% 80% MaxVO2	20% slowest (fit subjects) 40% fastest (unfit)

Significant effects of exercise on choice reaction time were demonstrated by Chmura et al. (1994), Levitt and Gutin (1971), Salmela and Ndoye (1986) and Delignières et al. (1994) but no effect was found by Côté et al. (1992), Meyers et al. (1969), Reynolds (1976), Williams et al. (1985) and Travlos and Marisi (1995). Salmela and Ndoye examined choice reaction time at rest and while exercising at heart rates of 115 beats/min, 145 beats/min, 160 beats/min and 180 beats/min. They found that performance at 115 beats/min was significantly better than that at rest. Performance at 145 beats/min was significantly quicker than that at 180 beats/min, but significantly slower than that at rest and 115 beats/min. However, when Côté et al. replicated this study they found no significant effects of exercise on choice reaction time. Levitt and Gutin tested subjects at rest and after exercising at heart rates of 115 beats/min, 145 beats/min and 175 beats/min. Reaction time was significantly better at 115 beats/min than at 145 beats/min, there were no other significant differences. Delignières et al. tested two and four choice reaction time at rest, 20%, 40%, 60% and 80% Max VO$_2$. They showed improvements in performance between rest and 20%, and 40% and 60% for the two choice test and between rest and 40%, and 40% and 60% for the four choice test.

The exercise protocols used by Meyers et al. (1969) and Williams et al. (1985) failed to take into account individual differences. It is, therefore, difficult to say what, if anything these studies revealed. The other studies have all tried to account for individual differences, but in different ways. Percentage of Max VO$_2$ (Chmura et al., 1994; Delignières et al., 1994) is a sound method of defining the individual's personal exercise intensity and exhaustion is by definition personal (Chmura et al., 1994; Travlos & Marisi, 1995). Although estimating maximum heart rate (Reynolds, 1976) has some merit it is based on an assumption that maximum heart rate is 220 - age. This is not always the case. Having subjects work at the same heart rates, however, (Levitt & Gutin, 1976; Salmela & Ndoye, 1986; Côté et al., 1992) can be misleading. As we have already seen, although all the subjects worked at the same heart rate, they would not all have the same maximum heart rate, therefore they were not all necessarily working at the same relative intensity.

Despite these reservations one could claim that exercise intensities were sufficient to constitute moderate and heavy exercise. The results, however, do not provide unequivocal support for exercise having an effect on performance. There is even less support for inverted-U and drive theories. Results would be best described as being somewhat equivocal.

Table 2. Research results concerning the effect of incremental exercise on choice reaction time

Author(s)	Exercise protocol	Results
Levitt & Gutin, 1971	rest, heart rates 115, 145, 175 beats/min	115 faster than 175 beats/min
Reynolds, 1976	rest, 75-80% max heart rate	no effect
Salmela & Ndoye, 1986	rest, heart rates 115, 145, 160, 180 beats/min	145 beats/min fastest
Côté et al., 1992	rest, heart rates 115, 145, 160, 180 beats/min	no effect
Chmura et al., 1994	rest, ~ 76%, 100% MaxVO2	inverted-U effect
Delignières et al., 1994	rest, 20%, 40%, 60% 80% MaxVO2	linear improvement rest to 60% MaxVO2
Davranche & Audiffren, 2004	rest, 20%, 50% MaxVO2	50% fastest

Research results examining the effect of exercise on coincidence anticipation are, also, somewhat contradictory. Isaacs and Pohlman (1990) found that performance on a Bassin anticipation timer was significantly poorer while exercising at 100% Max VO_2 compared to working at 25%, 40%, 75% Max VO_2 and while pedalling a cycle ergometer with no load. The dependent variables were constant error (CE), absolute error (AE), and variable error (VE). All were affected in the same way.

Research by Fleury and Bard (Bard & Fleury, 1978; Fleury, Bard & Carrière, 1981), however, does not fully support Isaacs and Pohlman (1990). Bard and Fleury measured AE on the Bassin anticipation timer at rest, immediately after exercising to exhaustion and 30 mins after exercise. They showed no significant effect of exercise on performance.

Table 3. Research results concerning the effect of incremental exercise on coincidence anticipation

Author(s)	Exercise protocol	Results
Bard & Fleury, 1978	rest & $\dot{W}_{max}$	no effect
Isaacs & Pohlman, 1991	no load, 25%, 40%, 75%, 100% MaxVO2	inhibition at 100% MaxVO2

Results of experiments into the effect of exercise on visual search are, also, somewhat equivocal. Bard and Fleury (1978) found no significant effect of fatiguing exercise on performance on, both, a central visual field and a peripheral visual field signal detection task. Allard et al. (1989) showed that speed of visual search was significantly faster during exercise at 60% of maximal workload, as predicted by the PWC 170 test, when compared to at rest and during exercise at 30% of maximal workload.

Table 4. Research results concerning the effect of incremental exercise on short-term memory

Author(s)	Exercise protocol	Results
Davey, 1973	420 kg/m (for 15 s), 840 (30 s), 2800 (120 s), 4200 (300 s), 7000 (600 s)	inverted-U effect
Sjöberg, 1980	rest, 25%, 50% & 100% $\dot{W}_{max}$	no effect

The position with regard to the effect of exercise on short-term memory tasks is not much clearer. Davey (1973) showed a facilitative effect of cycling on a cycle ergometer for 30 s at a constant speed to carry out 840 kg/m of work. In a follow up experiment (Davey, 1973) tested performance following exercise at 420 kg/m of work over 15 secs; 840 kg/m over 30 s; 2800 kg/m over 2 mins; 4200 kg/m over 5 mins; and 7000 kg/m over 10 mins. As we saw earlier, there are problems with the lack of control for individual differences in fitness in this experiment.

Furthermore, examination of the statistical treatment raises doubts about the experiment. Analysis of Covariance showed there to be a significant effect of exercise and Davey (1973) claimed that an inverted-U effect was demonstrated. He did not report any *post hoc* testing, however, and his final analysis appears to be based simply on observation of group means. To complicate matters further, Sjöberg (1980) examined subjects at rest and while working at 25%, 50% and 75% $\dot{W}_{max}$. He used three different tasks and fit and unfit subjects. Only one of the tasks was significantly affected by exercise and then only for the fit subjects. Again no *post hoc* results were reported, therefore one can not tell where the difference or differences lie.

Table 5. Research results concerning the effect of incremental exercise on simple arithmetic problems

Author(s)	Exercise protocol	Results
Flynn, 1972	rest, cycling at 150, 300 & 600 kpm/min	no effect accuracy speed facilitation
Gutin & Dui Gennaro, 1968	rest, $\dot{W}_{max}$	no effect

The effect of exercise on solving simple arithmetical problems is, also, inconclusive. McAdam and Wang (1967), Lawless (1988), and Zervas (1990) found no significant effect of exercise. Beh (1989) showed that accuracy of problem solving was not affected by exercise, but speed was significantly improved following 60 s of step ups. Flynn (1972) demonstrated that moderate intensity of exercise resulted in an improvement in speed of performance when compared to performance at rest and following low intensity exercise. Gutin and Di Gennaro (1968a) showed that both conditioned and unconditioned subjects performed better on an addition task following exercise than when at rest. However, Gutin and Di Gennaro (1968b) found that running to exhaustion had no effect on performance. What is more, only the latter experiment used an exercise protocol that has any validity.

Table 6. Research results concerning the effect of incremental exercise on judgement tasks

Author(s)	Exercise protocol	Results
McGlynn et al., 1977	40%, 54%, 71% & 97% max heart rate	no effect accuracy 97% fastest
McGlynn et al., 1979	40%, 54%, 71% & 97% max heart rate	no effect accuracy 97% fastest

McGlynn and his associates (McGlynn, Laughlin & Bender, 1977; McGlynn, Laughlin & Rowe, 1979) examined the effect of exercise on a discrimination task. Subjects had to match lines with a given line, which acted as the standard. The results showed that heavy exercise induced a significantly faster performance on a discrimination task than did exercise at a low level of intensity. There was no significant effect on accuracy of performance. Although the experiments could be questioned on the fact that they estimated maximum heart rates, the exercise protocols were sufficiently controlled to suggest that the results are valid. Obviously more than two experiments are required if one is to draw any definite conclusions.

Table 7. Research results concerning the effect of incremental exercise on decision making in soccer

Author(s)	Exercise protocol	Results
McMorris & Graydon, 1996a	rest, 70% & 100% $\dot{W}_{max}$	no effect accuracy rest slowest
McMorris & Graydon, 1996b experiment 1	rest, 70% & 100% $\dot{W}_{ma}$	no effect accuracy rest slowest
McMorris & Graydon, 1996b experiment 2	rest, 70% & 100% $\dot{W}_{max}$	no effect accuracy rest slower than $\dot{W}_{max}$
McMorris & Graydon, 1997a	rest, 70% & 100% $\dot{W}_{max}$	no effect accuracy rest slowest
McMorris & Graydon, 1997b	rest, 70% & 100% $\dot{W}_{max}$	accuracy $\dot{W}_{max}$ best rest slowest

McMorris and Graydon (1996a; 1996b; 1997a; 1997b) examining the effect of incremental exercise on decision making in soccer-specific tests unequivocally demonstrated a significant improvement in speed of decision during exercise at $\dot{W}_{max}$. Interestingly this was found even when subjects were told to concentrate on accuracy and that speed was not being assessed (McMorris & Graydon, 1996b). The situation with regard to speed of decision at 70% $\dot{W}_{max}$ is more complex. In all except the 1997b study there were no significant differences between speed at 70% $\dot{W}_{max}$ and that at $\dot{W}_{max}$. The authors concluded that this may have been due to the arbitrary nature of designating 70% $\dot{W}_{max}$ as representing moderate intensity exercise. As a result McMorris et al. (1999) used a more sophisticated design. Results of that study are examined later. There was no effect of any exercise intensity on accuracy of decision, except for a small improvement at $\dot{W}_{max}$ in the 1997a experiment. This is in line with the other research that places a stress on working memory (McGlynn, Laughlin & Bender, 1977; McGlynn, Laughlin & Rowe, 1977). This is also commented on in some detail later in the chapter.

Table 8. Research results concerning the effect of incremental exercise on visual search

Author(s)	Exercise protocol	Results
Allard et al., 1989	rest, 30%, 60% $\dot{W}_{max}$	60% fastest
McMorris & Graydon, 1997b	rest, 70% & 100% $\dot{W}_{max}$	rest slowest

Long Duration Exercise Results

Research examining long duration exercise on short-term memory tasks is limited and produces somewhat equivocal findings. Tomporowski et al. (1987) and Adam, Teeken, Ypellar, Verstappen and Paas (1997) found no significant effect but Paas and Adam (1991) showed an improvement in performance. Given that Paas and Adam, and Adam et al. used an identical exercise protocol, this is surprising. Also, Tomporowski et al.'s protocol was very similar. The situation is further complicated given the results of Marriott et al. (1993) and Tenenbaum et al. (1993) for decision making in soccer and team handball respectively. However, we may need to look more closely at those studies before making any decision on their merit.

Marriott et al. (1993) examined the performance of college soccer players (n = 8) and non-soccer players (n = 8) on a tachistoscopically presented test of decision making in soccer. Subjects ran on a treadmill at a heart rate of 157 beats/min, for two periods of 45 mins. The relationship between speed and heart rate was examined and the speed necessary to induce a heart rate of 157 beats/min was estimated. This figure was chosen as this was the mean value for a soccer game according to the findings of Reilly (1986). Subjects were tested before exercise and then after running for 45 mins on a treadmill. Following a 15 mins rest period (to simulate half-time in a soccer game), they ran for another 45 mins before being tested for the third time. On a separate day, subjects were again tested three times, on the decision-making test, over a 90 min period but undertook no physical activity.

The experienced group performed significantly better than the inexperienced group during the testing on the non-exercise day. On the exercise day the non-players performed significantly better after 45 mins of exercise than in the other two conditions. The experienced players were not significantly affected by exercise.

Tenenbaum et al. (1993) tested the decision-making performance of "experienced" (n = 39), "moderately experienced" (n = 37) and "novice" (n = 42) team handball players during exercise of different intensities. Although they used the terms "experienced", "moderately experienced" and "novice", the players were all of national standard. They did, however, have different lengths of experience, the "experienced" had played for M = 8.82 (SD = 4.24) years, the "moderately experienced" M = 6.22 (SD = 1.51) years and the "novices" M = 4.21 (SD = 1.79) years.

Table 9. Research results concerning the effect of long duration sub-maximal exercise on cognitive performance

Author(s)	Exercise protocol	cognitive performance	Results
Tomporowski et al., 1987	50 min at 80 MaxVO2	STM	no effect
Paas & Adam, 1991	20 min at 75% $\dot{W}_{max}$	STM visual search	improvement inhibition
Marriott et al., 199	90 min run at 157 beats/min	soccer decision making	no effect
Adam et al., 1997	20 min at 75% $\dot{W}_{max}$	information transfer STM	improvement no effect
Féry et al., 1997	13 min at 30% MaxVO2	choice reaction time	facilitation
Hogervorst, 1996	1 hour at 75% $\dot{W}_{max}$	simple reaction time choice reaction time Stroop colour test	facilitation facilitation facilitation
Tsorbatzoudis et al., 1998	30 min cycle at 160 180 beats/min heart rate	simple reaction time	no effect
Chmura et al., 1998, experiment 1	20 min at 10% < lactate threshold	choice reaction time	linear facilitation
experiment 2	60 min at 30% > lactate threshold	choice reaction time	facilitation up to 40 min
Collardeau et al., 2001	90 min at ventilatory threshold	simple reaction time	improvement

Subjects were tested on the decision-making test while walking on a treadmill at 5-6 km/h and while running on a treadmill at 80% of estimated maximum heart rate. Maximum heart rate was estimated by the 220 - age formula. The "novices" were significantly poorer than the other two groups. A main effect for exercise was, also, demonstrated, with decision making during running being significantly better than while walking. Unfortunately practical considerations meant that the exercise condition was taken second by all subjects, therefore a learning effect can not be ruled out. The authors tried to overcome this by using two different tests and counterbalancing their use between subjects.

Research examining the effect of long duration exercise on choice reaction time also provides mixed results (Hogervorst et al., 1996; Féry et al., 1997; Chmura, Krysztofiak, Ziemba, Nazar & Kaciuba-Uścilko, 1998; Tsorbatzoudis et al., 1998). If, however, we dismiss the research of Tsorbatzoudis et al. on the grounds that they did not take into account individual differences in fitness, it appears that choice reaction time is facilitated by long duration exercise. One should include Adam et al's (1997) information transfer task in this statement as it requires similar skills. Only one study has examined the effect of long duration exercise on simple reaction time and a significant facilitation in performance was demonstrated (Hogervorst et al., 1996).

Reaction Time Plus Movement Time Tasks

Although the aim of this chapter is to examine the effect of exercise on purely cognitive tasks, we should also make a brief mention of those protocols that required a movement response. Levitt and Gutin (1971) examined reaction and movement times on a 5-choice response task at rest and while walking/running on a treadmill at intensities which elicited heart rates of 115, 145 and 175 beats/min. Mean reaction time at 115 beats/min was significantly slower than that at 175 beats/min. There were no other significant differences for this variable.

Williams et al. (1985) compared reaction and movement times of three different groups of participants. Group one undertook a verbal task before being tested on an 8-choice response time test. Group two carried out an arm cranking activity that elicited a power output of 10 W before undertaking the task. Group three, also, carried out the arm cranking exercise, but at a power output of 75 W. The performance of the groups did not differ significantly. McMorris et al. (2003) examined participants on a 4-choice non-compatible response time task, while at rest and exercising at 70% and 100% $\dot{W}_{max}$. They found no effect of exercise on reaction time.

The types of psychomotor tasks used, in all of these experiments, required only a limited range of movement (between 11 cms and 44 cms) and only by the participant's arm. McMorris, Delves, Lauder, Sproule & Hale (2005) measured reaction time in a task that required a whole body response. They found that reaction time following exercise at 70% $\dot{W}_{max}$ was significantly faster than that at rest and $\dot{W}_{max}$. Reaction time following rest was significantly quicker than that following exercise at $\dot{W}_{max}$.

As we will see later, even when the response requires only a finger press as in the "normal" reaction time experiments, different neural pathways become involved compared to a voice response test. When a whole body or an arm movement is concerned there is such a great difference in pre-programming that it is not really sensible to compare reaction times in such experiments with those when only a cognitive response is required. Nevertheless, as with purely cognitive tasks, we can see that there is a failure to demonstrate unequivocal results.

Summary

To summarise, research results into the effect of incremental exercise on cognitive performance certainly do not provide unequivocal support for the hypothesis that exercise will affect cognitive functioning. Studies that have tested subjects' cognitive performance at various intensities of Max VO_2 and $\dot{W}_{max}$ have provided very little support for Tomporowski and Ellis' (1986) claim that exercise will affect cognitive performance in an inverted-U fashion.

There is, also, little support for the claims of Oxendine (1984) that complex tasks will be facilitated by moderate levels of arousal and inhibited by high levels, while simple tasks will be facilitated by high levels of arousal. The simple reaction time results demonstrated that high levels of arousal can cause a detriment in performance (McMorris, 1995; McMorris & Keen, 1994). While the results into the effect of exercise on solving arithmetical problems found no effect on accuracy (Gutin & Di Gennaro, 1968b; Lawless, 1985; McAdam & Wang, 1967; Zervas, 1990) yet improvements in speed of performance were observed, even following heavy exercise (Beh, 1989; Flynn, 1972).

There is some support for allocatable resources theories. McMorris and Graydon (2000) used Kahneman's (1973) theory to explain research results when cognitive performance during moderate intensity of exercise was not significantly better than that at rest. This they argued was particularly the case when the task was comparatively simple, e. g. simple reaction time. The amount of resources required for optimal performance are not great, therefore there are sufficient resources for optimal performance, even at rest, as long as effort allocates the resources to the task. When the task is more complex, optimal performance can only be experienced when arousal level is sufficient to increase the number of allocatable resources. This could also explain why Tomporowski (2003) found that, with complex cognitive tasks, there were improvements in performance when exercise was heavy and maximal. Kahneman would not have expected this. He believed that, at high levels of arousal, effort would not be able to control the allocation of resources sufficiently well to ensure optimal performance. He thought that resources would be diverted to feelings of anxiety and the individual might focus on their discomfort rather than the task in hand.

Eysenck and Calvo (1992) disagreed with this hypothesis. They asserted that, if cognitive effort can overcome low levels of arousal, it is possible that it can also overcome high levels of arousal. This they believed would be more likely to occur when the person was carrying out a well learned task. It could also occur if the individual was used to exercising maximally. Brisswalter et al. (1997) found that subjects unused to exercising maximally demonstrated an inverted-U effect of exercise on simple reaction time. Subjects, who trained regularly, were unaffected by exercise. McMorris and Graydon (2000) argued that this was because the regular exercisers did not perceive the exercise as being threatening, therefore resources were not allocated to feelings of distress. Instead they were allocated to the cognitive task.

Thus allocatable resources theories provide better explanations of research results than Yerkes and Dodson's (1908) and Easterbrook's (1959) theories. However, the fact that the success or failure of cognitive effort to allocate resources is difficult, if not impossible, to measure means that one can not be sure what the reasons are for any results. In fact, allocatable resources theory can explain away any results – significant improvements in performance are due to increases in arousal, while non-significant results are due to the failure of effort to allocate resources. There have been some attempts to measure how effort affects performance. Delignières et al. (1994), using a unidimensional rating of perception of task demands (Delignières, Famose, & Genty, 1994), found that perceptions of difficulty for 2-choice and 4-choice reaction time tests increased with exercise intensity. Moreover, they found that as perceptions of difficulty increased performance improved. Thus supporting the argument that cognitive effort can overcome the negative effects of high intensity exercise. In contrast, McMorris et al. (2003) found that effort, as measured by the National Aeronautics and Space Administration-Task Load Index (NASA-TLX) (Hart & Staveland, 1988), could not significantly predict non-compatible reaction time during exercise.

However, unpublished data from our laboratory provides some support for Delignières et al. (1994). We found that as exercise intensity increased so did perceptions of task demands, as measured by the NASA-TLX. This was the case for each of the sub-sections of the NASA-TLX, despite the fact that only the physical demands of the task that changed. The NASA-TLX is divided into the following sub-sections: - Mental Demand, Physical Demand, Temporal Demand, Performance, Effort and Frustration. Mental Demand refers to the individual's perception of how much mental and perceptual activity is required. Physical Demand examines perceptions of the amount of physiological effort required to perform the task. Temporal Demand is concerned with the time pressure that the performer believes he or she is under. Performance is concerned with the person's perception of how well they have completed the task. Effort is the perception of how hard, mentally and physically, the person had to work in order to complete the task. While Frustration refers to emotions of stress, relaxation, tension and complacency.

Hierarchical multiple regression analyses, with reaction time and intra-individual variations in reaction time (an individual's consistency over a number of trials) as the dependent variables and the sub-sections of the NASA-TLX as the independent variables were calculated. Effort was a significant predictor of intra-individual variations of reaction time, $R^2 = .21$ ($p < .05$), but there were no significant predictors for reaction time.

With regard to the effect of moderate to long duration, sub-maximal, steady state exercise on cognition, research results are somewhat equivocal. As far as I am aware, no attempt has been made to examine the effect of cognitive effort on these results. Based on Humphreys and Revelle's (1986) theory, it is tempting to argue that high levels of motivation would result in cognitive effort allocating resources to task relevant information, thus aiding cognition. On the other hand, low motivation would have the opposite effect. While this has strong intuitive appeal there is, as yet, no evidence to support it.

Development of a Neuroscientific Rationale for the Exercise-Arousal-Cognitive Performance Interaction

In order to explain how a neuroscientific rationale for the exercise-arousal-cognition interaction effect was developed, we must examine (a) how we process information; (b) the areas of the brain responsible for this process; (c) the effect of exercise on the neurotransmitters that serve these areas; (d) the interaction between the cognitive and emotional centres in the brain; and (d) the peripheral-central biochemical interaction during exercise.

Working Memory

As we have seen above, several different types of cognitive activity have been examined by researchers in this area. The majority have examined choice reaction time but also we have seen simple reaction time, coincidence anticipation, non-compatible choice reaction time, solving arithmetical problems, and decision making in soccer and team handball. Despite differences in the choice of type of cognitive activity, all of the researchers have taken an Information Processing Theory (e. g. Welford, 1968) approach with regard to the way in which the person controls their cognition. According to Information Processing Theory, information from the environment is relayed to the CNS by the senses. This information is meaningless in itself and has to be interpreted by the CNS. This is the role of *perception*. The interpretation is based on a comparison between what we hold in *Short-term memory* (*STM*) with what we hold in *Long-term memory* (*LTM*). The comparison of information, held in the STM and LTM, also allows the person to decide what action to take in any given situation – *Decision Making*. Once a decision of what action to make has been taken, the CNS has to organize the movement (*Efferent Organization*). This part of the Information Processing model is not of interest to us in this chapter. To summarize the cognitive aspects of the Information Processing model we can say that, first of all, information is taken in by the senses, this information is passed to the CNS where it is perceived (made sense of) due to a comparison of what the person holds in STM with their past experiences held in LTM. Based on this comparison a decision of what action to take is made.

Although what we have described above has intuitive appeal, Baddeley (1986) found some inconsistencies. Baddeley noted that some individuals where good at STM and/or LTM tasks but were not good on decision-making tests. Similarly accurate perception of objects and their position in space (spatial perception) was also not necessarily correlated to decision making. So the act of decision making must require something a little more than the simple transfer of information through the stages of the Information Processing model. Baddeley, therefore, put forward the notion of what he called *working memory*. Baddeley sees working memory as consisting of perception, STM, decision making and information recalled from LTM. The role of working memory is to integrate this information. So although perception,

STM and LTM are necessary for accurate decision making, working memory is the key because it is its responsibility to synthesize and evaluate this information. A very different task to simply recalling information as in STM and LTM tasks or recognizing features as in a perceptual task.

Baddeley (1986) argues that working memory consists of three separate but interdependent parts, the *central executive mechanism, the phonological loop and the visuospatial sketch pad*. The phonological loop is responsible for the encoding of acoustic and verbal information. The visuospatial sketchpad has the same role as the phonological loop except it processes visual and visuospatial information. The role of the central executive is to oversee and control the whole process. It ensures that integration of perceptual input and comparison of the present situation (held in STM) with recalled information from LTM occurs. Norman and Shallice (1980) used the term *Supervisory Attentional System (SAS)* to describe the central executive. They believe that the SAS is particularly active when the decision making is complex and when the correct response differs from a well learned habitual response.

Neuroscientific Evidence for the Existence of Working Memory

In this section we examine the evidence from neuroscience for the existence of working memory. This will allow us to better understand how exercise affects cognition. Baddeley's (1986) arguments came from his observation of human performance but evidence from neuroscience followed fairly quickly. This evidence comes from a variety of methods of measuring brain activity, the most common being *Positron Emission Tomography (PET)* and *functional Magnetic Resonance Imaging (fMRI)*. PET measures changes in cerebral blood flow and is particularly useful when trying to identify brain regions used during different tasks. It is even capable of showing functional variation within a given area. fMRI works in a similar way but measures the ratio between oxygenated and deoxygenated hemoglobin.

Evidence that the *prefrontal cortex* is responsible for working memory is very strong (e. g. Barbas, 2000; Critchley et al., 2003; Seamans, Nogueira & Lavin, 2003). Moreover, there is powerful evidence that the phonological and visuospatial loops are distinct. It would appear that the phonological loop involves the lateral frontal and interior parietal lobes of the left hemisphere. The visuospatial loop seems to be situated in the parieto-occipatal region of both hemispheres, although it is more active in the right hemisphere (Barbas, 2000). The role of the central executive would appear to be undertaken by almost all of the prefrontal cortex. However, there is evidence that many other parts of the brain are involved in working memory (Chudasama, Bussey & Muir, 2001; Critchley, et al., 2003). It seems that the prefrontal cortex is particularity responsible for recalling past experience from LTM and the integration of that information with perception of the present situation. The LTM information is probably held permanently in the post sensory regions of the temporal and parietal cortices. These areas are know to have strong connections with the prefrontal cortex (Gazzaniga, Ivry & Mangun, 2002). It appears that the prefrontal cortex is particularly active when decision making is complex and there is a necessity to recall information from LTM. The prefrontal cortex is less active in recognition tasks while the role of the parietal cortex stays the same for both tasks (Barbas, 2000; Seamans et al., 2003).

Reaction Time Tasks

Many researchers have claimed that the efficiency of the individual's ability to process information is best examined by the use of reaction time tasks. Hence the proliferation of studies using reaction time tasks to examine the effect of exercise on cognition. Reaction time is the time from the onset of a stimulus to the *beginning* of an overt response. As such it differs from working memory in that it includes some efferent organization. It is not surprising then to find that, during reaction time tasks, the basal ganglia are highly active (Rektor et al., 2003). The roles of the basal ganglia are to initiate the desired movement and to inhibit the initiation of unwanted movement. This is particularly important in choice reaction time tasks. An explanation often given to explain how the basal ganglia control this process is that the basal ganglia act like a dam controlling a river; the 'river' being the possible responses. The basal ganglia close the "locks" on the unwanted responses but allow the dominant response to "flow" through.

The claim that reaction time tasks are the best indicators of the proficiency of the information processing system is very dubious. As we saw earlier, Baddeley (1986) found that STM tasks did not explain the proficiency of decision making and hence working memory. Reaction time requires only recognition of the stimulus and then initiation of a pre-chosen response. As we saw above, recognition requires either the phonological or visuospatial loops but very little, if any, input from the executive control mechanism. Reaction time tasks are primarily controlled by the prefrontal cortex (Barbas, 2000) but less neural activity is demonstrated than for tasks involving a great deal of executive control. Indeed there is evidence to show that there is even a difference in prefrontal cortex activity levels during simple versus choice reaction time tasks (Babiloni et al., 2004). There is also evidence that other parts of the brain, including the basal ganglia, play a part in the processing of information when the response is a motor one (Bares, Rektor, Kanovsky & Streitova, 2003; Rektor et al., 2003).

In order to emphasize the limited amount of information that needs to be processed in reaction time tasks, Humphreys and Revelle (1986) labeled them "information transfer" tasks. To Humphreys and Revelle any tasks that simply require the individual to recognize the presence of a stimulus and then produce a predetermined response does not require a memory process therefore can not be equated with STM tasks. Humphreys and Revelle believe than the simplicity of such tasks means that as arousal increases so should performance on these tasks. This is very similar to drive theory and to Yerkes and Dodson's (1908) claim that easy tasks will demonstrate an inverted-U that is skewed towards the high side of arousal. To Humphreys and Revelle, STM tasks require more in the way of processing, therefore will demonstrate an inhibition in performance during high levels of arousal. This is similar to Yerkes and Dodson's claim that for complex tasks the inverted-U would be skewed towards the lower end of the arousal continuum. However, the types of tasks that Humphreys and Revelle see as being complex are dissimilar to those proposed by Yerkes and Dodson. The latter used tasks that had a large central executive component while Humphreys and Revelle talked about STM tasks. STM is normally examined by presenting the subject with a list of numbers or words and having them repeat them. This simply requires use of the phonological loop. Some researchers touch a number of objects in a given order and ask the subject to repeat the movement sequences. This tests the visuospatial sketchpad. As we have seen above, such tasks do not require as much activation of the prefrontal cortex as central executive tasks, therefore probably could not be classed as complex. We will further discuss this point when we examine neuroscientific explanations for research results.

Arousal and Cognition

In the first part of this chapter we highlighted the fact that the early researchers, such as Davey (1973), hypothesized that any effect of exercise on cognition would be due to exercise inducing increases in arousal level. We then outlined the major arousal-performance theories that have been used as underpinnings for an exercise-arousal-cognitive performance hypothesis. The most influential of recent theories has been that of Kahneman's (1973) allocatable resources theory. Following on from Kahneman, Pribram and McGuinness (1975) and, later, Sanders (1983) provided an explanation of the arousal-performance interaction that differed a little to Kahneman's. Pribram and McGuinness divided arousal into two separate factors. The first they termed "arousal" and the second "activation". They saw arousal as being a "phasic reaction to input". To them any input that broke the person's state of equilibrium, no matter how small, induced arousal. This takes place in the brainstem and is centered on the amygdala. It increases the organism's awareness of the presence of stimuli and hence the fact that, in order to re-establish equilibrium, a response may have to be made. Activation is the process by which this response is made. Activation is a "tonic readiness to respond". This means a readiness to perceive stimuli and to initiate movement. This takes place in the lateral hypothalamic region and is centered on the basal ganglia. The whole process is controlled by the hippocampal circuit and this action is similar to Kahneman's idea of cognitive effort.

Pribram and McGuinness' (1975) notion of what constitutes arousal is a little different from what is implied in the exercise-arousal-cognition literature. Recent researchers (e. g. Chmura et al., 1994; McMorris & Graydon, 1996a; 1996b) based their arguments on the physiological and biochemical similarities between exercise induced arousal and arousal induced by emotions such as anxiety. As emotional arousal has been seen to have an effect on cognition (Hagemann, Waldstein & Thayer, 2003), we will examine this factor here.

Emotion is difficult to define. According to Hagemann et al. (2003), emotion has been mostly described by the types of feelings displayed, e. g. "surprise, interest, happiness, rage fear, sadness, and disgust". Whether positive or negative, it has been shown that emotions affect many parts of the brain. MacLean (1949) identified the amygdala, orbitofrontal cortex and parts of the basal ganglia as being the most important areas. He called the interaction between these areas of the brain the *limbic system*. For many years it was thought that the limbic system was the only part of the CNS affected by arousal. More recent studies, however, have shown that many parts of the brain are activated by arousal. Hagemann et al. highlighted the frontal, temporal and parietal cortices, thalamus and hippocampus, as well as the basal ganglia and amygdala. Davidson, Putnam and Larson (2000) have shown that the orbitofrontal cortex and amygdala are probably the most important centers.

It would appear that, when activated by emotions, both the orbitofrontal cortex and amygdala are concerned with activities related to that arousal. The learning of responses to the stressor and memory for social repercussions of action are particularly affected. The amygdala, however, has also been shown to affect tasks that do not result in emotional changes. Whalen (1998) described the role of the amygdala as being to ready the organism for action. This is very similar to Pribram and McGuinness' (1975) idea of arousal. It would appear that, during moderate arousal, the amygdala can stimulate the hippocampus thus resulting in optimal performance. During high levels of arousal, however, increases in stress hormones negatively affect the hippocampus. Hence poor performance. There is also evidence to show that the amygdala influences the sensory cortical systems.

The synonymous use of the words emotion and arousal has come about because emotions induce not only a CNS response but also an Autonomic Nervous System response of which we are all aware during high emotions. Heart rate and respiratory rates increase, we sweat and blood pressure increases (Lacey & Lacey, 1970; Davidson, MacGregor et al., 2000). The link to exercise is obvious and we will examine this later in the chapter.

As we will see later, whether we perceive increases in arousal as being positive or negative may be as important as the fact that arousal levels have increased. The perception of arousal as being negative or positive will depend on many factors, e. g. past experience and personality. High sensation seekers may perceive jumping out of an aeroplane in a parachute as exhilarating, while low sensation seekers see it as being anxiety provoking. This is one way in which arousal and cognition interact. To Kahneman (1973), during high arousal, the person can not allocate resources efficiently. In negative situations they tend to focus on their fears while in very exciting situations they are enable to contain their enthusiasm. Although not coming from a neuroscientific approach, Landers (1980) suggested an explanation for poor performance during high levels of arousal as being due to "random firing of nerve cells". Although this is not a particularly accurate explanation of the brain's response to high levels of arousal, it does lead us to consider the possibility that the neural pathways involved with arousal interfere with those involved in working memory. Barbas (2000) explains the interaction by pointing to the dual role of many areas of the brain in both the regulation of emotion and of cognition. She also highlights the fact that areas involved in emotion and cognition are interconnected and often in close proximity to one another.

Neurotransmitters in the Brain

In the last two sections we outlined the areas of the brain responsible for working memory and the regulation of emotion. In this section we examine the role of the neurotransmitters norepinephrine, dopamine and 5-hydroxytryptamine (5-HT) in the excitation of these areas. The areas of the brain activated by each of these transmitters have been named the *noradrenergic, dopaminergic and serotonergic pathways*. The pathway for norepinephrine has been named noradrenergic as the term noradrenaline is often given to this transmitter. Just as epinephrine is often called adrenaline. Similarly the 5-HT pathway is given the title serotonergic based on the use of the word serotonin which is so often used instead of 5-HT.

The neurons serving the noradrenergic pathway are mainly found in the locus coeruleus. They enervate the dorsal raphe nucleus, thalamus, hypothalamus, hippocampus, septum, the entire cerebral cortex and the cerebellum. The dopaminergic pathway mainly serves the corpus striatum, where 80% of the brain's dopamine can be found (Kuhar, Couceyro & Lambert, 1999). This pathway also includes the frontal and cingulate cortex. Although the neurons containing 5-HT are almost entirely found in the brainstem their axons innervate nearly every area of the brain. They are strongly represented in the pons, midbrain, amygdala, hippocampus, hypothalamus and thalamus. "Intermediate" density is found in the cerebellum and cerebellar cortex (Loubinoux, Pariente, Rascol, Celsis & Chollet, 2002). Given the vast areas of the brain served by norepinephrine, dopamine and 5-HT, it is not surprising to find that they have been shown to be involved in the performance of cognitive skills and the regulation of emotion.

Synthesis of Norepinephrine, Dopamine and 5-Hydroxytryptamine in the Brain

Norepinephrine and dopamine, along with the hormone epinephrine, are called catecholamines. The synthesis of these neurotransmitters depends on the hydrogenation of phenylanine. This is converted to tyrosine with phenylalanine hydroxylase acting as a catalyst. This is further broken down into the metabolite 3, 4 dihydroxy–L-phenylalanine (L-DOPA) under the influence of tyrosine hydroxylase, which is found in all cells that synthesize catecholamines. L-DOPA is then catalyzed by DOPA decarboxylase and dopamine is formed. With the aid of dopamine-β-hydroxylase, norepinephrine is synthesized. Finally the N-methyleration of norepinephrine occurs and epinephrine is formed. Norepinephrine and dopamine, and a small amount of epinephrine, are secreted within the brain. We will examine secretion into the peripheral nervous system later in this chapter.

The synthesis of 5-HT begins with the transportation of the amino acid tryptophan from the blood into the brain. Under the influence of tryptophan hydroxylase, 5-hydroxytryptophan is formed. This is further broken down by aromatic L-amino acid decarboxyllase into 5-HT. This process takes place mainly in the raphe nuclei. This is the only place that 5-hydroxytryptophan is found.

Catecholamines and 5- Hydroxytryptamine During Cognition

fMRI and EEG studies provide evidence that the noradrenergic and dopaminergic pathways are involved in cognition. As the neurotransmitters for these pathways are norepinephrine and dopamine respectively, it is not surprising to find that there is evidence that these catecholamines play a part in cognitive functioning. Animal studies have shown increases in brain concentrations of norepinephrine and dopamine during mental stress (e. g. Eisenhofer et al., 1991). With humans the role of brain neurotransmitters can not be directly measured, nevertheless examination of catecholamine metabolites has provided strong evidence of the role of norepinephrine in mental activity (Peyrin, Pequinot, Lacour & Fourcade, 1987).

As brain concentrations of norepinephrine and dopamine can not be measured directly in humans one must rely on measurement of the metabolites which they produce during cognition. The main metabolite produced by norepinephrine activity in the brain is 3-methoxy-4-hydroxyphenyglycol (MHPG). While the main brain metabolites of dopamine are 3, 4-dihydroxyphenylacetic acid (DOPAC) and 4-hydroxy-3-methoxyphenylacetic acid, also known as homovanillic acid. These are produced by *O*-methylation and/or oxidative deamination, depending on the site where the metabolism takes place (Sian, Moussa, Youdim, Riederer & Gerlach, 1999). MHPG is formed by the *O*-methylation of norepinephrine.

A problem with using these metabolites as measures of brain use of catecholamines is the fact that they are also produced by peripheral activity. Therefore, measurement of plasma concentrations may be due to physical rather than mental changes. The best way to overcome this problem is to take an arterial blood sample and a venous blood sample. If catecholamine metabolites are higher in the venous outflow than in the arterial inflow, the brain must be using the catecholamines. If there is no difference then the concentrations are due to peripheral use. There is a problem, however. Arterial blood can be taken from any artery, as it has essentially the same composition throughout the body. Venous blood is specific to each tissue. In humans, cerebral venous blood taken from the internal jugular vein has less than 3% contamination from extracerebullar blood. As such, it is an ideal area from which to take the sample. It can not be taken unless under general anaesthetic. It is, therefore, a method of little use in practical terms. Moreover, as you can imagine, few individuals are keen to be subjects in such experiments. There is no fool proof way of overcoming this problem but a good attempt was made by Peyrin et al. (1987) and we will examine their research later in this chapter.

While the role of the neurotransmitter catecholamines in cognition is obvious, it is interesting to note that, in Peyrin et al.'s (1987) study, epinephrine also played a major role. Moreover, in animal studies, McGaugh (1983) has shown epinephrine to be a better predictor of performance than norepinephrine. It would appear that this is due to the fact that epinephrine is released from the adrenal medulla in response to stress. This secretion of epinephrine is also thought to affect the Sympathetic Nervous System (SNS) leading to a release of norepinephrine and dopamine into the brain by sympathetic neurons particularly in the hypothalamus (the process of how this occurs is explained later in this section). Thus plasma concentrations of epinephrine can be indicative of change in arousal and cognition.

As 5-HT is found in almost all areas of the brain it is not surprising to find that increases in concentrations have been shown to be related to cognitive performance (Bailey, Davis & Ahlborn, 1993a). It would appear that 5-HT also affects cognition in an inverted-U manner (Meneses, 1999; Loubinoux, et al., 2002). There is some doubt as to whether 5-HT directly affects cognition similar to norepinephrine and dopamine or whether its effect is one of increasing arousal similar to that of epinephrine (Loubinoux et al., 2002). The fact that it is heavily related to changes in anxiety (el Mansari, Bouchard & Bluer, 1995) and motivation (Montgomery, Rose & Herberg, 199) suggests that it may be the latter. Another effect of 5-HT is to inhibit dopamine synthesis (Freed & Yamamoto, 1985; Korsgaard, Gerlach & Christensson, 1985). Bailey, Davis and Ahlborn (1993b) argue that this interaction is the key rather than the action of 5-HT alone.

Catecholamines and 5-Hydroxytryptomine in the Brain During and Following Exercise

Given that the purpose of this chapter is to examine the effect of exercise on cognition we should look at research demonstrating changes in catecholamines and 5-HT in the brain during exercise. Obviously this is animal research. Early studies by McGaugh (1983) demonstrated increases in norepinephrine in rat brain during exercise. This was measured after decapitation. More recent research using the *in vivo* microdialysis method (see Meeusen, Piacentini & De Meirleir, 2001, for a description of microdialysis) has also shown increases in CNS concentrations of norepinephrine and dopamine during exercise (Meeusen, Sarre, Michotte, Ebinger & De Meirleir, 1994; Meeusen, Sarre & De Meirleir 1997). Prolonged exercise has also demonstrated increases in brain 5-HT (Chaouloff, Laude & Elghozi, 1989; Bailey et al., 1993a; 1993b; Meeusen et al., 1994; 1997).

In a review of brain neurotransmitters during exercise, Meeusen and De Meirleir (1995) provide a slightly different picture. They accept that whole brain norepinephrine concentrations show an increases with exercise, however this is not uniform throughout the brain. Indeed some areas demonstrate a decrease. In general they found that chronic exercise elevated brain concentrations of norepinephrine while acute exercise resulted in a depletion. They explain the latter, however, by pointing to an increase in norepinephrine turnover induced by increased tyrosine hydroxylase activity. They claimed that the situation with regard to brain dopamine concentrations and exercise is inconclusive and probably region dependent. With regard to 5-HT they argue that there is not unequivocal evidence of any effect but that there is some evidence of both acute and chronic exercise inducing increases in brain concentrations. In conclusion, they argue that overall the evidence is that exercise induces increases in brain concentrations of catecholamines.

Whether this increase is due directly to the activity of the peripheral nervous system or is an indirect result is somewhat debatable. Peripheral increases in catecholamines and 5-HT occur due to several reasons. Epinephrine and, to a lesser extent, norepinephrine play a major role in glycolysis. Epinephrine activates the enzyme adenyl cyclase thus increasing the intracellular concentration of adenosinemonophosphate. This increase results in the activation of phosphorylase and hence the break down of glycogen in active muscles. The catecholamines are also involved in lipolysis. Epinephrine and glucagons initiate the release of free fatty acids by binding to receptors that activate adenylate cyclase.

The process of secretion of catecholamines in the peripheral system are slightly different to those in the brain. While brain norepinephrine is released from vesicles, mainly in the hypothalamus and brainstem, peripheral secretion takes place in postganglionic nerves at the site of usage. Epinephrine on the other hand is released by the adrenal medulla directly into the blood stream. Some norepinephrine is also released in this way. It is generally thought that 80% of adrenal medulla release is epinephrine and 20% norepinephrine.

The difficulty in knowing whether changes in brain concentrations of catecholamines and 5-HT are directly or indirectly caused by peripheral activity is due to the action of the *blood brain barrier.* Brain endolethial cells differ from other endolethial cells in that they have tight junctions which prevent transcapillary movements of molecules. Nor do they contain transendolethial pathways, hence they form a barrier. Without the blood brain barrier we would be unable to control our emotions and cognition. It is essential, however, that some substances can cross the barrier. Crossing is mostly by diffusion and depends on the lipid solubility of the substance. 5-HT is less affected by the blood brain barrier than the catecholamines. Tryptophan, the precursor of 5-HT, is found in plasma either bound to albumin or unbound. Unbound tryptophan readily crosses the blood brain barrier. During exercise free fatty acids displace tryptophan from binding with albumin therefore there is an increase in unbound tryptophan. This crosses into the brain and forms 5-HT (Chaouloff, Kennett, Serrurrier, Merino & Curzon, 1986).

The way in which the catecholamines are affected, however, is very debatable. They do not readily crosses the blood brain barrier. Only a very small percentage can cross (see Oldendorf, 1977; Cornford, Braun, Oldendorf & Hill, 1982), therefore increases in plasma concentrations would have to be very high in order to make any effect. McGaugh (1983), however, argues that there may be sufficient transfer to affect cognition. McGaugh's research was with animals and he worked them to a level that is not viable with humans. It is very unlikely that, with humans, sufficient norepinephrine and dopamine cross the barrier during exercise to induce any significant effect on brain concentrations. The evidence for a direct effect of increases in plasma concentrations on brain concentrations is, therefore, limited.

The argument that there is an indirect effect is based on the relationship between the secretion of epinephrine into plasma by the adrenal medulla and the activation of the hypothalamus via the hypothalamic-pituitary-adrenocortical axis. During exercise, feedback from the cardiorespiratory system and muscles is detected by the SNS, which then stimulates secretion of epinephrine by the adrenal medulla (Pliszka, McCracken, and Maas, 1996). This, in turn, stimulates secretion of norepinephrine in the hypothalamus and brainstem (Genuth, 1998). Also, although the catecholamines can not readily cross the blood brain barrier, their precursors, tyrosine and L-Dopa do cross it. Thus, they may stimulate changes in brain catecholamine concentrations. Elam, Svensson and Thoren (1987) found increases in brain L-DOPA of rats during exercise. The evidence tends to support the argument that an indirect effect of peripheral changes in catecholamine concentrations is more likely than a direct one.

In long duration exercise we should not forget the effect of glucose concentrations. The brain derives almost all of its energy from the oxidation of glucose and increases in energy metabolism have been detected during mental activity (Sokoloff, 1969). As circulating plasma glucose increases during moderate exercise and glucose readily crosses the blood brain barrier then increases in brain glucose during moderate exercise is not surprising (Meeusen et al., 1994). However, long duration exercise, particularly heavy exercise, leads to glucose depletion in the musculature (Maughan et al., 2003), hence less for the brain. Therefore, a decrement in cognition will be expected. In extreme cases hypoglycaemia may result. Hypoglycaemia can vary from mild subjective perceptions of nausea, dizziness or confusion to coma. It should be noted that this will only occur due to exercise in very rare circumstances. When exercise intensity is above 75% of $\dot{W}_{max}$, which can only be tolerated for 1-1.5 hours, muscle glycogen stores become the limiting factor. Depletion of these stores will result in cessation of exercise before there is a fall in blood glucose concentrations (Åstrand & Rodahl, 2002).

Summary

The interaction between exercise and cognition from a neuroscientific perspective is based on the roles of the noradrenergic, dopaminergic and serotonergic pathways in cognition and emotion; and the increase, during exercise, of the CNS concentrations of the neurotransmitters that innervate these pathways. It is argued that during moderate exercise increases in catecholamines and 5-HT will raise arousal to an optimal level and that more norepinephrine and dopamine will be available for use by the prefrontal cortex, thus aiding the working memory performance. Further increases, resulting from high intensity exercise, will result in a detriment in performance as the emotional areas of the brain will become overstimulated at the expense of the cognitive areas. This hypothesis, however, fails to take into account the blood brain barrier. It may be that the interaction between the adrenal medulla, which is activated by exercise, and the hypothalamus may result in the secretion of catecholamines and 5-HT in the brain. The empirical evidence for this is examined below.

Plasma Catecholamine Thresholds and Cognitive Performance

Chmura et al. (1994) believed that, if there really was a link between peripheral changes in catecholamine concentrations and CNS increases, the point at which exercise would induce a significant improvement in cognitive performance, indeed optimal performance, would be related to observable changes in plasma concentrations of the catecholamines. Lehman, Schmid and Keul (1985) had shown that, when we exercise incrementally, plasma catecholamine concentrations rise exponentially. The point at which there is a significant increase in concentrations was termed the threshold. Although the thresholds of epinephrine and norepinephrine are highly correlated, and can be identical in some individuals, there are normally small differences, therefore we talk about the epinephrine threshold (T_E) and the norepinephrine threshold (T_{NE}). Moreover, lactate is affected by exercise in a similar way to the catecholamines (Beaver, Wassermann & Whipp, 1985; Lehman et al., 1985) and the lactate threshold (T_{LA}) is highly correlated to T_E and T_{NE} (Mazzeo & Marshall, 1989). This has led some researchers to examine the effect of exercise at T_{LA} on cognitive performance (Chmura et al., 1998; McMorris et al., 2004). This is favoured by some because the taking of samples of lactate can be done by finger prick rather than venepuncture or canulation. Moreover, methods of assaying the blood are cheaper and quicker than that for catecholamines.

Research Evidence

Chmura et al. (1994) examined subjects before, during and after a discontinuous incremental test to voluntary exhaustion using a cycle ergometer. Subjects rode for 3 mins with 1 min rest between each bout. Workload began at 50 W and was raised by 50 W for each increment. Choice reaction time was measured in the final minute of each ride. The authors claimed that reaction time had decreased linearly during exercise up to a workload that corresponded to 76% of the subjects MaxVO$_2$. They observed that each individual's minimum reaction time occurred at a workload that was above that which elicited the person's T_{LA} and T_E but not their T_{NE}. Each person's minimum reaction time was significantly lower than their reaction time at rest. While reaction time at 300W was also significantly higher than the minimal reaction time.

The authors demonstrated a relationship between reaction time and epinephrine, and reaction time and norepinephrine. This was in an inverted-U shape. However, they also claimed to show linear regressions of $r = 0.93$ and $r = 0.94$ between reaction time and epinephrine and norepinephrine, respectively. This is difficult to understand. If the relationship demonstrates an inverted-U effect how can a linear regression be so high? Observation of the graphs shown (Chmura et al., 1994, p. 175) suggest that there were no significant differences between the reaction times at each catecholamine value. No statistical analysis of this was made.

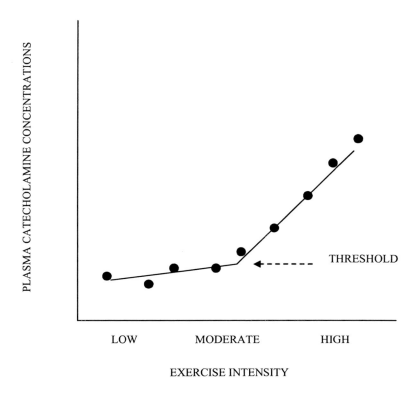

Figure 4. Graphical description of typical changes in catecholamine concentrations during incremental exercise.

This is not the only anomaly with the statistical treatment of the data. The authors did not compare reaction time at each of the workloads or rather do not report it. Instead they compared at rest values to the minimum reaction time found. They also compared minimum reaction time to the maximum reaction time observed. This is a strange statistical treatment. It is taking the dependent variable, reaction time, and using it as both an independent and a dependent variable at the same time. Furthermore, analysis was by Student t-tests with no Bonferroni correction factor. However, the probabilities given (p<.001) suggest that this would not have been an issue. Another problem with the data analysis is that exercise was until voluntary exhaustion yet we are not told when individuals dropped out or how many actually reached the 300 W stage, yet this is used in the regression analyses. Another major problem was the fact that subjects were only given 5–7 habituations trials on the reaction time test. This is not sufficient for such a test. McMorris et al. (2003) found that it was necessary to practise for 140–160 trials to eliminate a learning effect. Despite the problems with statistical treatment, Chmura et al. (1994) had presented a better rationale for an effect of exercise on cognitive performance than had hither to be seen. Moreover, even if we do not accept that the differences they claim to have shown are valid the authors still provide enough data to suggest that, with a larger sample size, significance may have been demonstrated.

McMorris et al. (1999) followed the example of Chmura et al. (1994) and compared performance of soccer players on a soccer-specific decision-making test at rest, a workload aimed to elicit T_E and $\dot{W}_{max}$. McMorris et al. used a test that had been shown to be reliable in a repeated measures protocol. They found that speed of decision at T_E and $\dot{W}_{max}$ was significantly faster than at rest. There was no effect of exercise on accuracy of decision. It should be noted that McMorris et al. examined subjects *at* T_E and not following T_E. Chmura et al. had shown that each individual's minimum reaction time was *following* T_E.

McMorris, Sproule, Draper and Child (2000) examined reaction time in a test requiring whole body movement following rest, exercise at T_E and $\dot{W}_{max}$. They found no significant effect. Similarly, McMorris et al. (2003) demonstrated no effect of exercise at 70% and 100% $\dot{W}_{max}$ on non-compatible choice reaction time. These authors reported that all except one subject had past their T_{NE} at 70% $\dot{W}_{max}$. Perhaps more importantly, McMorris et a. (2003) failed to demonstrate a significant linear regression between plasma concentrations of epinephrine and norepinephrine, and reaction time. However, McMorris et al. (2005) showed a significant regression ($R^2 = .40$) between lactate and reaction time. Thus the evidence that increases in plasma concentrations of epinephrine and norepinephrine affect cognition or are able to predict cognitive performance during and/or following incremental exercise to exhaustion is very dubious. This is further supported by the fact that examination of the empirical data from these studies (Chmura et al., 1994; McMorris et al., 1999; 2000; 2003; 2004) show only low to moderate effect sizes (d M = 0.20, SD = 0.17, range 0.09 to 0.53) when comparing performance at rest to that during exercise at the thresholds. When comparing the difference between rest and high intensity exercise, low to high effect sizes (d M = 0.31, SD = 0.26, range 0.12 to 0.79) are demonstrated but this is not unidirectional. Correlation coefficients between cognitive performance and plasma concentrations of epinephrine and norepinephrine show very low to moderate effect sizes (r^2 M = 0.28, SD = 0.21, range 0.001 to 0.46*)*.

Evidence for a relationship between plasma concentrations of catecholamines and cognition during sub-maximal exercise of comparatively long duration is a little more positive. Peyrin et al. (1987) examined word discrimination, STM and solving simple arithmetical problems in a control condition and during 1 hour of cycling at 70% MaxVO$_2$. They found no significant effect of cycling on STM and the arithmetical test but word discrimination was significantly better during exercise. More interestingly, they showed significant regression correlations between performance on the discrimination task during exercise and changes, from resting values, in plasma concentrations of the norepinephrine metabolite MHPG ($r = .63$), and epinephrine and metanephrine combined ($r = .61$). Metanephrine is a metabolite of epinephrine.

The most important finding of Peyrin et al. (1987) was that plasma concentrations of the metabolites MHPG, metanephrine and normetanephrine were significantly higher when exercising *and* undertaking the cognitive tests than when doing the mental tests without exercising. While epinephrine, metanephrine and MHPG were higher while exercising *and* carrying out the cognitive tests compared to when exercising without a mental task. Taken together these results point to an interaction between exercise and cognition.

Chmura et al. (1998) also examined cognition during exercise at moderate duration sub-maximal exercise. They had one group ($T_{LA}+$ group) of subjects exercise for 20 mins at a workload that meant that the person was exercising at 10% above their T_{LA}. Another group (75% T_{LA} group) exercised for 60 mins at 75% of the workload required to elicit T_{LA}. For the $T_{LA}+$ group, reaction time was examined every 5 mins and for the other group every 10 mins. For the 75% T_{LA} group significant decreases from choice reaction time at rest were observed for each of the other measurements, while the $T_{LA}+$ group demonstrated significant improvements from 10 mins onwards. Significant correlations were found between choice reaction time and plasma concentrations of epinephrine ($r = -.65$), and norepinephrine ($r = -.68$) for the $T_{LA}+$ group only. Once again there were design problems. Habituations were only 5-7 trials and the statistical analysis between reaction times was by a series of Wilcoxon tests with no correction factor, hence the possibility of a compound error.

Summary

Chmura et al. (1994) and McMorris et al. (1999) showed respectively that reaction time and decision time at the catecholamine thresholds were significantly faster than at rest or during exercise at $\dot{W}_{max}$. This was in tasks where the response was purely verbal or a finger press. In tasks where the response was whole body the results are equivocal. McMorris et al. (2000; 2003) demonstrated no effect while McMorris et al. (2005) found faster reaction times at T_{LA}. Perhaps of greater importance is the comparatively low effect sizes for differences and correlations demonstrated by the research. However, the work of Peyrin et al. (1987) strongly suggests that there is some relationship between plasma concentrations of catecholamines or more likely their metabolites and cognitive performance. To summarize we could say that the there is some support for a claim that increases in peripheral and central neurotransmitters during exercise are related. The strength of that relationship and whether or not a cause and effect exists requires a great deal more research.

Discussion

Examination of the research literature reviewed in this chapter provides very little support for an inverted-U effect of exercise, incremental or long term, on cognitive performance. There is not even unequivocal evidence that exercise has any effect at all. With regard to those tasks that Humphreys and Revelle (1986) termed information transfer tasks, e. g. simple and choice reaction time, the situation is particularly confusing. The Poitiers group (Delignières et al., 1994; Brisswalter et al., 1997; Arcelin et al., 1998) have generally found that there is a linear improvement in information transfer tasks, however other researchers have failed to support these findings. This may be due to the methodology used by the Poitiers group. They have used a variation of a dual task paradigm. Subjects were asked to pedal on a cycle ergometer at a given cadence and concentrate equally on maintaining the cadence and carrying out the cognitive task. Other researchers have instructed the subjects to focus on the cognitive tasks and have let the exercise "take care of itself". McMorris and associates (McMorris & Graydon, 1996a; 1996b; 1997a; 1997b; McMorris et al., 1999) followed this protocol but compared power output in an exercise only condition with that while exercising and undertaking the cognitive test. They found no significant effect, on the power output, of carrying out the two tasks simultaneously. This, of course, does not mean that the different instructions did not have different effects. The conscious attempt to maintain the cadence and the possibility, or likelihood, of divided attention may make results from the two protocols impossible to compare.

There does appear to be some agreement concerning the effect of exercise on the more complex, working memory tasks, used by several researchers. McMorris and Graydon (2000), Brisswalter, Collardeau and Rene (2002), and Tomporowski (2003) concluded that there is a linear improvement in performance during incremental exercise for such tasks. It may, however be better described as being exponential in nature. Undoubtedly low levels of exercise intensity have no effect. Following the catecholamine thresholds, it would appear that there is a significant improvement in speed of performance. This does not appear to be the case for accuracy. The improvement appears to continue up to $\dot{W}_{max}$.

The fact that speed improves, but not accuracy, in these tasks may appear surprising, at first. However, closer observation of the nature of the tasks and the effects of exercise induced increases in brain concentrations of catecholamines may cast some light on these findings. The processing of these more complex tasks takes place in the prefrontal cortex. They require not only the use of the visuospatial sketchpad and phonological loop, but also place a strain on the executive control system. In particular information recalled from LTM is a key factor. Exercise and probably any form of arousal affects the speed at which this information can be recalled from the temporal and parietal cortices, and the speed of processing in the parietal lobes. It is logical to suppose that increases in available neurotransmitters results in increases in the speed of brain functioning. More transmitters should result in faster processing. If the individual is focussing correctly on the task relevant information - correct use of cognitive effort - then the accuracy of the response will remain the same regardless of the number of transmitters. Increases in neurotransmitters will improve speed but can not improve accuracy. Accuracy would only be affected if the individual's selective attention was disrupted. This may well happen when the display facing the subject contains a great deal of irrelevant information. However, in the types of task used in most experiments the display is comparatively limited. McMorris and associates (McMorris and Graydon, 1996a; 1996b; 1997a; 1997b; McMorris et al., 1999) used the most complex of displays so far used in this area of research but the task was familiar to subjects, therefore selective attention was presumably automatic and unlikely to be disrupted by high arousal (Eysenck & Calvo, 1992).

McMorris and Graydon (1996a) supply some support for this claim. They found that, for experienced soccer players, speed of performance on a soccer-specific decision-making task improved with increases in exercise intensity. However, for inexperienced performers there was no effect on speed. McMorris and Graydon had expected to find a negative effect of exercise at $\dot{W}_{max}$ on accuracy in the inexperienced group. They hypothesised that limited experience would result in inappropriate selective attention and incorrect recall from LTM. The problem with such a theory is that, with an inexperienced group, poor selective attention is occurring even during optimal arousal, therefore no significant effect of maximal exercise will be demonstrated. This is in line with drive theory.

While McMorris and Graydon (1996a) based their hypothesis on the experience of the subjects on the cognitive task, the results of Brisswalter et al. (1997) suggest that the problem may be the experience of the subjects in undertaking high intensity exercise. Brisswalter et al. found that fit subjects were unaffected by exercise intensities of 20%, 40%, 60% and 80% MaxVO$_2$. Unfit subjects, however, showed an inverted-U effect. The authors put the difference in the results down to the effect of fitness. This appears to be a somewhat illogical conclusion. As the subjects all exercised at the same intensity with regard to their own MaxVO$_2$ it is difficult to sustain a claim that fitness was the key factor. For the unfit group, one would expect a decrement in performance during heavy exercise because they were exercising at an intensity of which they had no previous experience. Thus cognitive effort would have great difficulty in focusing attention to task relevant information. For the fit group, who were used to such an exercise intensity, this would not be a problem.

The results concerning performance at 40% MaxVO$_2$ are also interesting. It is unlikely that, at this intensity, any of the fit subjects would have reached their catecholamine thresholds, while some of the unfit group may well have done so. These thresholds rise with training (Kjaer, 1989). This may account for the significant improvement in performance for the unfit group and failure of the fit group to show a significant improvement. If the threshold is the key then the fit group should have demonstrated a significant improvement at 80% MaxVO$_2$, as most subjects would have reached their T_{NE} by then (McMorris, Sproule, Draper, Child, Sexsmith et al., 2000).

This latter point brings us to the problem of what constitutes moderate intensity exercise. The most commonly held belief is that the lactate and catecholamine thresholds are the best indicators. This is an objective measure and takes into account individual differences in fitness. Moreover, as we saw in the previous section of this chapter, there is evidence to support the claim that this intensity has an effect on cognition. However, the evidence is not unequivocal. The reason for this may be due to the nature of the link between what is happening peripherally with what is happening centrally. Research with animals has undoubtedly shown that as exercise intensity increases so do central concentrations of catecholamines and 5-HT. The way in which this occurs is debatable, however. How this occurs may be the key to determining how exercise affects cognition.

Despite the findings of studies with animals that have shown some crossing of the blood brain barrier by peripherally circulating epinephrine and norepinephrine (Brown et al., 1979; McGaugh, 1983), there is little support in the neurochemistry community for such an argument with humans (Kuhar et al., 1999). There would appear to be little doubt that adrenal medulla secretion of epinephrine and norepinephrine stimulates the secretion of the catecholamines into the prefrontal cortex, hypothalamus and brainstem (Genuth, 1998). The relationship between peripheral and central concentrations, however, is unknown. The research of Peyrin et al. (1987), with sub-maximal, steady state exercise, provides circumstantial evidence for a fairly high correlation between central and peripheral concentrations. McMorris et al. (2003), using incremental exercise, did not support such a relationship. Furthermore, if we accept that improvements in cognitive performance following the catecholamine thresholds, as found by Chmura et al. (1994) and McMorris et al. (1999), are indicative of significant central increases in catecholamines then the circumstantial evidence for a relationship between peripheral and central concentrations is high. At first it may look sound to argue that the peripheral changes *directly* cause the central changes. This I believe is not proven.

Two factors with regard to the secretion of catecholamines within the brain and the take up of the neurotransmitters within the noradrenergic and dopaminergic pathways need to be considered. That the action of the adrenal medulla stimulates catecholamine secretion in the brain is unquestionable, but the SNS is also directly affected by the CNS response to stress (Sothmann et al., 1991). In fact, just as adrenal medulla activity triggers off a response by the hypothalamus, this also works the other way round (Genuth, 1998).

The way in which the individual perceives the situation will affect the response of the SNS and perhaps more importantly the way in which increases in CNS neurotransmitters are used. Increases in secretion of catecholamines in the brain will occur if the person perceives the situation as being stressful. This increase in catecholamine concentrations in the brain may be directly and/or *indirectly* induced by exercise. If the person perceives exercise as being stressful, the uptake of these neurotransmitters will be in the areas of the brain responsible for emotions. However, if the exercise is seen as neutral (i. e. something that the person does often, without distress), it is likely that the increased neurotransmitters will be used by the cognitive areas of the brain. This is akin to Kahneman's (1973) notion of the role of cognitive effort. If the person perceives the task as stressful, the increase in arousal may lead to a greater binding of catecholamines to neurons in the emotional areas of the brain resulting in a negative effect on cognitive performance. In other words, cognitive effort will not be able to allocate resources to the task. If, however, the person sees the situation as a neutral or positive one, increases in arousal may lead to better allocation of resources and the catecholamines will bind to areas involved in cognition. These factors taken together may explain the somewhat equivocal nature of research results.

The situation may be further complicated by the role of 5-HT, especially during long term exercise. Increases in 5-HT undoubtedly affect emotion. Their effect on cognition is debatable, however. There is some evidence to show that very high concentrations can have a negative effect on the synthesis of dopamine but the major effect seems to be the stimulation of arousal. As 5-HT affects almost all parts of the brain, its effect on arousal may be particularly important. Increases in 5-HT concentrations have been shown to be indicative of both positive and negative emotions (Barchas & Altemus, 1999). It would appear that if the person is concerned about the nature of the stressor, 5-HT stimulates that concern.

The reader may well have noted that the above arguments combine neuroscientific and cognitive psychology approaches to explaining the affect of exercise on cognition. I believe that, at this moment in time, this is the best way in which research results can be explained. As we saw earlier in the chapter, cognitive psychology theories provide a very poor explanation for research results. While the neuroscientific theories provide a better explanation, they are still far from convincing. It would appear fair to state that there is sufficient evidence to claim that exercise does affect cognition. It would also appear that, when the exercise is incremental in nature, different cognitive tasks are affected differently. Surprisingly, it appears that complex tasks are the most likely to be affected positively and that all tasks appear to benefit from high exercise intensities. For long duration, sub-maximal, steady state exercise the situation is also unclear.

Evidence for a direct effect of biochemical changes in the periphery on central changes exists but the extent of this direct effect may be very limited. While the argument that the interaction between the adrenal medulla and the hypothalamus, in response to exercise, is the main cause of changes in performance has intuitive appeal, there is no direct evidence and the circumstantial evidence is somewhat flimsy. However, I believe that this interaction can explain the equivocality of the research findings. Moreover, it fits in with both neuroscientific and cognitive theories. The neuroscientific theories and research can point to central–peripheral interactions during exercise, the dual roles of norepinephrine and dopamine in cognition and emotion and the effect of 5-HT on emotional responses. While the cognitive psychologists can point to allocation of resources and, in particular, the role of cognitive effort to explain both positive and negative effects of exercise.

Towards a Cognitive Psychology/Neuroscientific Model

In this section, I outline my initial thoughts on the proposal of a model to explain the arousal-exercise-cognition interaction. The model takes primarily a neuroscientific approach but also calls on Kahneman's (1973) notion of cognitive effort. The initial decision to undertake exercise is taken by the CNS. This results in feedforward initiating the release of epinephrine and a small amount of norepinephrine into the blood stream by the adrenal medulla. It is generally thought that this is part of the organisms response to stress. It is a warning to the peripheral system to be ready to "fight or flee". At the same time, the interaction between the adrenal medulla and other parts of the SNS leads to secretion of norepinephrine, dopamine and a very small amount of epinephrine in the brain. When exercise is the stressor this is unlikely to have any significant effect on cognition or emotion in the early stages. As the person continues to exercise increases in muscle metabolism and cardiorespiratory responses lead to a build up of blood pH which triggers off the secretion of more epinephrine and norepinephrine by the adrenal medulla (Chwalbińska-Moneta, Robergs, Costill & Fink, 1989). This in turn initiates a central response by the hypothalamus (Genuth, 1998). The action of the hypothalamus is not only determined by direct responses to adrenal medulla activity but it is also affected by perceptions of the nature and intensity of the stressor. If the person perceives increases in exercise intensity as being distressful then the there will be increases in brain catecholamine concentrations.

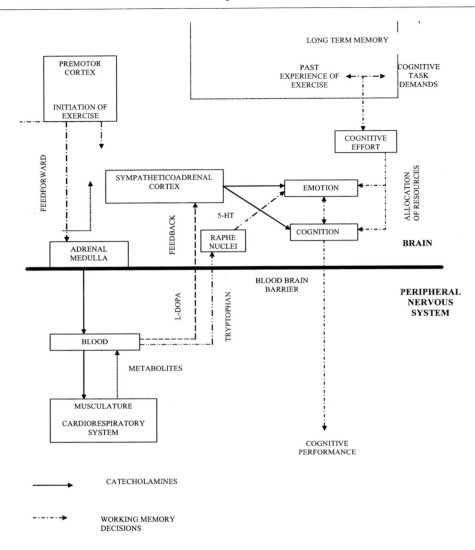

Figure 5. Proposed model for the exercise-arousal-cognitive performance interaction

CNS catecholamines serve both emotional and cognitive areas of the brain. Thus the possibility that both emotional and cognitive responses will be facilitated is possible. Classical inverted-U theories suggest that cognitive areas are stimulated at moderate levels of arousal but as arousal rises the emotional areas become innervated at the expense of the cognitive. As we have already seen, research does not support an inverted-U effect therefore something else must be occurring. I believe that the key factor is the person's perception of the nature and intensity of the stressor and how cognitive effort allocates resources. It would appear that, if the exercise is moderate in intensity, effort can allocate resources to the task demands. As exercise intensity increases, however, the situation changes. If the person perceives exercise as stressful, it is most likely that the neurotransmitters will bind to neurons involved in the control of emotions, at the expense of those involved in cognition. The result being a deterioration in performance. If the person perceives exercise as being neutral or positive, more neurotransmitters will be available to the cognitive areas of the brain and effort will have little difficulty in allocating attention to the task demands. Hence performance will be facilitated.

If exercise continues over a period of time, increases in unbound tryptophan will cross the blood brain barrier resulting in the synthesis of 5-HT. This will further stimulate the emotional centres of the brain, positively or negatively depending on the individual's perception of the stressor. However, even if the individual perceives exercise as being exciting, there may be a negative effect of increases in 5-HT concentrations. It may be that there comes a point when the stimulation of the emotional centres of the brain by 5-HT is such that cognitive effort can not control the allocation of resources. This is in line with the claims of Pribram and McGuinness (1975) and Sanders (1983). There is, however, little evidence to support such a claim.

The situation is further complicated by the nature of the cognitive task. In line with allocable resources theories I believe that different tasks require different amounts of resources to be performed effectively. If a task requires only limited resources then it can be successfully performed, even if other resources are directed towards non-task relevant information e. g. perceptions of distress. Thus not all tasks will be negatively affected by even high intensity exercise. This is supported by the fact that, for complex tasks, it is speed of performance rather than accuracy that is affected. It would appear that the individual has sufficient resources to ensure the accuracy of the tasks, so far examined by research, regardless of arousal level. However, increases in the number of neurotransmitters available in the CNS appears to a ensure faster responses.

References

Adam, J. J.; Teeken, J. C.; Ypellar, P. J. C.; Verstappen, F. T. J. & Paas, F. G. W. (1997). Exercise-induced arousal and information processing. *International Journal of Sports Psychology*, *26*, 2217-220.

Allard, F.; Brawley, L. R.; Deakin, J. & Elliott, D. (1989). The effect of exercise on visual attention performance. *Human Performance, 2*, 131-145.

Arcelin, R.; Delignières, D. & Brisswalter, J. (1998). Effects of physical exercise on choice reaction processes. *Perceptual and Motor Skills, 87*, 175-185.

Åstrand, P-O. & Rodahl, K. (1977) *Textbook of work physiology* (1st edition). New York: McGraw.

Åstrand, P-O. & Rodahl, K. (2002). *Textbook of work physiology* (4th edition). New York, McGraw.

Babiloni, C.; Babiloni, F.; Carducci, F.; Cappa, S. F.; Cincotti, F.; Del Percio, C. et al. (2004). Human cortical responses during one-bit short-term memory. A high-resolution EEG study on delayed choice reaction time tasks. *Clinical Neurophysiology*, *115*, 161-170.

Baddeley, A. D. (1986). *Working memory,* New York: Oxford University Press.

Bailey, S. P.; Davis, J. M. & Ahlborn, E. N. (1993a). Neuroendocrine and substrate responses to altered brain 5-HT activity during prolonged exercise to fatigue. *Journal of Applied Physiology, 74*, 3006-3012.

Bailey, S. P.; Davis, J. M. & Ahlborn, E. N. (1993b). Serotonergic agonists and antagonists affect endurance performance in the rat. *International Journal of Sports Medicine, 14,* 330-333.

Barbas, H. (2000). Connections underlying the synthesis of cognition, memory, and emotion in primate prefrontal cortices. *Brain Research Bulletin, 52,* 319-330.

Barchas, J. D. & Altemus, m. (1999). Biochemical hypotheses of moods and anxiety disorders. In G. J. Siegel, B. W. Agranoff, R. W. Albers, S. K. Fisher, & M. D. Uhler (Eds.), *Basic neurochemistry: molecular, cellular and medical aspects.* 6th edition (pp. 1073-1094). Philadelphia: Lippincott, Williams & Wilkins.

Bard, C. & Fleury, M. (1978). Influence of imposed metabolic fatigue on visual capacity components. *Perceptual and Motor Skills, 47,* 1283-1287.

Bares, M.; Rektor, I.; Kanovsky, P. & Streitova, H. (2003). Cortical and sub-cortical distribution of middle and long latency auditory and visual evoked potentials in a cognitive (CNV) paradigm. *Clinical Neurophysiology, 114,* 2447-2460.

Beaver, W. L.; Wasserman, K. & Whipp, B. J. (1985). Improved detection of lactate threshold during exercise using a log-log transformation. *Journal of Applied Physiology, 59,* 1936-1940.

Beh, H. C. (1989). Mental performance following exercise. *Perceptual and Motor Skills, 69,* 42.

Brisswalter, J., Arcelin, R., Audiffren, M., & Delignières, D. (1997). Influence of physical exercise on simple reaction time: effect of physical fitness. *Perceptual and Motor Skills, 85,* 1019-1027.

Brisswalter, J.; Collardeau, M. & Rene, A. (2002). Effects of acute exercise characteristics on cognitive performance. *Sports Medicine, 32,* 555-566.

Brown, B. S.; Payne, T.; Kim, C.; Moore, G.; Krebs, P. & Martin, W. (1979). Chronic response of rat brain norepinephrine and serotonin levels to endurance training. *Journal of Applied Physiology, 46,* 19-23.

Chaouloff, F.; Kennett, G. A.; Serrurrier, B.; Merino, D. & Curzon, G. (1986). Amino acid analysis demonstrated that increased plasma tryptophan causes the increase in brain tryptophan during exercise in the rat. *Journal of Neurochemistry, 46,* 1647-1650.

Chaouloff, F.; Laude, D. & Elghozi, J. L. (1989). Physical exercise: evidence for differential consequences of tryptophan on 5-HT synthesis and metabolism in central serotonergic cell bodies and terminals. *Journal of Neural Transmission, 78,* 121-130.

Chudasama, Y.; Bussey, T. J. & Muir, J. L. (2001). Effects of selective thalamic and prelimbic cortex lesions on two types of visual discrimination and reversal learning. *European Journal of Neuroscience, 14,* 1009-1020.

Chmura, J.; Krysztofiak, H.; Ziemba, A. W.; Nazar, K. & Kaciuba-Uścilko, H. (1998). Psychomotor performance during prolonged exercise above and below the blood lactate threshold. *European Journal of Applied Physiology, 77,* 77-80.

Chmura, J.; Nazar, K. & Kaciuba-Uscilko, H. (1994). Choice reaction time during graded exercise in relation to blood lactate and plasma catecholamines thresholds. *International Journal of Sports Medicine, 15,* 172-176.

Chwalbińska-Moneta, J.; Roberts, R. A.; Costill, D. L. & Fink, W. J. (1989). Threshold for muscle lactate accumulation during progressive exercise. *Journal of Applied Physiology, 66,* 270-2716.

Collardeau, M.; Brisswalter, J. & Audiffren, M. (2001). Effects of a prolonged run on simple reaction time of well trained runners. *Perceptual and Motor Skills, 93,* 679-689.

Cooper, C. J. (1973). Anatomical and physiological mechanisms of arousal, with special reference to the effects of exercise. *Ergonomics, 16,* 601-609.

Cornford, E. M.; Braun, L. D.; Oldendorf, W. H. & Hill, M. A.(1982). Comparison of lipid mediated blood-brain barrier after intraperitoneal administration in the rat. *American Journal of Physiology, 243,* C161-C168.

Côté, J.; Salmela, J. & Papathanasopoulu, P. (1992). Effects of progressive exercise on attentional focus. *Perceptual and Motor Skills, 75,* 351-354.

Critchley, H. D.; Matthias, C. J.; Josephs, O.; O'Doherty, J.; Zanini, S.; Dewar, B-K. et al. (2003). Human cingulate cortex and autonomic control: converging neuroimaging and clinical evidence. *Brain, 126,* 2139-2152.

Davey, C. P. (1972). Mental performance after physical activity. *Australian Journal of Sports Medicine, 4,* 25-33.

Davey, C. P. (1973). Physcial exertion and mental performnce. *Ergonomics, 16,* 595-599.

Davidson, K.; MacGregor, M. W.; Stuhr, J.; Dixon, K. & MacLean, D. (2000). Constructive anger verbal behavior predicts blood pressure in a population-based sample. *Health Psychology, 19,* 55-64.

Davidson, R. J.; Putnam, K. M. & Larson, C. L. (2000). Dysfunction in the neural circuitry of emotion regulation - A possible prelude to violence. *Science, 289,* 591-594.

Davranche, K. & Audiffren, M. (2004). Facilitating effects of exercise on information processing. *Joiurnal of Sports Sciences, 22,* 419-428.

Delignières, D.; Brisswalter, J. & Legros, P. (1994). Influence of physical exercise on choice reaction time in sports experts: the mediating role of resource allocation. *Journal of Human Movement Studies, 27,* 173-188.

Delignières, D.; Famose, J. P. & Genty, J. (1994). Validation d'une echelle de categories pour la perception de la difficulté (Validation of a rating scale to measure perceived difficulty). *STAPS: Revue des Sciences et Techniques des Activités Physiques et Sportive, 15,* 77-88.

Douchamps, J. (1988). A metatheoretical approach of operational performance. In J. P. Leonard (Ed.), *Vigilance: methods, models and regulation* (pp. 23-34). Frankfurt: Long.

Easterbrook, J. A. (1959). The effect of emotion on cue utilization and the organization of behavior. *Psychological Review, 66,* 183-201.

Edwards, R. H. T. (1983). Biochemical bases of fatigue in exercise performance: catastrophe theory of muscular fatigue. In H. Knuttgen, J. Vogel, & J. Poortmans (Eds.), *International series on sports sciences. Vol. 13. Biochemistry of exercise* (pp. 3-28). Champaign, Il: Human Kinetics.

Eisenhofer, G.; Meredith, I. T.; Ferrier, C.; Cox, H. S.; Lambert, G.; Jennings, G. L. et al. (1991). Increased plasma dihydroxyphenylalanine during sympathetic activation in humans is related to increased norepinephrine turnover. *Journal of Laboratory and Clinical Medicine, 117,* 266-273.

Elam, M.; Svensson, T. & Thoren, P. (1987). Brain monoamine metabolism is altered in rats following spontaneous long-distance running. *Acta Physiologica Scandinavica, 130*, 313-316.

el Mansari, M.; Bouchard, C. & Blier, P. (1995). Alteration of serotonin release in the guinea pig orbitofrontal cortex by selective serotonin reuptake inhibitors. Relevance to treatment of obsessive-compulsive disorder. *Neuropsychopharmacology, 13*, 117-127.

Eysenck, M. W. & Calvo, M. G. (1992). Anxiety and performance: the processing efficiency theory. *Cognition and Emotion, 6*, 409-434.

Féry, Y. A.; Ferry, A.; Vom Hofe, A. & Rieu, M. (1997). Effect of physical exhaustion on cognitive functioning. *Perceptual and Motor Skills, 84*, 291-298.

Fleury, M. & Bard, C. (1990). Fatigue métabolique et performance de tâches visuelle (Metabolic fatigue and performance of visual tasks). *Canadian Journal of Sports Science, 15*, 43-50.

Fleury, M.; Bard, C. & Carrière, L. (1981). Effects of physical or perceptual loads on a coincidence timing task. *Perceptual and Motor Skills, 53*, 843-850.

Fleury, M.; Bard, C.; Jobin, J. & Carrière, L. (1981). Influence of different types of physical fatigue on a visual detection task. *Perceptual and Motor Skills, 53*, 723-730.

Flynn, R. B. (1972). Numerical performance as a function of prior exercise and aerobic capacity for elementary schoolboys. *Research Quarterly for Exercise and Sport, 43*, 16-22.

Freed, C. R. & Yamamoto, B. K. (1985). Regional brain dopamine metabolism: a marker for speed, direction, and posture of moving animals. *Science, 229*, 62-65.

Gazzaniga, M. S.; Ivry, R. B. & Mangun, G. R. (2002). *Cognitive neuroscience: the biology of the mind*, 2nd edition. New York: Norton

Genuth, S. M. (1998). The endocrine system. In R. M. Berne; M. N. Levy, B. M. Koepen, & B. A. Stanton (Eds.), *Physiology* (pp. 779-1013). St. Louis, MO: Mosby.

Gutin, B. & Di Gennaro, J. (1968a). Effect of one-minute step-ups on performance of simple addition. *Research Quarterly for Exercise and Sport, 39*, 81-85.

Gutin, B. & Di Gennaro, J. (1968b). Effect of a treadmill run to exhaustion on performance of long addition. *Research Quarterly for Exercise and Sport, 39*, 958-964.

Hagemann, D.; Waldstein, S.R. & Thayer, J. F. (2003). Central and autonomic nervous system integration in emotion. *Brain and Cognition, 52*, 79-87.

Hart, S .G. & Staveland, L. E. (1988). Development of NASA-TLX (Task Load Index): results of empirical and theoretical research. In P.A. Hancock, & N. Meshkati (Eds.), *Human mental workload* (pp. 239-250). Amsterdam, North Holland Press.

Hogervorst, E.; Riedel, W. J.; Jeukendrup, A. & Jolies, J. (1996). Cognitive performance after strenuous physical exercise. *Perceptual and Motor Skills, 83*, 479-488.

Hull, C. L. (1943). *Principles of behavior*, New York: Appleton.

Humphreys, M. S. & Revelle, W. (1984). Personality, motivation and performance: a theory of the relationship between individual differences and information processing. *Psychological Review, 91*, 153-184.

Isaacs, L. D. & Pohlman, E. L. (1991). Effects of exercise intensity on an accompanying timing task. *Journal of Human Movement Studies, 20*, 123-131.

Kahneman, D. (1973) *Attention and effort.* Englewood Cliffs, NJ: Prentice-Hall.

Kjaer, M. (1989). Epinephrine and some other hormonal responses to exercise in man: with special reference to physical training. *International Journal of Sports Medicine, 10*, 2-15.

Korsgaard, S.; Gerlach, J. & Christensson, E. (1985). Behavioral aspects of serotonin-dopamine interaction in the monkey. *European Journal of Pharmacology, 118*, 245-252.

Kuhar, M. J.; Couceyro, P. R. & Lambert, P. D. (1999). Catecholamines. In G. J. Siegel, B. W. Agranoff, R. W. Albers, S. K. Fisher, & M. D. Uhler (Eds.), *Basic neurochemistry: molecular, cellular and medical aspects.* 6th edition (pp. 243-262). Philadelphia: Lippincott, Williams & Wilkins.

Lacey, J. L. & Lacey, B. C. (1970). Some autonomic central nervous system interrelationships. In P. Black (Ed.), *Physiological correlates of emotion* (pp. 205-208). New York: Academic Press.

Landers, D. M. (1980). The arousal-performance relationship revisited. *Research Quarterly for Exercise and Sport, 51*, 77-90.

Lawless, W. F. (1988). Effect of arousal on mathematic scores. *Perceptual and Motor Skills, 67*, 318.

Lehman, M.; Schmid, P. & Keul, J. (1985). Plasma catecholamine and blood lactate cumulation during incremental exhaustive exercise. *International Journal of Sports Medicine, 6*, 78-81.

Levitt, S. & Gutin, B. (1971). Multiple choice reaction time and movement time during physical exertion. *Research Quarterly for Sport and Exercise, 42*, 405-410.

Loubinoux, I.; Pariente, J.; Rascol, O.; Celsis, P. & Chollet, F. (2002). Selective serotonin reuptake inhibitor paroxetine modulated motor behavior through practice. A double-blind, placebo-controlled, multi-dose study in healthy subjects. *Neuropsychologia, 40*, 1815-1821.

MacLean, P. D. (1949). Psychosomatic disease and the "visceral brain": recent developments bearing on the Papez theory of emotion. *Psychosomatic Medicine, 11*, 338-353.

Marriott, J.; Reilly, T. & Miles, A. (1993). The effect of physiological stress on cognitive performance in a simulation of soccer. In T. Reilly, J. Clarys, & A. Stibbe (Eds.), *Science and football II* (pp. 262-264). London, Spon.

Maughan, R.; Gleeson, M. & Greenhaff, P. L. (2003). *Biochemistry of exercise and training*. Oxford: Oxford University Press.

Mazzeo, R. S. & Marshall, P. (1989). Influence of plasma catecholamines on the lactate threshold during graded exercise. *Journal of Applied Physiology, 67*, 1319-1322.

McAdam, R. E. & Wang, Y. K. (1967). Performance of a simple mental task following various treatments. *Research Quarterly for Sport and Exercise, 38*, 208-212.

McGaugh, J. L. (1983). Preserving the presence of the past: hormonal influence on memory storage. *American Psychologist, 38*, 161-174.

McGlynn, G. H.; Laughlin, N. T. & Bender, V. L. (1977). Effect of strenuous to exhaustive exercise on a discrimination task. *Perceptual and Motor Skills, 44*, 1139-1147.

McGlynn, G. H.; Laughlin, N. T. & Rowe, V. (1977). The effects of increasing levels of exercise on mental performance. *Ergonomics, 22*, 407-414.

McMorris, T. (2004). *Acquisition and performance of sports skills*. Chichester, Wiley.

McMorris, T.; Delves, S.; Lauder, M.; Sproule, J. & Hale, B. (2005). Effect of incremental exercise on initiation and movement times in a whole-body repsons time task. *British Journal of Sports Medicine*, , in press.

McMorris, T. & Graydon, J. (1996a). Effect of exercise on the decision-making performance of experienced and inexperienced soccer players. *Research Quarterly for Exercise and Sport, 67*, 109-114.

McMorris, T. & Graydon, J. (1996b). Effect of exercise on soccer decision-making tasks of differing complexities. *Journal of Human Movement Studies, 30*, 177-193.

McMorris, T. & Graydon, J. (1997a). Effect of exercise on cognitive performance in soccer-specific tests. *Journal of Sports Sciences, 15*, 459-468.

McMorris, T. & Graydon, J. (1997b). Effect of exercise on the decision-making performance of college soccer players. In T. Reilly, J. Bangsbo, & M. Hughes (Eds.), *Science and football III* (pp. 290-294). London: E. & F. N. Spon. .

McMorris, T. & Graydon, J. (2000). The effect of incremental exercise on cognitive performance. *International Journal of Sport Psychology, 31*, 66-81.

McMorris, T. & Keen, P. (1994) Effect of exercise on simple reaction times of recreational athletes. *Perceptual and Motor Skills, 78*, 123-130.

McMorris, T.; Myers, S.; MacGillivary, W.W.; Sexsmith, J. R.; Fallowfield, J.; Graydon, J. et al. (1999). Exercise, plasma catecholamine concentrations and decision-making performance of soccer players on a soccer-specific test. *Journal of Sports Sciences, 17*, 667-676.

McMorris, T.; Sproule, J.; Draper, S. & Child, R. (2000). Performance of a psychomotor skill following rest, exercise at the plasma epinephrine threshold and maximal intensity exercise. *Perceptual and Motor Skills, 91*, 553-562.

McMorris, T.; Sproule, J.; Draper, S.; Child, R.; Sexsmith, J. R.; Forster, C. D. et al. (2000). The measurement of plasma catecholamine and lactate thresholds: a comparison of methods. *European Journal of Applied Physiology, 82*, 262-267.

McMorris, T.; Tallon, M.; Williams, C.; Sproule, J.; Draper, S.; Swain, J. et al. (2003). Incremental exercise, plasma concentrations of catecholamines, reaction time, and motor time during performance of a noncompatible choice response time task. *Perceptual and Motor Skills, 97*, 590-604.

Meeusen, R. & De Meirleir, K. (1995). Exercise and brain neurotransmission. *Sports Medicine, 20*, 160-188.

Meeusen, R. & Piacentini, M. F. (2003). Exercise, fatigue, neurotransmission and the influence of the neuroendocrine axis. *Advances in Experimental Medicine and Biology, 57,* 521-525.

Meeusen, R.; Piacentini, M. F. & De Meirleir, K.(2001). Brain microdialysis in exercise research. *Sports Medicine, 31,* 965-983.

Meeusen, R.; Roeykens, J.; Magnus, L.; Keizer, H. & De Meirleir, K. (1997). Endurance performance in humans: the effect of a dopamine precursor or a specific serotonin (5-HT $_{2A/2C}$) antagonist. *International Journal of Sports Medicine, 18,* 571-577.

Meeusen, R.; Smolders, J.; Sarre, S.; De Meirleir, K.; Keizer, H.; Serneels, N. et al. (1997). Endurance training effects on neurotransmitter release in rat striatum: an *in vivo* microdialysis study. *Acta Physiologica Scandinavica, 159* 335-341.

Meneses, A. (1999). 5-HT system and cognition. *Neuroscience and Biobehavioral Reviews, 23,* 1111-1125.

Meyers, C. A.; Zimmerli, W.; Farr, S. D. & Baschnagel, N. A. (1969). Effect of strenuous physical activity upon reaction time. *Research Quarterly for Exercise and Sport, 40,* 333-337.

Montgomery, A. M. J.; Rose, I. C. & Herberg, L. J. (199). 5-HT agonists and dopamine: the effects of 8-OH-DPAT and busoprin on brain-stimulation reward. *Journal of Neural Transmission, 83,* 139-148.

Norman, D. A. & Shallice. T. (1986). Attention to action: willed and automatic control of behavior. In R. J. Davidson, G. E. Schwarz, & D. Shapiro (Eds.), *Consciousness and self-regulation* (pp. 1-18). New York: Plenum Press.

Oldendorf, W. H. (1977) The blood-brain barrier. *Experimental Eye Research, 25,* 177-190.

Oxendine, J. B. (1984). *Psychology of motor learning.* 1st edition. Englewood Cliffs, NJ: Prentice-Hall.

Paas, F. G. W. C. & Adam, J. J. (1991). Human information processing during physical exercise. *Ergonomics, 34,* 1385-1397.

Peyrin, L.; Pequinot, J. M.; Lacour, J. R. & Fourcade, J. (1987.) Relationships between catecholamine or 3-methoxy 4-hydroxy phenylglycol changes and mental performance under submaximal exercise in man. *Psychopharmacology, 93,* 188-192.

Pliszka, S. R., McCracken, J. T., & Maas, J. W. (1996) Catecholamines in attention-deficit hyperactivity disorder: Current perspectives. *Journal of the American Academy of Child and Adolescent Psychiatry, 35,* 264-272.

Pribram, K. H. & McGuinness, D. (1975) Arousal, activation, and effort in the control of attention. *Psychological Review, 82,* 116-149.

Reilly, T. (1986). Fundamental studies in soccer. In R. Andresen (Ed.), *Sportswissenschaft und Sportpraxis* (pp. 114-121). Hamburg: Ingrid Czvalina.

Reilly, T. & Smith, D. (1986). Effect of work intensity on performance in a psychomotor task during exercise. *Ergonomics, 29,* 601-606.

Rektor, I.; Kanovsky, P.; Bares, M.; Brazdil, M.; Streitova, H.; Klajblova, H. et al. (2003). A SEEG study of ERP in motor and premotor cortices and in the basal ganglia. *Clinical Neurophysiology, 114,* 463-471.

Reynolds, H. L. (1976). The effect of augmented levels of stress on reaction time in the peripheral visual field. *Research Quarterly for Exercise and Sport, 47,* 768-775.

Salmela, J. & Ndoye, O. D. (1986). Cognitive distortions during progressive exercise. *Perceptual and Motor Skills, 63,* 1067-1072.

Sanders, A. F. (1983). Towards a model of stress and human performance. *Acta Psychologica, 53,* 61-97.

Seamans, J. K.; Nogueira, L. & Lavin, A. (2003). Synaptic basis of persistent activity in prefrontal cortex *in vivo* and in organotypic cultures. *Cerebral Cortex, 13,* 1242-1250.

Sian, J.; Youdim, M. B. H.; Riederer, P. & Gerlach, M. (1999). Neurotransmitters and disorders of the basal ganglia. In G. J. Siegel, B. W. Agranoff, R. W. Albers, S. K. Fisher, & M. D. Uhler (Eds.), *Basic neurochemistry: molecular, cellular and medical aspects.* 6th edition (pp. 917-948). Philadelphia: Lippincott, Williams & Wilkins.

Sjöberg, H. (1980). Physical fitness and mental performance during and after work. *Ergonomics, 23,* 977-985.

Sokoloff, L. (1969). Cerebral circulation and behavior in man. Strategy and findings. In A. J. Mandell, & M. P. Mandell (Eds.), *Psychochemical research in man* (pp. 237-252). New York: Academic Press.

Sothmann, M. S.; Hart, B. A. & Horn, T. S. (1991). Plasma catecholamines response to acute psychological stress in humans: relation to aerobic fitness and exercise training. *Medicine and Science in Sports and Exercise, 23,* 860-867.

Spence, (1958). A theory of emotionally based drive (d) and its relation to performance in simple learning situations. *American Psychologist, 13,* 131-141.

Tenenbaum, G.; Yuval, R.; Elbaz, G.; Bar-Eli, M. & Weinberg, R. (1993). The relationship between cognitive characteristics and decision making. *Canadian Journal of Applied Physiology, 18,* 48-62.

Tomporowski, P. D. (2003). Effects of acute bouts of exercise on cognition. *Acta Psychologica, 112,* 297-394.

Tomporowski, P. D. & Ellis, N. R. (1986) Effects of exercise on cognitive processes: a review. *Psychological Bulletin, 99,* 338-346.

Tomporowski, P. D.; Ellis, N. R. & Stephens, R. (1987). The immediate effects of strenuous exercise on free recall memory. *Ergonomics, 30,* 121-129.

Travlos, A. K. & Marisi, D. Q. (1995). Information processing and concentration as a function of fitness level and exercise induced activation to exhaustion. *Perceptual and Motor Skills, 80,* 15-26.

Tsorbatzoudis, H.; Barkoukis, V.; Danis, A. & Grouios, G. (1998). Physical exertion in simple reaction time and continuous attention of sport participants. *Perceptual and Motor Skills, 86,* 571-576.

Welford, A. T. (1968). *Fundamentals of skill.* London: Methuen.

Whalen, P. J. (1998). Fear, vigilance, and ambiguity: initial neuroimaging studies of the human amygdala. *Current Directions in Psychology, 7,* 177-188.

Williams, L. R. T.; Pottinger, P. R. & Shapcott, D. G. (1985). Effects of exercise on choice reaction latency and movement speed. *Perceptual and Motor Skills, 60,* 67-71.

Yerkes, R. M. & Dodson, J. D. (1908). The relation of strength of stimulus to rapidity of habit formation. *Journal of Comparative Neurology and Psychology, 18,* 459-482.

Zervas, Y. (1990). The effect of a physical exercise session on verbal, visuospatial, and numerical ability. *Perceptual and Motor Skills, 71,* 379-383.

Chapter III

Exercise-Induced Oxidative Stress and Lipid Peroxidation: The Exercise Paradox

David Alexander Leaf[*,1] *and Michael Kleinman*[2]

[1]Departments of Medicine, U.C.L.A. School of Medicine and Greater Los Angeles V.A. Healthcare System, Los Angeles, California

[2]Department of Community and Environmental Medicine, University of California, Irvine, Irvine, California

Abstract

The pathogenesis of coronary artery disease (CAD), the leading cause of morbidity and mortality in the United States, is characterized by an underlying inflammatory response that generates free radicals and associated oxidative stress. Although participation in aerobic physical exercise is recommended to reduce CAD risk, a single bout of acute physical exercise generates free radicals and causes oxidative stress that can be measured as increased levels of lipid peroxides. In accordance with the role of oxidative stress in the pathogenesis of CAD we have found that exercise-induced oxidative stress (measured as lipid peroxides) is greater among high risk patients than healthy individuals without CAD. These findings suggest the following paradox; if aerobic exercise causes potentially deleterious oxidative stress, should physical exercise be recommended as a public health measure? Our finding in high risk populations and studies in healthy subjects by other investigators show physical exercise training reduces oxidative stress. Hence the paradox is solved. Participation in regular physical exercise reduces exercise-induced oxidative stress. This effect should lower the risk for CAD and other disease conditions related to oxidative stress by reducing cumulative burden of oxidative stress

---

[*] Address correspondence to: David Alexander Leaf, M.D., M.P.H., Division of General Internal Medicine, 111G, Greater Los Angeles V.A. Healthcare System, Wilshire & Sawtelle Blvds. , Los Angeles, California, 90073. Tel (310) 268-3254; Fax (310) 268-4933; David.Leaf@med.va.gov.

accrued during a lifetime of activities of daily living. The mechanism(s) by which aerobic physical exercise causes this effect are numerous and include both exogenous factors such as diet as well as endogenous anti-oxidant systems that may be up-regulated in response to exercise-induced oxidative stress. Further studies are warranted to evaluate the 'anti-oxidant' role of role of physical exercise in reducing CAD risk, and identify the mechanism(s) by which exercise exerts this effect.

Key Words: Oxidative Stress, Lipid Peroxidation, Physical Exercise, Coronary Artery Disease.

Introduction

The pathogenesis of coronary artery disease (CAD), the leading cause of morbidity and mortality in the United States, is characterized by an underlying inflammatory response that generates free radicals and associated oxidative stress [1-5]. The term 'free radical' denotes a molecule or molecular fragment (atom or groups of atoms) with an unpaired electron in the valence shell [6]. Free radical injury occurs after localized oxidative stress, which is caused by excessive production and release of reactive oxygen species (ROS) and free radicals [7] that interact with proteins, lipids, nucleic acids and cellular membranes. Oxidative stress results in free radical-generated cellular injury [8], and can promote atherogenic oxidative modification of low-density lipoprotein (LDL_{ox}) [9,10]. LDL_{ox} plays a pivotal role in atherogenesis.

Oxidative stress has been said to occur when "pro-oxidant capacity exceeds antioxidant capacity" and can contribute to an overall decline in health status and increase the prevalence of diseases such as CAD among susceptible individuals [11]. Antioxidant systems can be grossly dichotomized as exogenous (see Table 1) and endogenous (see Table 2). Depression of anti-oxidant defenses in some individuals can lead to increased susceptibility to oxidative stress. In addition oxidative stress can be increased by exposure to a number of exogenous pro-oxidants including tobacco smoke.

Table 1. Selected exogenous nutrients and their primary food sources

Water-soluble nutrients	Food sources
Ascorbate (Vitamin C)	Fresh fruits and vegetables
Glutathione	Liver
Fat-soluble nutrients	
Tocopherols (Vitamin E)	Grains and oils
Carotenoids (alpha-carotene, beta carotene, lycopene, lutein)	Fresh fruits and vegetables
Ubiquinol 10 (Coenzyme Q_{10})	Liver, yeast

Table 2. Endogenous antioxidant systems

Class
Primary
Peroxidases
Catalases
Superoxide dismutases
Secondary
Ubiquinol (Coenzyme Q_{10})
Uric Acid
Metal binding proteins

This presentation integrates findings from our laboratory involving exercise-induced oxidative stress, which we have measured using lipid peroxidation as a biomarker, with relevant findings from other studies that show physical exercise exerts both pro-oxidative and antioxidant effects. In order to reduce redundancy we present our laboratory techniques at this time. Interested readers can obtain the original publications for further details. The Institutional Review Boards and Human Subjects Protection Committee from U.C.L.A. School of Medicine and the VA Greater Los Angeles Healthcare Center, approved all protocols discussed in this presentation according to guidelines adopted from the Helsinki Declaration.

Oxidative Stress and Measurements of Lipid Peroxidation

Superoxide free radicals, the source of oxidative stress, can be directly measured in tissues using electron spin resonance (ESR) and paramagnetic resonance spectometry. This technique measures transition states of the free radicals. However, the application of this technique has generally been limited to animal studies. Davies et. al. [12] were the first group to demonstrate that the rate of free radical generation increases during exercise using paramagnetic spin resonance to measure the production of free radicals in rat muscle. Following an endurance exercise stress test a 2 to 3 fold increase in free radical formation occurred that was related to an increase in lipid peroxidation. These findings indicate that the amount of free radicals produced during physical exercise is sufficient to overwhelm the free radical scavenging systems. Animal studies show that increased work of breathing by experimentally-induced respiratory failure is associated with increased diaphramatic ROS [13-15].

Lipid peroxidation is one of the best understood reactions induced by free radicals. Halliwell and Gutteridge [11] suggest the use of two or more assays to increase one's ability to interpret the results of studies attempting to assess the extent of oxidative stress in humans and animals. The markers of lipid peroxidation employed in our studies include breath ethane and pentane and plasma malonadehyde (MDA). In vitro studies of lipid peroxidation in homogeneous solutions indicate that oxidative susceptibility increases with the number of double bonds of fatty acids [16,17]. Studies of acqueous micelles suggest that oxidative susceptibility is influenced by additional factors such as polarity of lipid peroxides formed from specific fatty acids [18]. The measurement of lipid peroxidation *in vivo* is relevant because oxidative conditions that are used to determine oxidative susceptibility *in vitro* may not be relevant *in vivo* [19]. *In vivo* assessments of lipid peroxidation are complicated by a number of issues discussed below.

We have measured markers of lipid peroxidation non-invasively *in vivo* by measuring the secondary lipid peroxidation by-products ethane and pentane in samples of expired breath. Ethane and pentane are end products of beta scission of alkoxy radicals arising from free-radical-induced oxidative degradation of polyunsaturated fatty acids (PUFAs). The majority of PUFAs in the body are comprised of the n-3 and n-6 series. Ethane is produced by the peroxidation of n-3 fatty acids (i.e., linolenic, eicosapentanoic, and docosahexanoic fatty acids) [20-22], while pentane is derived from peroxidation of n-6 fatty acids (i.e., linoleic and arachidonic fatty acids) [23,24]. In a validation study we demonstrated the reproducibility of breath ethane and pentane samples in subjects taken at rest, during and after maximal aerobic exercise 12 weeks apart showing little within-individual variation in the values [25].

MDA is an adlehyde by-product largely derived from tissue polyunsaturated fatty acids that are susceptible to fragmentation from ROS. These include conjugated dienes and thiobarbituric acid-reactive substances (TBARS). Conjugated dienes, which absorb light at 230-235 nm are among the initial products of lipid peroxidation [26]. Because conjugated dienes can be introduced in the diet, the interpretation of this measurement must be viewed with caution. Moreover, technical issues are controversial because of non-specificity of the TBARS test [27]. Although MDA has been widely used as a measure of lipid peroxidation, its use as a biomarker of lipid peroxidation has been challenged [28-30]. Reasons include the lack of a standard assay [27], significant subject to subject variation, and non-specificity of the measurement. Halliwell and Chirico [31] suggest that separation of peroxidation products using high-pressure liquid chromatography improves the accuracy of this measurement and further specificity can be obtained by separation using monoclonal antibody techniques. A additional problem in interpreting different exercise studies involving MDA is that it has been measured from different blood constituents including serum [32], plasma [25], red blood cells [33], and platelets [34].

Measurements of Lipid Peroxidation Markers

Breath ethane and pentane flux measurements obtained in our studies were performed in conjunction with cardiopulmonary exercise stress (CPX) testing as will be described, then analyzed according to the following methods [25]. Breath samples containing picomole quantities of ethane and pentane were collected onto an adsorbent column (Carbotrap 200, Supelco, Bellefonte, PA). A sampling line was inserted into the expired breath line of the 2 way respiratory valve used for O_2 and CO_2 measurements. Samples were collected for 1 minute at 1 liter/min using carbotrap tubes. Tubes were shipped on ice for ethane and pentane analysis and analyzed within 8 hours of collection. Samples were heat-desorbed directly onto the analytic column of a 5840 A gas chromatograph (Hewlett-Packard) and analyzed using a stainless steel carbopack 60/80 column (Supelco). The analytic conditions were; carrier gas = He (20 mL/min); flame ionization detector (FID) temperature = 150°C, starting temperature = 45°C, rate = 18°C to a final temperature of 225°C in 20 minutes. The gas chromatograph was standardized using NIST-traceable gas standards. The ethane and pentane concentrations in picomoles/L were multiplied by the Ve in L/min, obtained at a given workload, to compute the flux in picomoles/min.

Plasma MDA was determined as TBARS before and 5 minutes post CPX-testing. Blood was allowed to clot, the clot was carefully separated from the walls of the tube, the tube was centrifuged at 400 X g for 10 minutes. The plasma was removed, and stored, frozen (-80°C) until analyzed. Serum (50 uL) was added to 4 mL N/12 H_2SO_4 and 0.5 mL 10% phosphotungstic acid. The resulting precipitate was isolated by centrifugation (700 g for 5 minutes), washed with 2 mL N/12 H_2SO_4 plus 0.3 mL 10% phosphotungstic acid, and recentrifuged. The precipitate was resuspended with 1 mL TBA reagent (0.7% thiobarbituric acid in water and glacial acetic acid 1:1) and heated at 95°C for 1 hour. After cooling under tap water, 5 mL n-butanol was added and vigorously shaken. The absorbance of the n-butanol layer at 525 nm was determined. A calibration curve was constructed using known amounts of 1,1,3,3 tetraethoxypropane as a source of MDA.

Physical Exercise and Oxidative Stress

Maximal aerobic capacity (VO_{2max}) is associated with decreased CAD and total mortality [35]. Physical activity is recommended as a public health measure to reduce CAD risk [36]. Although participation in aerobic physical exercise is recommended to reduce CAD risk, as is subsequently discussed a single bout acute physical exercise generates free radicals and causes oxidative stress that can be measured as increased levels of lipid peroxides.

Although physical exercise itself represents a spectrum of forms of muscle function, these functions can be grossly dichotomized as 1.) concentric (i.e. dynamic or aerobic) exercises such as stationary cycling or jogging and 2.) eccentric (i.e. resistive) exercises such as heavy lifting and resistive/strength training. Both forms of physical exercise contribute to exercise-induced oxidative stress and are described in the context of 3 models of exercise-induced oxidative stress: Model I.) Aerobic exercise: O_2 flux; Model II.) Aerobic exercise: ischemia/reperfusion; and Model III.) Resistive exercise: injury/repair.

Model I.) Aerobic exercise: O_2 flux. According to this hypothesis, increasing workloads with aerobic exercise generate increased oxygen needs. As discussed previously, the increased electron 'leakage' from the mitochondrial electron transport chain during aerobic exercise exacerbated by the presence of lactic acidosis creates conditions of increased production of ROS [11,25,37,38,39] This model has been studied primarily in young, healthy athletes exercising to maximal levels of aerobic work performance [40,41,42]. Studies generally have evaluated markers of lipid peroxidation. Breath concentrations of expired ethane and pentane are increased 100-fold above resting levels at the lactic acidosis threshold (LAT) and increase dramatically by 1,000-fold above resting levels at peak exercise [25]. LAT is the point at which lactate begins to accumulate above resting levels during exercise of increasing intensity. VO_{2LAT} is the oxygen consumption level at which LAT occurs and is considered one of the best determinants of an individual's ability to perform endurance exercise.

Yet it is notable that significant increases in breath ethane and pentane levels are already occurring during exercise at approximately 50 percent of maximal aerobic capacity [25,43,44]. The clinical relevance of this mechanism is that exercise-induced oxidative stress is substantial at lower levels of physical activity that occur with levels of exertion incurred during many activities of daily living [45]. Recently, Child et. al examined the effects of a structured half marathon run on markers of muscle injury and oxidative stress in a group of highly fit, young athletes [41]. During exercise, serum anti-oxidant capacity increased but not sufficiently enough to protect against exercise-induced muscle injury (i.e. increased plasma creatinine kinase [CK] levels) and oxidative stress (i.e., increased plasma MDA levels). This finding is consistent with the hypothesis that exercise-induced oxidative stress is of physiological importance and is not totally eradicated even in highly conditioned athletes.

Model II.) aerobic exercise: ischemia/reperfusion. Early in the ischemic (or hypoxic) episode ATP is used faster than it is synthesized. Although the cytoplasmic ATP/ADP·Pi ratio is considered the primary sensing mechanism for changes in cellular energy requirements, the mitochondrial NAD/NADH ratio allows the rate of ATP production to change at a given ATP/ADP·Pi ratio [46]. Depletion of oxygen and mitochondrial carbon substrates during ischemia inhibits electron transport and reoxidation of NADH, thereby making the mitochondrial redox state more reduced. Thus, mitochondrial respiration fails and electrons increasingly leak from the respiratory chain during ischemia, due to the combined consequences of hypoxia and damage to the mitochondrial respiratory chain proteins. This results in an imbalance in ATP production relative to ATP consumption, and culminates with failure to maintain a normal intra-mitochondrial redox state.

This phenomenon of ischemia/reperfusion-induced oxdiative stress has been noted in cardiac patients where increased O_2 flux following a period of reduced tissue perfusion leads to a burst of ROS and oxidative stress. This aspect of ROS injury is a well-recognized phenomenon in invasive cardiology procedures where increased blood flow following a successful percutaneous transthoracic coronary angioplasty (PTCA) procedure has been shown to increase plasma MDA levels [47-49]. Physical exercise training can mitigate this effect as shown by a study of Sprague Dawley rats [50]. Animals given a 10 week endurance exercise training (4 day/week for 90 minutes/day at 75 percent of VO_{2max}) then undergoing coronary artery occlusion followed by reperfusion had significantly lower levels of left ventricular MDA content compared with non-exercise-trained controls [50]. This effect was associated with increased myocardial levels of heat shock protein (HSP) 72 but not glutathione peroxidase (GSH) or superoxide dismutase (SOD).

Model III.) Resistive exercise: ischemia/reperfusion and injury/repair. Resistive exercise has generally been believed to have little direct effect on oxidative stress [51,52]. Perhaps this is because initial studies had been done using low intensity workloads exercising a limited number of muscle groups. More recently, McBride et al. [53], have shown that young, healthy adults undergoing higher intensity levels of resistive exercise employing large muscle groups experienced increased plasma MDA levels at 6 and 24 hours following resistive exercise. Resistive exercise may cause oxidative stress by two mechanisms.

i) Because resistive exercise rapidly produces extreme lactic acidosis, one might expect evidence of oxidative stress immediately post-exercise as is noted with the ischemia/reperfusion model of aerobic exercise. This condition creates ischemia-reperfusion-induced activation of the xanthine oxidase pathway during resistance exercise [54,55,56]. Formation of superoxide in this pathway can cause inflammation, damage to cells, oxidation of protein channels and transporters, and adhesion of leukocytes to the endothelium [57]. Alessio et. al [58] recently found that non-aerobic isometric exercise increased immediate post exercise lipid hydroperoxides despite increasing VO_2 by only twofold from rest compared to exhaustive aerobic exercise that increased VO_2 by 14 fold.

ii) In resistive exercise, such as weightlifting, the production of ROS is delayed from the time of actual exercise and occurs as the result of the biological processes of inflammation and repair by monocytes in response to eccentric exercise. Physical exercise can lead to direct muscle injury which has been documented directly histologically by myofibrillar disruption and indirectly by the perception of muscle soreness and a prolonged loss of strength and range of motion [59,60]. CK is often used as a biochemical marker of muscle damage after exercise. Among the various CK isoforms CK-MM1 is the only gene product found within the muscle, and has been shown to increase in the circulation following muscle injury [61,62]. McBride et. al. [53] showed resistive exercise increased plasma CK levels as well as plasma levels of MDA, and that this response was reduced following vitamin E supplementation(1,200 I.U./day for 2 weeks). Potential sources of ROS in muscle are neutrophils and monocytes. These cells may enter a muscle as part of the immune response to micro damage of the muscle cell. Once inside, the neutrophils and monocytes utilize a 'respiratory burst' (i.e., rapid production of superoxide and H_2O_2) to aid in breaking down the damaged myofibril during phagocytosis. The ROS released during this process are essential to the inflammatory response, as well as being important in the removal of the damaged myofibrils. Furthermore, ROS released during the phagocytosis process may, hypothetically, be important in the activation of satellite cells for the regeneration of the fibril and the development of stronger fibers.

Exercise-Induced Oxidative Stress in Health

Aerobic physical exertion can induce oxidative stress through mitochondrial production of oxygen-derived free radicals as has been demonstrated in studies using ESR in rats showing stimulation of gastrocnemius muscle increases the ESR signal by $70 \pm 20\%$ [63]. The chain of events that follows the initial production of free radicals culminates in lipid peroxidation [64]. We [25] and others [42,43,65,66] have shown that lipid peroxide markers of oxidative stress increase after intensive physical exercise.

Healthy Adults

We evaluated exercise-induced lipid peroxidation in 7 healthy men (N = 5) and women (N = 2) who regularly engaged in regular physical exercise training [25]. All subjects reported no tobacco use within 6 months prior to entry and did not consume ethanol-containing beverages 1 week before CPX testing, and were not consuming antioxidant compounds including vitamins and medications, and had not participated in physical exercise training at least 2 days before CPX testing. Subjects' clinical characteristics (mean ± standard deviation) included age = 36.4 ± 3 years, height = 171 ± 7.2 cm, body weight = 60 ± 8.2 Kg, and VO_{2max} = 56.6 ± 5.5 ml/Kg/min.

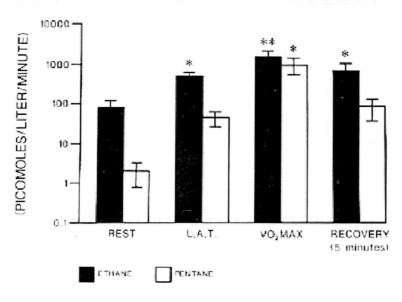

Figure 1. Time course of ethane and pentane flux in expired breath of 7 healthy subjects.

CPX stress testing employing a modified Bruce protocol was conducted using a treadmill apparatus (Quinton, Seattle, WA). Breath ethane and pentane samples were collected before exercise, at one minute following the attainment of LAT, at VO_{2max}, and after 5 minutes of post-exercise recovery. Plasma MDA was measured at rest before exercise and after 5 minutes of post-exercise recovery. Respiratory gases were continuously measured during exercise with a Hans Rudolf two-way valve and analyzed on a breath-by-breath basis using a Sensor Medics 4400 TC Metabolic Measurement Cart. The V-slope method was employed as an *a priori* criteria to identify LAT [67]. An R value > 1.0 was used to indicate the onset of LAT and trigger the initiation of expired ethane and pentane collection. LAT was later confirmed for each subject using the "V-slope" method, which is more widely accepted as an indicator of LAT. During the 1 minute breath sampling period the treadmill was held at constant speed and grade; the Bruce protocol was then completed after each sample was completed. ANOVA was conducted using log transformations for expired ethane and pentane levels and differences between group means measured at each time interval were tested using the Tukey Studentized range method. Paired t-test comparisons were made for plasma MDA levels before and after exercise.

Both expired ethane and pentane flux levels, shown in Figure 1, increased from rest to maximal exercise, then declined to baseline during recovery. Group mean values the differed significantly (as per the Tukey method) as indicated in Figure 1. Ethane levels at 5-minute recovery declined from level at peak exercise by 55.8% and pentane levels at 5-minute recovery declined by 89.9% from, peak levels. There was no significant ($p \leq 0.05$) difference between pre- and post-exercise plasma MDA levels ($32.6 \pm$ to 35.8 ± 5.3 nanomoles/mL).

The changes in breath ethane and pentane flux from rest to peak exercise reveal a large, yet transient increase in exercise-induced lipid peroxidation that rapidly attenuates during recovery. The results of our findings regarding breath ethane and pentane flux differ from those of plasma MDA that did not increase as anticipated with exercise. Although others have shown that a bout of high intensity physical exercise raises plasma MDA levels [42] and in contrast to the large increase in breath ethane and pentane flux we noted, the lack of exercise-induced increases in plasma MDA in our study suggests that these compounds are cleared from the plasma by several mechanisms, including excretion, catabolism, or redistribution to body tissues.

Healthy Children Compared with Children with Cystic Fibrosis

During mild exercise, healthy children showed a significant increase in concentrations of ethane and pentane compare to their pre-exercise resting levels as shown in Figure 2. They showed a small increase in both ethane and pentane exhalation 30 and 60 minutes after cessation of exercise, however the changes were not significantly different from their resting pre-exercise levels. Thus mild exercise probably does not induce oxidative stress in healthy children. The children with cystic fibrosis, on the other hand, showed a markedly different pattern of responses. Expired ethane levels from the children with cystic fibrosis were significantly (approximately 3 fold) lower than those for healthy children . However, the resting expired pentane flux levels for the children with cystic fibrosis were approximately 50% higher than those for the healthy children.

Exercise-Induced Oxidative Stress in Disease

Our previous studies in healthy adult individuals show breath ethane and pentane flux were increased even at levels of exertion comparable to those used in simple activities of daily living, such as walking up a flight of stairs and doing household chores [68]. Oxidative stress occurred even at submaximal levels (i.e. VO_{2LAT}) of exercise and therefore could be exacerbated in older, deconditioned individuals and among patients with chronic disease conditions such as CAD who may have impaired anti-oxidant capacity.

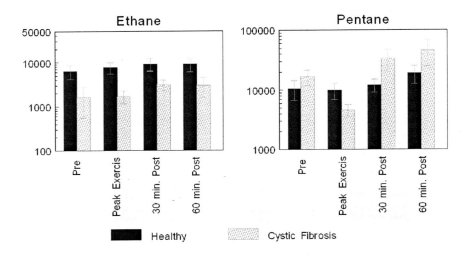

Figure 2. Breath ethane and pentane flux levels of exercising healthy children and children with cystic fibrosis.

CAD Patients and O_2 Flux

To evaluate this hypothesis we compared the previous findings in the 7 healthy subjects with the effects of exercise-induced oxidative stress in 12 patients with CAD (10 men and 2 women) [69]. The patients' clinical characteristics (mean ± standard deviation) included: age = 63 ± 8 years, height = 175 ± 7 cm, weight = 89 ± 147 Kg, and aerobic capacity at LAT (ie. VO_{2LAT}) = 21.6 ± 9.4 ml O_2/Kg/minute. 7 had cardiac artery bypass grafting (CABG) procedures and 3 had PTCA procedures. Medication use included 6 angiotensin converting enzyme inhibitor, 7 beta-adrenergic receptor blocker, 5 calcium channel blocker, 7 diuretic, 1 amiodarone, 2 nitrate, and 5 lipid-lowering medication recipients.

The exercise protocol differed from that previously employed in healthy subjects because the cardiac patients were physically deconditioned and were unable to tolerate high intensity levels of exercise. The cardiac patients were therefore exercised only to VO_{2LAT} using the previously described exercise methods, and not continued to VO_{2max}. As shown in figure 3, the healthy subjects experienced substantial increases in breath ethane and pentane flux from rest to peak exercise with the greatest increase occurring between LAT and peak aerobic exercise. Once these subjects stopped exercising, oxidative stress rapidly declined to baseline. The cardiac patients experienced increased breath ethane and pentane flux levels from rest to VO_{2LAT} (i.e. LAT) that declined only slightly after exercise ceased. Although the magnitude of the increase in breath ethane and pentane flux at VO_{2LAT} was lower among cardiac patients, this may reflect lower levels of peak exercise intensity achieved during CPX testing.

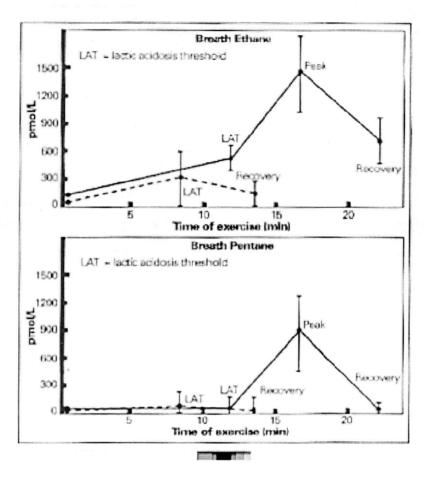

Figure 3. Time course of ethane and pentane flux in expired breath measured at rest, during exercise, at peak exercise and recovery in 7 young, healthy subjects (———) and 12 older patients who had CAD (----------).

These findings might be taken to mean that the deconditioned cardiac patients had less oxidative stress. Our important finding, however, is that the healthy subjects actually had faster recovery from much higher levels of exercise-induced oxidative stress compared with the cardiac patients. This suggests that aerobic fitness promotes an oxidative advantage that allows rapid clearance of free-radical species as they are generated.

CAD Patients, Ischemia Reperfusion, and Cigarette Smoking

Although we have previously considered CAD-related oxidative stress according to the O_2 flux hypothesis we have also evaluated the ischemia/reperfusion hypothesis in the setting of exercise-induced myocardial ischemia. Another potential mechanism whereby oxidative stress can be increased in cardiac patients is from reperfusion injury as previously described [47,48,49].

We evaluated 18 patients referred for exercise stress testing with thallium imaging (ETT-thallium) [70]. Exclusion criteria included ethanol abuse, and the use of antioxidant compounds including vitamins. Monitored exercise exercise testing was conducted using a symptom-limited standard Bruce protocol. Immediately post-exercise, single photon emission computed tomography (SPECT) imaging was performed (ADAC Laboratories, Milpitas, CA). Image acquisition was 180^0 using a 64 (ts) 16 matrix with 20 seconds of stop. Redistribution images were obtained 4 hours later. Number, location, and degree of reversibility of defects were reported. Plasma MDA samples were collected and measured immediately prior to and following completion of exercise stress testing.

Based on thallium stress testing subjects were divided into 2 groups. Group A (n = 8, all male) had reversible thallium defects and Group B (n = 10; nine male, 1 female) had normal thallium studies. Patient profiles revealed similar clinical characteristics (Group A vs. Group B) including; age (62 ± 13 vs. 56 ±10 years), personal history of myocardial infarction (4 vs. 3), diabetes mellitus (1 vs. 2), hypertension (4 vs. 6) and/or dyslipidemia (4 vs. 3); and cardiac medications: beta blockers (4 vs. 3), calcium channel blockers (5 vs. 4), and angiotensin converting enzyme inhibitors (3 vs. 4) recipients. The groups had similar levels of exercise tolerance including duration of exercise, percent maximal predicted heart rate, and peak rate-pressure product. A significantly greater increase in plasma MDA levels was noted among Group A patients (46 ± 12%, i.e. from 3.45 ± 1.50 to 5.47 ± 1.02 nanomoles/mL) than in Group B patients (-16.8 ± 6%, i.e. from 5.32 ± 1.02 to 4.07 ± 0.96 nanomoles/mL) whose plasma MDA levels decreased in response to exercise.

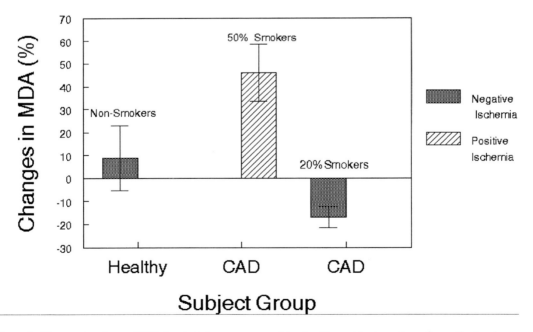

Figure 4. Changes in plasma MDA levels between non-smoking healthy subjects, and cardiac patients who are cigarette smokers with positive and negative thallium tests.

Smoking is prevalent among CAD patients and represents a potential confounding factor in this study. We compared pre- and post exercise stress testing changes in plasma MDA levels measured in the 7 healthy non-smoking subjects described in our previous study [25] with the cardiac patients sub-grouped on the basis of the presences or absence of myocardial ischemia as previously described and characterized according to cigarette smoking status. Our findings shown in Figure 4 reveal that healthy, non-smoking individuals did not significantly ($p \geq 0.05$) increase plasma MDA levels from resting pre-exercise levels during and after CPX testing after exercise while the CAD patients with myocardial ischemia significantly increased their plasma MDA levels following exercise stress testing. CAD patients without myocardial ischemia experienced decreased levels of plasma MDA in response to CPX testing. The group of patients with myocardial ischemia had a greater percentage of cigarette smokers than did the group without myocardial ischemia. The study results suggest that the exercise-induced effects of myocardial ischemia/reperfusion increases exercise-induced oxidative stress, and that exposure to environmental agents that produce ROS (i.e. cigarette smoking) can exacerbate the susceptibility to oxidative stress.

Chronic Maintenance Dialysis (CMD) Patients

In accordance with the etiologic role of oxidative stress in the pathogenesis of CAD we hypothesized patients at high risk for CAD would have also increased levels of exercise-induced oxidative stress compared with healthy individuals because they may have impaired ability to limit exercise-induced lipid peroxidation. Chronic maintenance dialysis (CMD) patients are a high-risk population for CAD [71,72] and oxidative stress [73]. Spittel et al. [74] have shown breath ethane levels are greater among CMD patients than control subjects. Hemodialysis alone is not an effective tool for reducing oxidative stress as Capodicasa et. al. [75] have shown that hemodialysis does not modify breath ethane and pentane production. Some suggested oxidative stress-inducing mechanisms specific to CMD patients include: i) neutrophil activation during dialysis [73,76-78]; ii) alterations in erythrocyte pentose-phosphate shunt activity [79]; iii) depletion of internal anti-oxidant capacity from (a) reduced anti-oxidant enzyme systems (SOD, and GSH) [80,81] and/or anti-oxidant compounds (vitamins E and C, and carotenoids) [82,83], or (b) a direct pro-oxidant effect from the uremic condition [84,85].

We conducted a cross-sectional study to compare the susceptibility to exercise-induced lipid peroxidation between CMD patients (Group A) and an age-, gender-, medical diagnosis-, smoking-, and ethanol consumption-matched comparison group (Group B). The clinical characterists of these subjects are shown in Table 3. CPX testing conducted to symptom-limited maximal functional capacity was administered using an rpm independent workload on an upright Lode stationary cycle according to our previous studies [20]. Pulmonary gas exchange values were continuously measured breath-by-breath during CPX using a Sensor Medics 4400 TC Metabolic Measurement System (Kalamazoo, MI). CPX was performed to VO_{2LAT} as determined by an on-line R value measurement (VCO_2/VO_2) > 1.0, and was later confirmed using the 'V-slope' Method [67] and by measurements of serum lactic acid. Blood samples were immediately analyzed after retrieval in duplicate for whole blood lactate using a YSI lactate analyzer (Yellow Springs, Ohio). Breath ethane and pentane were measured at rest before exercise, at VO_{2LAT}, and at 5 minutes post CPX test.

Because of the wide variation in subjects' breath ethane and pentane levels analysis employed nonparametric ANOVA (Two-factor ANOVA of ranks with replication) between Group A and Group B subjects' measurements of breath ethane and pentane flux taken before CPX testing, at VO_{2LAT}, and following CPX testing.

Group comparisons (see Table 3) reveal that the groups were similar in terms of age, ethnicity, and co-morbid diagnoses as well as cigarette smoking and ethanol consumption behaviors. Although diet was not explicitly considered in this study, CMD patients were receiving a standard low fat diet and no subject was receiving antioxidant-containing supplements (i.e., vitamins E and C). The prevalence of medication use appears to be similar in both groups (angiotensin converting enzyme inhibitors [Group A = 4, Group B = 5], alpha receptor-blockers [Group A = 1, Group B = 1], calcium channel blockers [Group A = 6, Group B = 4], beta receptor- blockers [Group A = 2, group B = 2], and glyburide [Group A = 2, Group B = 2.]). Although Group B subjects have a higher prevalence of obesity, their body mass index (BMI) values were not significantly different than Group A subjects. No differences were noted in measurements of aerobic exercise performance (i.e., VO_{2LAT}, VO_{2peak}, and peak workload).

Table 3. Clinical characteristics of study groups

Group A

Subject	Age	Ethnicity	Diagnosis	Smoker	Ethanol	Medications	BMI	VO_{2LAT}	VO_{2peak}	Peak Work
1.	61	A.A.	HTN	No	No	F, N	24.7	9	13.4	30
2.	55	C	HTN	No	No	A	34.2	9.2	13.2	82
3.	46	C	HTN	No	No	F,N, S	26.8	14.4	20.7	112
4.	73	A.A.	HTN	No	Yes	C, Dilt	24.4	14.2	21.3	96
5.	53	A.A.	DM	Yes	Yes	Am, G, M	31.1	14.3	17.3	112
6.	41	A.A.	HTN	Yes	Yes	F	20.3	18.9	26.5	112
7.	39	A.A.	DM	No	No	D,F,G,N	24.5	14.1	25.3	132
Mean	52.6						26.6	13.4	19.7	96.6
± S.D.	± 11.9						±4.7	±3.4	±5.3	±33.2

Group B

Subject	Age	Ethnicity	Diagnosis	Smoker	Ethanol	Medications	BMI	VO_{2LAT}	VO_{2peak}	Peak Work
1.	62	A.A.	HTN	No	No	Dilt, M	24.2	14.9	25.1	158
2.	61	C	HTN	No	No	F, Felo, T	23.8	18.3	31.1	170
3.	33	A.A.	HTN	No	No	Dilt, M	36.3	20	22.8	158
4.	69	A.A.	HTN	No	Yes	Am,F	32.4	12.1	16.5	82
5.	53	A.A.	DM	Yes	Yes	A,F,G	32.2	17.2	18.4	152
6.	43	A.A.	HTN	Yes	Yes	F	28.4	18.9	25.3	107
7.	58	C	DM	No	No	F,G	30.2	12.9	17.5	82
Mean	54.1						34.3	16.3	22.4	129.9
± S.D.	±12.4						±4.6	± 3.0	±5.2	±38.3

A.A. = Afro-American, C = Caucasian, HTN = Hypertension, DM = Diabetes Mellitus, A = aspirin, Am = amlopidine, C = clonidine, D = digitalis, Dilt = diltiazem, F = fosinopril, Felo = felodipine, G = glyburide, M = metoprolol, N = nifedipine, S = sotalol, T = terazocin.

Group A = patients receiving chronic maintenance dialysis (CMD) (N = 7), and Group B = control patients (N = 7). Age is measured in years, peak workload is measured in watts, and VO_{2peak} and VO_{2LAT} are measured in ml O_2/Kg body weight / minute.

All subjects successfully completed the CPX protocol achieving LAT (documented by post exercise increases in serum lactic acid). Table 4 shows breath ethane and pentane flux levels (mean ± standard deviation) in CMD patients and control subjects at rest, VO_{2LAT}, and post exercise recovery. Because of the wide variation in these mean ± SD, values reflect absolute rather than relative group values. The results of nonparametric ANOVA (Two-factor ANOVA of ranks with replication) showed significant (F value = 6.44, P < 0.015) differences between Group A and Group B subjects with increased pre-, VO_{2LAT}, and post-exercise ethane levels in and post-exercise pentane levels in Group A compared with Group B subjects. These findings indicate that CMD patients are more susceptible to exercise-induced lipid peroxidation than non-CMD control subjects, and implies that CAD may be linked to this phenomenon.

Table 4. Breath ethane and pentane flux ($pmolL^{-1}Min^{-1}$) at rest, VO_{2LAT}, and 5 minutes post-exercise in Group A = patients receiving chronic maintenance hemodialysis (n = 7) and Group B = control patients (n=7). (ND = non-detectable)

Group A

Subject	Ethane			Pentane		
	rest	VO_{2LAT}	recovery	rest	VO_{2LAT}	recovery
1	91,297	2,404,160	46,678	4,195	11,520	3,153,146
2	239,091	313,044	60,088	32,205	10, 032	8,937,713
3	68,052	29,484	7,847,145	2,567	764,634	18,077
4	28,039	871,055	5,191	81,613	170,925	54
5	121,556	261,632	306, 203	142,187	3,278	968,400
6	90, 229	8,383	124, 802	535	54, 015	8,285
7	0 (ND)	2,322	5,951	299,832	675	727,236
Mean	91,181	555,726	1,199,437	80,448	145,011	1,973,273
± S.D.	77,068	870,277	2,933,210	109,951	279,835	3,266,891

Group B

Subject	Ethane			Pentane		
	rest	VO_{2LAT}	recovery	rest	VO_{2LAT}	recovery
1	0(ND)	0 (ND)	0(ND)	69,416	388,938	3, 036
2	0(ND)	3,320	0(ND)	1,564,000	0 (ND)	18,276
3	1,634,000	617,400	171,212	1,194,024	2,196,600	548,550
4	77,225	2,945	0 (ND)	10,451	39,486	0 (ND)
5	32,559	140,180	55,764	205, 351	8,084	467,369
6	0(ND)	3,320	240,321	0 (ND)	2,470,080	813,800
7	7,320	740	239,145	31,600	31,561	61,318
Mean	250,158	109,701	100,920	439,263	733, 536	273, 193
± S.D.	610,871	229,719	112,601	654,372	1,104,062	332,484

Obese Patients

Vincent et. al. [86] have shown that both resistive and aerobic exercise exacerbate lipid peroxidation in obese individuals. Compared to 29 non-obese subjects (mean body fat = 20.8%), obese subjects (mean body fat = 35.0%) experienced greater post exercise increases in plasma lipid peroxides and MDA following both resistance and aerobic exercise sessions.

We evaluated the relationship of BMI and breath ethane and pentane flux levels at rest, at VO_{2LAT}, and recovery in the 7 subjects who served as the matched 'control' group for CMD patients (see Table 3, Group B) and found a highly significant Spearman correlation (rank order) of 0.9643 between increasing BMI and increasing breath ethane flux levels at rest in this group. These finding have important clinical relevance as the prevalence of overweight/obesity and diabetes mellitus, a common sequelea of obesity, continue to increase [87].

The Exercise Paradox

These findings suggest the following paradox; if aerobic exercise causes potentially deleterious oxidative stress, should physical exercise be recommended as a public health measure? We hypothesized that participation in regular physical exercise reduces the risk for exercise-induced oxidative stress.

Aerobic Exercise

In order to evaluate the effects of physical exercise training on exercise-induced lipid peroxidation we compared measurements of breath ethane and pentane flux and plasma MDA in response to CPX testing between cardiac patients before and after they had completed a 12 week aerobic-based physical exercise training program in a cardiac rehabilitation setting (Group A, n = 10; 9 male, 1 female) or had remained as a non-exercising control group (Group B, n = 10; 9 male, 1 female) [88]. Groups characteristics were similar (Group A vs. Group B) with respect to age (64 ± 10 vs. 62 ± 6 years), height (174 ± 7 vs. 177 ± 7 cm), weight (90 ± 19 vs. 89 ± 7 Kg), cardiac procedures (4 vs. 3 CABGs, and 1 vs. 3 PTCAs), medications (3 vs. 4 angiotensin converting enzyme inhibitor, 3 vs. 5 beta-adrenergic receptor blocker, 2 vs. 5 calcium channel blocker, 7 vs. 1 diuretic, 1 vs. 0 amiodarone, 0 vs. 2 nitrate, and 2 vs. 3 lipid-lowering medication recipients) and VO_{2LAT} (18.7 ± 12.0 vs. 23.6 ± 7.3 ml O_2/Kg/minute).

CPX-testing using a modified Bruce protocol was conducted on a treadmill apparatus to VO_{2LAT} before and after completion of the 12 weeks study according to our previously described methods [25]. Breath ethane and pentane flux values were obtained at rest before exercise, at VO_{2LAT}, and 5 minutes following exercise and plasma MDA levels were measured before and 5 minutes after completion of CPX testing. After completing physical exercise training Group A patients experienced a significant ($P = 0.02$) increase in VO_{2LAT} ($17.5 + 1.0$ to $21.1 + 5.2$ ml O_2/Kg/minute) while Group B patients remained the same (26.4 ± 2.0 vs. 26.9 ± 5.1 ml O_2/Kg/minute). Although resting plasma MDA levels did not differ between the groups at entry, following physical exercise training Group A significantly decreased in resting (25.3 ± 24.3 to 12.7 ± 6.0 nmol/mL) and post CPX-testing (25.3 ± 24.3 to 12.7 ± 6.0 nmol/mL) plasma MDA levels compared with entry values while Group B patients experienced increased plasma MDA levels before (4.3 ± 2.2 to 15.6 ± 11.3 nmol/mL) and post CPX-testing (7.9 ± 3.0 to 22.8 ± 11.8 nmol/mL) compared with entry values. A Spearman rank-order correlation between entry VO_{2LAT} levels and resting plasma MDA levels for all subjects (shown in Figure 5) revealed a significant negative relationship (r = -0.476, P < 0.01). This suggests that the presence of physical deconditioning at entry, as indicated by a low VO_{2LAT} levels among subjects, might be a contributing factor to increased lipid peroxidation in response to exercise.

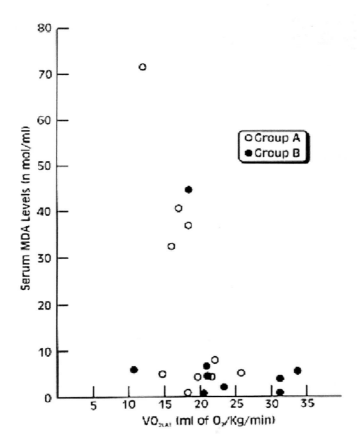

Figure 5. Correlation between entry resting plasma MDA levels before CPX testing and VO_{2LAT} levels.

As shown in figure 6, although both groups had increased breath ethane and pentane flux levels in response to exercise, exercise-induced increases in pentane tended to persist during recovery, whereas ethane levels returned toward baseline more rapidly. Patterns of change of expired ethane and pentane during exercise were similar for entry and 12-week follow-up. Despite their increased VO_{2LAT} levels following physical exercise training in Group A patients, their breath ethane and pentane flux levels at VO_{2LAT} were not increased above entry levels although at the 12-week follow-up CPX testing although they exercised to a high intensity level of VO_{2LAT}. This represents a training-related reduction in free radical flux relative to absolute exertion levels.

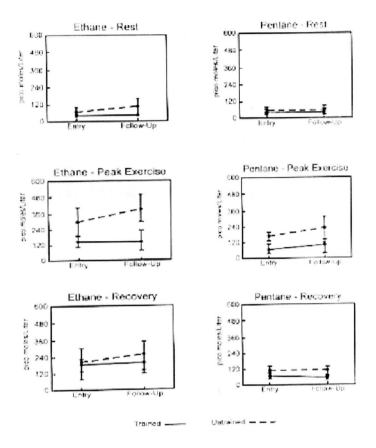

Figure 6. Exercise-induced ethane and pentane flux levels in cardiac patients measured at rest, during and following CPX testing before and after completing a physical exercise training program (Group A) and non-exercising controls (Group B).

Resistive Exercise Training

Vincent et. al. [89] have shown that resistance exercise training reduces the amount of exercise-induced lipid peroxidation. We also evaluated the exercise paradox hypothesis in CMD patients randomized for enrollment in 8 week conventional physical exercise training programs of either aerobic-based or strength- plus aerobic-based physical exercise training. Participation in the study protocol was offered to all CMD patients receiving hemodialysis 3 times per week at the Greater Los Angeles Healthcare System Dialysis Center during a one-year period of time. Specific exclusion criteria for CMD patients included disorders that would exclude them from safely participating in physical exercise training. The exclusion criteria included: 1) Cardiovascular diseases of a significant nature such as angiographic documentation of greater than 70 percent stenosis of a major epicardial vessel; recent myocardial infarction or cardiac procedure (CABG, PTCA), dilated cardiomyopathy (ejection fraction < 20 percent), and cerebrovascular accident or peripheral arterial disease impairing ability to exercise; 2) Orthopedic conditions including rheumatoid arthritis and limb amputation; and 3) Mental incapacity, or known non-compliance issues, which might prevent the ability to understand and follow directions while participating in the physical exercise training programs. Eleven male volunteers who met the entry criteria received an 8-week program of either strength- plus aerobic-based or aerobic-based only physical exercise training.

Before entering and after competing the 8- week physical exercise training programs these patients underwent CPX testing as previously described [25]. Markers of lipid peroxidation and oxidative stress (i.e., breath ethane and pentane flux levels were measured at rest before exercise, at VO_{2LAT}, and at 5 minutes post-CPX testing).

The entry CPX test established that most subjects were very physically deconditioned and only able to complete 30 minutes of aerobic exercise at a zero workload. Hence, all aerobic PET subjects initiated at this level with incremental workload increases made when subjects were able to perform at a particular workload for 30 minutes. The strength- based exercise training sessions lasted approximately 15 minutes and were conducted prior to the aerobic exercise training component. The training program used a leg curl and leg extension apparatus (Pacific Gym). The specific exercises included leg presses, knee extensions, knee flexions, hamstring curls, and ankle plantar and dorsiflexions. Subjects attempted to do 3 sets of 10 repetitions of exercise for each muscle group, with 2-minute rest intervals between sets. The initial amount of weight was set at 70 % of the initial 1 repetition maximum (1 RM = the maximum amount of weight that could be lifted 1 time as determined by the best of three trials) for each exercise. Once subjects were able to complete 3 sets of 10 repetitions for 2 sessions in a row at a particular weight, a new 1 RM was established for the strength exercise. The subjects then continued with the protocol as before at 70% of 1 RM until they were able to complete 3 sets with 10 repetitions for the exercise. Adherence to the PET training programs was defined as having completed more than 70 percent of the 24 scheduled sessions during the 8-week period (i.e. more than 17 sessions) and completion of follow-up exercise testing.

Table 5. Clinical characteristics of patients receiving chronic maintenance dialysis (CMD) at entry (N = 6)

Subject	Age	Ethnicity	Diag-osis	Smo-er	Etha-ol	Medi-ations	BMI	VO_{2LAT}	VO_{2peak}	Peak Work
1.	61	A.A.	HTN	No	No	F, N	24.7	9	13.4	30
2.	55	C	HTN	No	No	A	34.2	9.2	13.2	82
3.	73	A.A.	HTN	No	Yes	C, Dilt	24.4	14.2	21.3	96
4.	53	A.A.	DM	Yes	Yes	Am, G, M	31.1	14.3	17.3	112
5.	41	A.A.	HTN	Yes	Yes	F	20.3	18.9	26.5	112
6.	39	A.A.	DM	No	No	D,F,G,N	24.5	14.1	25.3	132
Mean	52.6						26.6	13.4	19.7	96.6
± S.D.	± 11.9						±4.7	±3.4	±5.3	±33.2

A.A. = Afro-American, C = Caucasian, HTN = Hypertension, DM = Diabetes Mellitus, A = aspirin, Am = amlopidine, C = clonidine, D = digitalis, Dilt = diltiazem, F = fosinopril, Felo = felodipine, G = glyburide, M = metoprolol, N = nifedipine, S = sotalol, T = terazocin.

Note: Age is measured in years, peak workload is measured in watts, and VO_{2peak} and VO_{2LAT} are measured in ml O_2/Kg body weight / minute.

Six of 11 patients who entered were able to complete the 8-week physical exercise training programs. Their characteristics are shown in Table 5. Because of the small numbers in the final group they were combined for further analysis. Because breath ethane and pentane flux values were not symmetrically distributed nonparametric ANOVA was employed to test for significant differences between pre- and post-exercise training measurements of breath ethane and pentane flux measurements measured in conjunction with CPX testing.

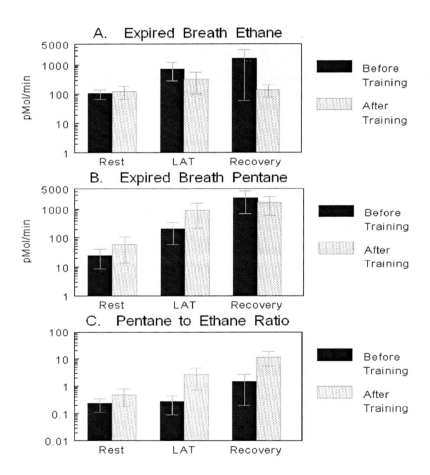

Figure 7. Breath ethane and pentane flux and pentane/ethane flux ratio values measured at rest, VO_{2LAT}, and 5 minutes post-CPX testing in patients receiving chronic maintenance dialysis before and after completing a physical exercise training program.

Figures 7A and B show breath ethane and pentane flux values (mean ± standard deviation) measured at rest, VO_{2LAT}, and 5 minutes after completing CPX testing at entry and after completing the physical exercise training programs. There was a small, but not significant (p ≥ 0.1), decrease in the mean flux of ethane before and after physical exercise training averaged over the three measurement periods. As shown in Figure 7A, before training ethane production during and after CPX testing was slightly increased above resting levels measured before CPX testing. After physical exercise training ethane production during and after CPX testing was not different from the pre-CPX testing resting values. These differences were not statistically significant (p=0.26). As shown in Figure 7B, during and after CPX testing expired pentane flux levels increased (p = 0.06) from resting levels measured before CPX testing both at entry and after completing the physical exercise training programs. These findings indicate that physical exercise training has a role in reducing exercise-induced oxidative stress as shown by the reduced levels of breath ethane flux in response to CPX testing following physical exercise training.

Effects of Exercise Training on Peroxidation of Fatty Acid Classes

Fatty acids have been gaining recognition for specific effects they exert in health and disease including modulation of peroxisome proliferation-activated receptor activity [90], hepatic lipoprotein assembly [91], and cytokine production [92]. N-3 fatty acid classes appear to have an important role in reducing CAD risk [93]. Therefore increased peroxidation of n-3 fatty acids as we noted among obese patients reflected by their increased levels of resting breath ethane flux may indicate increased disease risk due to selective oxidative damage to this important fatty acid series.

We employed the breath ethane/pentane flux ratio to evaluate the effects of physical exercise on the relative peroxidation of these two fatty acid series. We hypothesized that a high ratio, indicating greater relative peroxidation of the n-3 fatty acid series, would reflect greater disease risk. Table 6 shows breath ethane/pentane ratio values (mean ± standard error) in CMD patients and non-CMD control subjects at rest, VO_{2LAT}, and post-CPX recovery. Nonparametric ANOVA showed significant group differences (F value = 8.83, p = 0.005) between these measurements with breath ethane/pentane flux ratios higher at rest, VO_{2LAT}, and post-CPX recovery in CMD (Group A) than in non-CMD control (Group B) patients. These findings suggest CMD causes a deleterious selective peroxidation of the n-3 fatty acids.

There are no prior reports of the effects of physical exercise training on selective changes in ethane and pentane production in CMD patients during acute exercise. In order to evaluate the possibility that physical exercise training could selectively affect fatty acid susceptibility to exercise-induced peroxidation we evaluated the effect of CPX testing on breath pentane/ethane flux ratio values in CMD patients before and after completing the previously described 8 week physical activity programs. Our hypothesis is that a larger breath pentane/ethane flux ratio value, i.e. increased n-6 fatty acid peroxidation relative to n-3 fatty acid peroxidation, is favorable because it reflects selective peroxidation of n-6 to n-3 fatty acids indicating that n-3 fatty acids are 'spared' from exercise-induced oxidative stress.

Table 6. Breath ethane and pentane flux ratios at rest,
VO$_{2LAT}$, and 5 minutes post-exercise in Group A =patients receiving
chronic maintenance hemodialysis (n = 7) and Group B = control patients (n=7)

Group A

Subject	Breath ethane-pentane flux ratio		
	Rest	VO$_{2LAT}$	Recovery
1	21.76	208.67	0.01
2	3.82	31.20	0.01
3	26.50	0.04	434.07
4	0.34	5.10	94.38
5	0.85	79.80	0.32
6	168.65	0.16	15.06
7	0	3.43	0.01
Mean	31.66	46.91	77.69
± S.D.	61.25	76.94	160.88

Group B

Subject	Breath ethane-pentane flux ratio		
	Rest	VO$_{2LAT}$	Recovery
1	0	0	0
2	0.36	3,320.00	0
3	1.36	0.28	0.31
4	7.38	0.07	0
5	0.16	17.34	0.12
6	0	0.001	0.30
7	0.23	0.02	3.90
Mean	1.30	476.82	0.66
± S.D.	2.72	1,253.74	1.43

Shown in Figures 7A and 7B physical exercise training significantly reduced the production of ethane relative to that of pentane in response to CPX testing. This is reflected by the increases in breath pentane/ethane flux ratio values as shown in figure 7C. Physical exercise training induced changes in breath pentane/ethane flux ratios indicate that physical exercise training resulted in a preferential shift from n-3 fatty acid peroxidation (whose by-product is breath ethane) to increased n-6 fatty acid peroxidation (whose by-product is breath pentane). The mean ± standard error values of pentane/ethane flux ratios before physical exercise training (mean ± standard error; at rest before CPX testing = 0.23 ± 0.12, at VO$_{2LAT}$ = 0.27 ± 0.18, and following CPX testing = 1.5 ± 1.3) and after physical exercise training (mean ± standard error; rest before CPX testing = 0.48 ± 0.3, at VO$_{2LAT}$ = 2.7 ± 0.2, and following CPX testing = 11.9 ± 6.5) were clearly different. The 2-way nonparametric ANOVA confirmed that post-physical exercise training breath ethane-pentane flux ratios were significantly reduced from the pre-training levels at VO_{2LAT}, and recovery following PET (F=6.01, p = 0.02).

Because these subjects were on stable therapeutic diets throughout the course of this study it is unlikely that nutritional factors caused this effect. The cause(s) of this phenomenon could result from exercise-induced changes in endogenous fatty acid synthesis recently shown in rats [94] and /or selective changes in fatty acid susceptibility to oxidative stress resulting from exercise-induced mobilization of endogenous anti-oxidants recently shown in dialysis patients [95] and/or exercise-induced adaptive changes in internal anti-oxidant defense systems. Because of the importance of the n-3 to n-6 fatty acid balance with respect to health and disease, our findings suggesting that PET promotes a favorable 'endoperoxide shift' [96] deserve further study.

Discussion

Current evidence indicates that participation in both aerobic- and resistance-based PET reduce exercise-induced oxidative stress. This evidence is suggested by findings in human [88] and animal studies [66]. Ginsberg et al. have shown that in highly trained athletes, susceptibility to lipid peroxidation (serum MDA) is reduced following ultra-endurance competition [97]. The study we conducted shows that following physical exercise training cardiac patients are able to exercise to greater VO_{2peak} levels without increasing exercise-induced lipid peroxidation [88]. Recently Vasankari et. al. [98] showed that a 10 month aerobic-based physical exercise training program given to 34 sedentary men and 70 women reduced plasma LDL's susceptibility to lipid peroxidation. The recent findings of Meijer et al. [99] also show that regular physical exercise in older adults reduces exercise-induced oxidative stress.

Hence the paradox is solved. Participation in regular physical exercise reduces exercise-induced oxidative stress. This should lower the risk for CAD and other disease conditions related to oxidative stress by reducing cumulative burden of oxidative stress accrued during a lifetime of activities of daily living.

Mechanisms

The mechanism(s) by which physical exercise training reduces exercise-induced oxidative stress are numerous and include both exogenous factors such as diet (summarized in Table 1) as well as endogenous anti-oxidant systems (summarized in Table 2) that may be up-regulated in response to exercise-induced oxidative stress.

Our findings among CMD patients indicate that exercise training-induced changes in exercise-induced oxidative stress are not a direct result of lifestyle changes because our subjects did not use tobacco products and were maintained on a constant diet during the course of the study. Although antioxidant supplementation can reduce exercise-induced oxidative stress [44,53], clinical trials with vitamin E supplementation have not been shown to reduce CAD risk [100,101]. On the other hand, a recent study by Cesari et. al. [102]

indicates that increased levels of muscle strength and physical performance in older individuals are associated with increased levels of plasma alpha tocopherol and daily dietary intake of vitamin C and Beta-carotene. We interpret these findings to suggest that increased aerobic capacity may have a sparing effect on some dietary antioxidants such as alpha tocopherol so that their levels are increased in body tissues.

Endogenous factors could include a number of constituent antioxidant systems such as superoxide dismutase and glutathione. Animal studies indicate that adaptive up-regulation of endogenous antioxidant systems occurs with regular physical exercise [66,103]. Changes in the glutathione anti-oxidant system are considered indicative of oxidative stress. GSH is oxidized to GSSG in cells in response to an increase in free radicals and the resulting GSSG effluxes from the cell into the plasma [104] and reflects oxidative stress. Decreased plasma GSH after exercise may reflect its consumption by skeletal muscles that results in its reduced export rate into plasma [105]. Hence an increase in plasma GSSG or a change in glutathione redox status in the blood (decreased GSH and increased GSSH, i.e. reduced GSH/GSSH ratio) indicate increased oxidative stress. GSSH and SOD are polymorphic, hence constituent isoforms of these compounds may modulate inherent susceptibility to oxidative stress.

The effect of physical exercise training on the GSH redox system has mainly been studied in animal models that examine skeletal muscle anti-oxidant systems including GSH and SOD [66]. Although these findings in aggregate indicate that physical exercise training results in an elevation in the activities in these antioxidant systems, these results are not shown in all studies.

The effect of an acute bout of exercise in blood-related samples on GSH redox status shows conflicting results. Studies by Sastre et. al. [106] and Tessier et. al. [107] in athletes show a post-exercise increase in plasma GSSH levels but GSH levels did not change. On the other hand, Camus et. al. [108] and Marin et. al. [109] found that healthy fit subjects completing exercise protocols of approximately 30 minutes showed no change in blood GSH or GSSG levels. Tiides et al. [110] found no effect of an 8 week aerobic-based physical exercise training program on the plasma GSH/GSSH ratio in young (19-23 years of age) men ($N = 7$), and women ($N = 6$). Because these studies have been performed in athletes the interpretation of these outcomes may not extend to sedentary individuals. This issue is exemplified by a study of Ortenblad et. al. [111] that compared measurements of internal antioxidant systems(SOD, GPX, GR, and magnesium SOD) between 8 sedentary men and 8 male Danish trained elite volleyball players before and after a strenuous aerobic exercise bout based on a jumping protocol. Although internal anti-oxidant status was greater in the trained athletes than the sedentary men, the acute exercise event did not affect these measurements. This suggests a more protracted bout of exercise may be necessary to elicit this effect. Gohil et. al. [112] showed that prolonged submaximal exercise resulted in decreased plasma GSH and increased plasma GSSH levels. Similar findings suggesting an exercise-related effect of GSH redox status were shown by Laires et. al. [113], and Viguie et al. [114]. The study of Viguie et. al. [114] administered exercise sessions on consecutive days. Physical exercise training may increase chronic shear stress on the endothelium, which can induce cytosolic Cu/Zn superoxide dismutase and endothelial cell nitric oxide synthase [115-117].

Conclusions

This 'exercise paradox' may be explained by various metabolic adaptations known to occur when patients participate in regular exercise programs to reduce exercise-related Further studies are warranted to evaluate the 'anti-oxidant' role of role of physical exercise in reducing CAD risk, and identify the mechanism(s) by which exercise exerts this effect.

References

[1] Taubes G. Does inflammation cut to the heart of the matter? *Science* 2002;296:242-245.
[2] Ridker PM. On evolutionary biology, inflammation, infection, and the causes of atherosclerosis. *Circulation* 2002;105:2-4.
[3] Buffon A, Biasucci LM, Liuzzo G, D'Onofrio G, Crea F, Maseri A. Widespread coronary inflammation in unstable angina. *N Engl J Med.* 2002;347:5-12.
[4] Libby P, Ridker PM, Maseri A. Inflammation and atherosclerosis. *Circulation* 2002;105:1135-1143.
[5] Ridker PM, Rifai N, Rose L, Buring JE, Cook NR. Comparison of C-reactive protein and low-density lipoprotein cholesterol levels in the prediction of first cardiovascular events. *N Engl J Med.* 2002;347:1557-1565.
[6] Holmberg P. The physics and chemistry of free radicals. *Medical Biology* 1984; 62:68070.
[7] Buege JA, Aust SD. Microsomal lipid peroxidation. *Methods Enzymol.* 1978; 52:302-310.
[8] McCord JM. The evolution of free radicals and oxidative stress. *Am J Med* 2000;108:652-659.
[9] Witzum JL. The oxidation hypothesis of atherosclerosis. *Lancet* 1994; 334:793-795.
[10] Steinberg D, Parathasarathy S, Carew TE, Khoo, JC, Witzum JL. Beyond cholesterol: modifications of low-density lipoprotein that increase its atherogencity. *N Engl J Med.* 1989; 320:915-924.
[11] Halliwell B, Gutteridge JMC. *Free Radicals in Biology and Medicne.* 2nd Edition, Clariton Press: Oxford 1989.
[12] Davies KJ, Quintanilha AT, Brooks GA, Packer L. Free radicals and tissue damage produced by exercise. *Biochem Biophys Res Commun* 1982;107:1198-1205.
[13] Borzone G, Zhao B, Merola AJ, Berliner L, Clanton TL. *Detection of free radicals by electron spin resonance in rat diaphram after resistive loading.*
[14] Reid MB, Haack KE, Franchek KM, Valberg PA, Kobzik L, West MS. Reactive oxygen in skeletal muscle. I. Intracellular oxidant kinetics and fatigue in vitro. *J Appl Physiol* 1992;73(5):1797-1804.
[15] Reid MB, Shoji T, Moody MR, Entman ML. Reactive oxygen in skeletal muscle. II. Extracellular release of free radicals. *J Appl Physiol* 1992;73(5):1805-1809.
[16] Cosgrove JP, Church DF, Pryor WA. The kinetics of autooxidation of polyunsaturated fatty acids. *Lipids* 1987;22;299-304.

[17] Liu J, Yeo HC, Doninger SJ, Ames BN. Assay of aldehydes from lipid peroxidation: gas chromatography-mass spectrometry compared to thiobarbituric acid. *Anal Biochme* 199;245:161-166.

[18] Bruna E, Petit E, Beljean-Leymarie M, Huynh S, Nouvelot A. Specific susceptibility of docosahexanoic acid and eicosapentanoic acid to peroxidation in acqueous solutions. *Lipids* 1989;24:970-975.

[19] Upston JM, Terentis AC, Stocker R. Tocopherol-mediated peroxidation of lipoproteins: implications for vitamin E as a potential antiatherogenic supplement. *Faseb J* 1999;13:977-994.

[20] Horvat RJ, Lane WG, Shepherd AD. Saturated hydrocarbons from autooxidizing methyl linoleate. *Nature* 1964; 203:523-524.

[21] Dumelin EE, Tappel AL. Hydrocarbons gases produced during in vitro peroxidation of polyunsaturated fatty acids and deomposition of preformed hydroperoxides. *Lipids* 1977; 12:894-900.

[22] Evans CD, List GR, Doley A, McConel DG, Hoffman RL. Pentane from thermal decomposition of lixidase derived products. *Lipids* 1967; 2:432-434.

[23] Riely CA, Choen G, Liberman M. Ethane evolution: A new index of lipid peroxidation. *Science* 1974; 182:208-210.

[24] Lawrence GD, Choen G. Ethane exhalation as an index of lipid peroxidation: Concentrating ethane from a breath collection chamber. *Ann Biochme* 1982; 1222:283-290.

[25] Leaf DA, Kleinman MT, Hamilton M, Barstow TJ. The effect of exercise intensity on lipid peroxidation. *Med Sci Sports Exerc* 1997;29:1039-1043.

[26] Frankel EN. Recent advances in lipid peroxidation. *J Sci Food Agric* 1991;54:495-511.

[27] Esterbauer H, Cheeseman KH. Determination of aldehydic lipid peroxidation products: malonaldehyde, and 4-hydroxynonenal. *Methoids Enzymol* 1990;186:504-508.

[28] Kikagawa K, Kojima T, and Kosugi H. Major thoibarbituric acid-reasctive substances of liver homogenate are alkakienals. *Free Radical Res Commun* 1990;28:107-113.

[29] Lapenna D, Cuccurullo. TBA test and "free' MDA assay in evaluation of lipid peroxidation and oxidative stress in tissue systems (Letter). Ceconi C. (Reply). *Am J Physiol* 1993;265:H1030-H1032.

[30] Lee HS, Casallany AS. Measurement of free and bound malondialdehyde in vitamin E-deficient and supplemented rat liver tissues. *Lipids* 1987;22:104-107.

[31] Halliwell B, Chirco S. Lipid peroxidation: its mechanism, measurement and significance. *Am J Clin Nutr* 1993;57(suppl):S715-724.

[32] Balke PO, Snider MT, Bull AP. Evidence for lipid peroxidation during moderate exercise. *Med Sci Sports Exerc* 1984;16:181.

[33] Koz M, Erbas D, Biligihan AQ, Aricioglu A. Effects of acute swimming exercise on muscle and erythrocyte malonaldehyde, serum myoglobin, and plasma ascorbic acid concentrations. *Can J Physiol Pharmacol* 1992;70:1392-1395.

[34] Buczynski A, Kedziora J, Tkaczewski W, Wachowicz B. Effect of submaximal physical exercise on antioxidant protection of human blood platelets. *Int J Sports Med* 1991;12:52-54.

[35] Myers J, Prakash, M, Froelicher V, Do D, Partington S, Atwood JE. Exercise capacity and mortality among men referred for exercise testing. *N Engl J Med* 2002; 346:793-801.

[36] *Healthy People 2010: Volume II.* Conference Edition. Washington DC: US Dept Health and Human Services:2002.

[37] Wallace DC, Mitochondrial diseases in man and mouse. *Science* 1999;283:1482-1488.

[38] McCord JM, Turrens JF. Mitochondrial injury by ischemia and reperfusion. *Curr Topics Bioenerg* 1994;17:225-239.

[39] Stacpoole PW, Lactic acidosis and other mitochondrial disorders. *Metabolism* 1997;46:306-321.

[40] Keul J, Doll E. Oxidative energy supply. *Energy Metabolism Of Human Muscle,* E. Jokl(Ed.). Basel: Karger, 1972.

[41] Child RB, Wilkinson DM, Fallowfield JL, Donnelly AE. Elevated serum antioxidant capacity and plasma malonaldehyde concentration in response to a simulated half marathon. *Med Sci Sports Exerc* 1998;30:1603-1607.

[42] Kanter M, Lesmes GR, Kaminsky LA, La Ham-Saeger J. Serum creatinine kinase and lactate dehydrogenase changes following an eighty kilometer race. *Eur J Appl Physiol* 1988;57:60-63.

[43] Balke PO, Snider MT, Bull AP. Evidence for lipid peroxidation during moderate exercise. *Med Sci Sports Exerc* 1984;16:181.

[44] Dillard CJ, Litor RE, Sabvin WM, Dumelin EE, Tapel AL. Effects of exercise, vitamin E, and ozone on pulmonary function and lipid peroxidation. *J Appl Physiol* 1978;45:927-932.

[45] Powers SK, Ji LL, Leeuwenburgh C. Exercise training-induced alterations in skeletal muscle antioxidant capacity: a brief review. *Med Sci Sports Exerc* 1999;31:987-997.

[46] Erecinska M, Silver IA. ATP and brain function. *J Cereb Blood Flow Metab.* 1989;9:2-19.

[47] DeSheeder IK, Van deKray AMM, Lamers JMJ, Koster JF, de Jong JW, Serruys PW. Myocardial malonaldehyde and uric acid release after short-term coronary artery occlusion during coronary angioplasty: potential mechanisms of free radical generation. *Am J Cardiol* 1991;68:392-395.

[48] Davies SW, Ranjadayalan K, Wickens DG, Dormandy TL, Timmis AD. Lipid peroxidation associated with successful thrombolysis. *Lancet* 1990;336:741-743.

[49] Roberts MJD, young IS, Trouton TG, Trimble ER, Khan MM, Webb SW, et. al. Transient release of lipid peroxides after coronary artery balloon angioplasty. *Lancet* 1990;336:143-145.

[50] Demirel HA, Powers SK, Caillaud C, Coombes JS, Naito H, Fletcher LA, Vrabas I, Jessup JV, and Li JJ. Exercise training reduces myocardial lipid peroxidation following short-term ischemia-reperfusion. *Med Sci Sports Exerc.* 1998;30:1211-1216.

[51] Sahlin KS, Czinsky S, Warholm M, Hoberg J. Repetitive static muscle contractions in humans: a trigger of metabolic and oxidative stress. *Eur J Appl Physiol* 1992;64:189-236.

[52] Saxton JM, Donnely AE, Roper HP. Indices of free radical-mediated damage following maximum voluntary eccentric and concentric muscular work. *Eur J Appl Physiol* 1994;21:189-193.

[53] McBride JM, Kraemer WJ, Triplett-McBride, Travis ED, Sebastianelli W. Effect of resistive exercise on free radical production. *Med Sci Sports Exerc* 1998;30:67-72.

[54] Chevon S, Moran DS, Heled Y, et. al. Plasma antioxidant status and cell injury after sever physical exercise. *Proc Natl Acad Sci* 2003;100:5119-5123.

[55] Johnson P. Antioxidant enzyme expression in health and disease: effects of exercise and hypertension. *Comp Biochem Physiol* 2002;133:493-505.

[56] Yu B. Cellular defenses against damage from reactive oxygen species. *Phs Rev* 1994;74:139-162.

[57] Kukreja RC, Heiss ML. The oxygen free radical system: from equations through membrane-protein interactions to cardiovascular injury and protection. *Cardiovasc Res* 1992;26:641-655.

[58] Alessio HM, Hagerman AE, Fulkerson BK, Ambrose J, Rice R, Wiley RL. Generation of reactive oxygen species after exhaustive aerobic and isometric exercise. *Med Sci Sports Exerc* 2000;32:1576-1581.

[59] Clarkson PM, Nosaka K, Braum B. Muscle function after exercise-induced muscle damage and rapid adaptation. *Med Sci Sports Exerc* 1992;24:512-520.

[60] Newham DJ, Jones DA, Clarkson PM. Repeated high-force eccentric exercise: effects on muscle pain and damage. *J Appl Physiol* 1987;63:1381-1386.

[61] Apple FS, Rogers MA, Ivy J. Creatinine kinase isoenzyme MM variants in skeletal muscle and plasma from marathon runners. *Clin Chem* 1986;32:41-44.

[62] Page S, Jackson MJ, Coakley J, Edwards RHT. Isoforms of creatinine kinase: MM in the study of skeletal muscle damage. *Eur J Clin Invest* 1989;19:185-191.

[63] Jackson MJ, Edwards RHT, Symons MCR. Electron spin resonance studies of intact mammalian skeletal muscle. *Biochimica Et Bioph"Ysica Acta* 1985;847:185-190.

[64] Jenkins RR. Free radical chemistry, relationship to exercise. *Sports Med* 1988; 5:156-170.

[65] Ji LL. Exercise and oxidative stress: role of the cellular antioxidant systems. *Exercise Sports Sci Rev* 1995; 23:135-166.

[66] Allessio HM. Exercise-induced oxidative stress. *Med Sci Sports Exerc* 1993; 252:218-224.

[67] Wasserman K, Hansen JE, Sue DY, Whipp BJ. *Principles Of Exercise Testing And Interpretation*. Lea & Febiger: Philadelphia. 1987, Chapter 5. Protocols for exercise testing pp. 62-71.

[68] Wilke NA, Sheldahl LM, Dougherty SM, et al. Energy expenditure during household tasks in women with coronary artery disease. *Am J Cardiol* 1995; 75:670-674.

[69] Leaf DA, Glassman PA, Deitrick RW, Kleinman MT. Regular exercise as an antioxidant. *Your Patient & Fitness* 1999; 4:6-13.

[70] Leaf DA, Yusin M, Gallik D, Kleinman MT. Exercise-induced oxidative stress in patients during thallium stress testing. *Am J Med Sci* 1998; 315:185-187.

[71] Lindner A, Charra B, Sherrard DJ, Scribner BH. Accelerated atherosclerosis in prolonged maintenance dialysis. *N Engl J Med* 1974; 290:697-701.

[72] Bonomini V, Feleth C, Scolari MP, Stefoni S, Vangelista A. Atherosclerosis in uremia: A longitudinal study. *Am J Clin Nutr* 1980; 33:1493-1500.

[73] Galli F, Ronco C. Oxidant stress in hemodialysis. *Nephron* 2000; 84:1-5.

[74] Spittle MA, Hoenich NA, Handelman GJ, Adhikarla R, Homel P, Levin NW. Oxidative stress and inflammation in hemodialysis patients. *Am J Kidney Dis* 2001; 38:1408-1413.

[75] Capodicasa E, Trovarelli G, DeMedio GE, Pelli AM, Lippi G, Verdura C, Timio M. Volatile alkanes and increased concentrations of isoprene in exhaled air during hemodialysis. *Nephron* 1999; 82:331-337.

[76] Westhuyzen J, Adams CE, Fleming SJ. Evidence for oxidative stress during in vitro dialysis. *Nephron* 1995; 70:49-54.

[77] Dasgupta A, Hussain S, Suhail A. Increased lipid peroxidation in patients on maintenance hemodialysis. *Nephron* 1992; 60:56-59.

[78] Giardinin O, Taccone-Gallucci M, Lubrano R, et. al. Evidence of red blood cell membrane lipid peroxidation in haemodialysis patients. *Nephron* 1984; 36:235-237.

[79] Taccone-Gallucci M, Giardini O, Lubrano R, et. al. Red blood cell lipid peroxidation in predialysis chronic renal failure. *Clinical Nephrology* 1987; 27:238-241.

[80] Toborek M, Wasik T, Drozdz M, et. al. Effect of hemodialysis on lipid peroxidation and antioxidant system in patients with chronic renal failure. *Metabolism* 1992; 41:1229-1232.

[81] Richard MJ, Arnaud J, Jurkovitz C, et al. Trace elements and lipid peroxidation abnormalities in patients with chronic renal failure. *Nephron* 1991; 57:10-15.

[82] Taccone-Gallucci M, Lubrano R, Bandino D, et. al. Discrepancies between serum and erythrocyte concentrations of vitamin E in hemodialysis patients: Role of HDL-Bound fraction of vitamin E. *Artificial Organs* 1988;12:379-381.

[83] Rock CL, Jahnke MG, Gorenflo DW, Swartz RD, Messana JM. Racial group differences in plasma concentrations of antioxidant vitamins and carotenoids in hemodialysis patients. *Am J Clin Nutr* 1997; 65:844-850.

[84] Kuroda M, Asaka S, Tofuku Y, Takeda R. Serum antioxidant activity in uremic patients. *Nephron* 1985; 41:293-298.

[85] Maggi E, Bellazzi R, Falaschi F, et. al. Enhanced LDL oxidation in uremic patients: An additional mechanism for accelerated atherosclerosis? *Kidney International* 1994; 45:876-883.

[86] Vincent HK, Morgan JW, Vincent KR. Obesity exacerbates oxidative stress levels after acute exercise. *Med Sci Sports Exerc* 2004;36:772-779.

[87] Flegal KM, Carrol MD, Ogden CL, Johnson CL. Prevalence and trends in obesity among US Adults, 1999-2000. *JAMA* 2002;288:1723-1727.

[88] Leaf DA, Kleinman MT, Hamilton M, Deitrick RW. The exercise-induced oxidative stress paradox: The effects of physical exercise training. *Am J Med Sci* 1999; 317:295-300.

[89] Vincent KR, Vincent HK, Braith RW, Lennon SL, Lowenthal DT. Resistance exercise training attenuates exercise-induced lipid peroxidation in the elderly . *Eur J Appl Physiol* 2002;87:416-423

[90] Ricote M, Valledor AF, Glass CK. Decoding transcriptional programs regulated by PPARs and LXRs in the macrophage: Effects on lipid homeostasis, inflammation, and atherosclerosis. *Arterioscler Thromb Vasc Biol* 2004;24:230-239.

[91] Pan M, Cederbaum AI, Zhang Y-L, Ginsberg HN, Williams KJ, Fisher EA. Lipid peroxidation and oxidant stress regulate hepatic apolipoprotein B degradation and VLDL production. *J Clin Invest* 2004;113:1277-1287.

[92] ADD Cytokine paper here

[93] Whelton SP, He J, Whelton PK, Munter P. Meta-analysis of observational studies on fish intake and coronary heart disease. *Am J Cardiol* 2004;93:119-1123

[94] Fiebig RG, Hollander JM, Ney D, Boileau R, Jeffery E, Ji LL. Training down-regulates fatty acid synthase and body fat in Zucker rats. *Med Sci Sports Exerc* 2002; 34:1106-1114.

[95] Jimenez L, Lefevre G, Richard R, Couderc R, Saint George M, Duvallet A, Rieu M. Oxidative stress in hemodialyzed patients during exhaustive exercise. *J Sports Med Phys Fitness* 2001; 41:513-520.

[96] Force, T, Milani R, Hibbard P, Lorenz R, Vedelhover W, Leaf A, Weber P. Aspirin-induced decline in prostacyclin production in platelets with coronary artery disease is due to decreased endoperoxide shift. Analysis of the effects of a combination of aspirin and n-3 fatty acids on the eicosanoid profile. *Circulation* 1991; 84:2286-2293.

[97] Ginsberg GS, Agil A, O'Toole, et al. Effects of a single bout of ultraendurance exercise on lipid levels and susceptabililty of lipids to peroxidation in triathletes. *JAMA* 1996; 276:221-225.

[98] Vasankari TJ, Kujala UM, Vasankari TM, Ahotupa M. Reduced oxidized LDL levels after a 10-month exercise program. *Med Sci Sports Exerc* 1998; 30:1496-1501.

[99] Meijer EP, Goris AHC, van Dongen JLJ, Bast A, Westerterp KR. Exercise-induced oxidative stress in older adults as a function of habitual activity level. *J Am Geriatr SOC* 2002; 50:349-353.

[100] The Heart Outcomes Prevention Evaluation Study Investigators. Vitamin E supplementation and cardiovascular events in high-risk patients. *N Engl J Med* 2000;342:154-160.

[101] GISSI-Prevenzione Investigators. Dietary Supplements with n-3polyunsaturated fatty acids and vitamin E after myocardial infarction: results of the GISSI-Prevention Trial. *Lancet* 1999;354:447-455.

[102] Cesari M, Pahor M, Bartali B, Cherubini A, Penninx BWJH, Williams GR, Atkinson H, Martin A, Guralnik JM, and Ferrucci L. antioxidants and physical performance in elderly persons: the Invecchiare in Chianti (InCHIANTI) study. *Am J Clin Nutr* 2004;79:289-294.

[103] Meilhac O, Ramachandran S, Chiang K, Santanam, Parthasarathy S. Role of arterial wall antioxidant defense in beneficial effects of exercise on atherosclerosis in mice. *Arterioscl Thromb Vasc Biol* 2001; 21:1681-1688.

[104] Sahlin K, Ekberg K, Cizinsky S. Changes in plasma hypoxanthine and free radical markers during exercise in man. *Acta Physiol Scand* 1991;142:273-281.

[105] Powers SK, Ji LL, Leeuwenburgh C. Exercise training-induced alterations in skeletal muscle antioxidant capacity: a brief review. *Med Sci Sports Exerc* 1999;31:987-997.

[106] Sastre J, Aseni M, Gasco E, et al. Exhaustive physical exercise causes oxidation of glutathione status in blood : prevention by antioxidant administration. *Am J Physiol* 1992;263:R992-R995.

[107] Tessier F, Margaritis I, Richard M, Moynot C, Marconnet P. Selenium and training effects of the glutathione system and aerobic performance. *Med Sci Sports Exerc* 1995;27:390-396.

[108] Camus G, Felekidis A, Pincemail J, et. al. Blood levels of reduced/oxidized glutathione and plasma concentrations of ascorbic acid during eccentric and concentric exercises of similar energy cost. *Arch Int Physiol Biochim Biophys* 1994;102:67-70.

[109] Marin E, Hanninen O, Muller D, Klinger W. Influence of acute physical exercise on plasma glutathione and lipid peroxides. *Sports Med* 1993;15:196-209.

[110] Tiidus PM, Pushkarenko J, Houston ME. Lack of antioxidant adaptation to short-term aerobic traing in human muscle. *Am J Physiol* 1996;271:R832-R836.

[111] Ortenblad N, Madsen K, Djurhuus MS. Antioxidant status and lipid peroxidation after short-term maximal exercise in trained and untrained humans. *Am J Physiol* 1997;272:R1258-R1263.

[112] Gohil K, Viguie C, Stanley WC, Brooks GA, Packer L. Blood glutathione oxidation during human exercise. *J Appl Physiol* 1988;64:115-119.

[113] Laires MJ, Madeira F, Sergio J, et. al. Preliminary study of the relationship between plasma and erythrocyte magnesium variations and some circulating pro-oxidant and antioxidant indices in a standardized physical effort. *Magnes Res* 1993;6:233-238.

[114] Vigue CA, Frei B, Shigenaga MK, Ames BN, Packer L, Brooks GA. Antioxidant status and indexes of oxidative stress during consecutive days of exercise. *J Appl Physiol* 1993;75:566-572.

[115] Uematsu M, Ohara Y, Navas JP, et. al. Regulation of endothelial cell nitric oxide synthase mRNA expression by shear stress. *Am J Physiol* 1995; 269:C1371-1378.

[116] Inoue N, Ramasamy S, Fukai T, et. al. Shear stress modulates expression of Cu/Zn superoxide dismutase in human aortic endothelial cells. *Circ Res* 1996; 79:32-37.

[117] Sessa WC, Pritchard K, Seyedi N, et. al. Chronic exercise in dogs increases coronary vascular nitric oxide production and endothelial cell nitric oxide synthase gene expression. *Circ Res* 1994; 74:349-353.

Chapter IV

Postprandial Lipid Metabolism and Exercise: Recent Findings and Future Directions

*Christina Koutsari**

Department of Internal Medicine; Endocrine Research Unit; 5-194 Joseph
Mayo Clinic; 200 First St. SW; Rochester, MN 55905; USA

Abstract

In the past two decades, there has been a wealth of evidence for a link between postprandial triacylglycerol (TAG) metabolism and atherosclerosis. Postprandial lipemia predominantly represents the presence in plasma of large TAG-rich lipoproteins (TRL) produced from the intestine (chylomicrons), but also reflects the accumulation of TRL particles of hepatic origin (very low density lipoproteins; VLDL). The precise mechanisms by which postprandial TAG metabolism affect the pathogenesis and progression of coronary heart disease (CHD) have not been elucidated yet but it seems that a constellation of potentially atherogenic lipoprotein changes is involved, including increases in plasma TRL particles and their remnants, decreases in HDL-cholesterol and formation of small dense LDL particles. This review will present an overview of the current knowledge on postprandial lipid and lipoprotein metabolism, its regulation and link between its impairment and CHD. Exercise performed 12-16 h before a high- or normal-fat mixed meal ameliorates fasting and postprandial TAG concentrations. Important determinants of exercise-induced decreases in postprandial lipemia appear to be exercise timing and the total energy expended during exercise. The reduction in postprandial lipemia is transient, independent of qualitative differences in substrate utilisation during exercise and greater than that attributable to the energy deficit incurred. Although significant progress has been made on the effects of exercise on postprandial

---

* Telephone: +1 507 255 1488; Fax: +1 507 255 4828; E-mail: koutsari.christina@mayo.edu

lipid metabolism, there are still many questions to be answered. Future directions of research in this important field of human metabolism will be discussed.

Introduction

For many years, atherosclerosis research mainly focused on low-density lipoproteins (LDL). However, results from a number of studies the last two decades have revealed that triacylglycerol (TAG)-rich lipoprotein (TRL) metabolism is also implicated in the development of coronary heart disease (CHD). Exercise has been shown to decrease the postprandial plasma TAG excursion. The aim of this invited review is to provide an update on the effects of exercise on TAG and TRL metabolism. The first three sections consider the postprandial metabolism of TRL particles, its regulation and association with atherosclerosis. The fourth section deals with the effects of exercise, focusing mainly on recent findings and studies that have substantially contributed to our understanding in this area. Lastly, future directions for research are discussed.

Triacylglycerol-Rich Lipoproteins

Plasma lipoproteins are a heterogeneous group of particles with different lipid and protein compositions, and different sizes. They have the major function of transporting the hydrophobic lipids in blood. They are particles with a relatively hydrophilic outer surface (unesterified cholesterol and a monolayer of phospholipids) and a highly hydrophobic lipid core (TAG and cholesteryl esters). Each particle has also associated with it one or more protein molecules, the apolipoproteins (apo). Chylomicrons and very-low density lipoprotein (VLDL) particles are rich in TAG and are referred to as the TAG-rich lipoproteins (TRL).

Metabolism of Chylomicrons and their Remnants

Chylomicrons are secreted by the intestine after fat intake and provide the means to introduce newly absorbed dietary fat and fat soluble vitamins into the systemic circulation. Triacylglycerols represent by far the major dietary lipid and may amount to 100-150 g/day. Triacylglycerol digestion takes place mainly in the duodenum with hydrolysis by pancreatic lipase. Gastric predigestion facilitates the digestion process in the duodenum, so that gastric lipase can be responsible for ~30% of the fat digestion processes occurring in humans. The products of hydrolysis (monoacylglycerols and fatty acids) are taken up by endothelial cells in the small intestine, and subsequently TAG are resynthesized and packaged into chylomicrons. For an extensive review on TAG digestion, the interested reader is referred to the recent publication by Mu & Høy [1].

The assembly and secretion of chylomicrons in the intestine requires the presence of one molecule of apoB-48 as the structural protein [2]. This apo B variant comprises the N-terminal 48% of the liver-derived variant of apoB (apoB-100), and is formed after tissue-specific posttranscriptional editing of the apo B100 mRNA [3]. In addition to apoB-48, nascent chylomicrons also contain apo A-I, A-II and A-IV that are *de novo* synthesized by intestinal cells [4]. It seems that apoB-48-containing particles are continuously secreted from the enterocyte and at times of excessive TAG availability (i.e. in the postprandial state) the size, but not number, of particles increases resulting in the secretion of large chylomicrons [5].

Hussain [6] recently proposed a model with three discrete and independent steps to explain the assempy of chylomicrons. The first step is the assempy of "primordial lipoproteins" which involves the release to the endoplasmic reticulum (ER) lumen of nascent apoB associated with phospholipids present in the rough ER membrane. The microsomal TAG transfer protein (MTP) plays a critical role in the formation of primordial lipoproteins. Membane-bound apoB that does not form primordial particles is degraded intracellularly. The second step involves the formation of TAG-rich lipid droplets in the smooth ER during the postprandial state, and occurs independent of apoB synthesis. The third step involves fusion of primordial lipoproteins with lipid droplets resulting in the expansion of the lipoprotein core. This core expansion takes place at a junction between the smooth and the rough ER and renders TAG-rich lipid droplets secretion-competent. The rare MTP-493G variant of a functional polymorphism in the promoter region of the MTP gene has been shown to confer higher transcriptional activity *in vitro* and be associated with increased postprandial plasma levels of very small apoB-48-containing particles in humans *in vivo* [7]. These findings suggest that increased MTP transcriptional activity may induce enhanced production of the smallest chylomicron particles.

Experiments in differentiated Caco-2 cells, an established model to study intestinal lipid metabolism *in vitro*, have shown that nascent, rather than preformed, TAG are preferentially used for chylomicron assembly [8]. This observation agrees with early feeding studies reporting that the fatty acid composition of human thoracic duct and serum chylomicrons reflects the fatty acid composition of the test meal [9]. Interestingly, postprandial studies with sequential meals have shown appearance of chylomicrons in the circulation within 1 hour of consuming the second meal regardless if the latter contains fat [10, 11] or not [12]. These chylomicrons carry fatty acids of similar composition with those consumed with the first meal [10]. This rapid appearance of chylomicrons suggests that part of the dietary fat consumed with the first meal is stored in chylomicrons in a location (enterocytes and/or lymph) from which it can be released on consuming a second meal. What provokes its release is currently unknown.

Chylomicrons are transported into the systemic circulation via the lymphatics and enter the blood stream via the thoracic duct in the left subclavian vein. Once the chylomicron has reached the blood stream, several compositional changes take place. ApoA-I is transferred to circulating high-density lipoprotein (HDL) particles with reciprocal transfer of apoC-I, C-II, C-III and apoE. ApoC-II is the essential activator of lipoprotein lipase (LPL), the key-enzyme for chylomicron-TAG hydrolysis, located on the endothelial surfaces of capillaries, especially in adipose tissue, skeletal and heart muscle. Some TAG is transferred to HDL and LDL particles in exchange for cholesteryl esters, catalyzed by cholesteryl ester transfer protein (CETP). During the time they spend in the circulation, chylomicrons become smaller in size (remnants). During this catabolism, the surface apoAs and almost all apoCs, together with cholesterol and phospholipids, are released and transferred to HDL [2]. Chylomicron remnants are rich in cholesteryl ester and contain two major protein components: apoB-48 and apoE.

Remnant particles are removed from plasma mainly by the liver. The LDL receptor and the LDL receptor-related protein (LRP) are the two receptors that appear to have a significant role in the removal process (for review [13]). ApoE is the key ligand mediating the binding of the remnant particles to these receptors. Heparan sulfate proteoglycans appear to fulfill a major role in sequestration of the particles, but also in the internalization step, either in association with the LRP or acting alone as a receptor [13]. Hepatic lipase can enhance the uptake of remnants by facilitating their lipolytic processing after sequestration, but also by exerting ligand-binding activity. A recent *in vivo* study in humans [14] confirmed the findings of previous *in vitro* studies that hepatic lipase plays a role in apoB-containing lipoprotein removal, independent of its lipolytic activity. Similarly, it has been shown *in vivo* that TRL-associated LPL facilitates TRL removal independent of its lipolytic activity [15]. Obviously, this function would require detachment of LPL from its endothelial binding site and association with the lipoprotein particles. Indeed, the study by Heeren *et al* demonstrated a significant postprandial increase in endothelial-derived LPL bound to TRL particles in humans [15]. Once within the hepatocyte, chylomicron remnants are subject to lysosomal degradation, which releases their components for further degradation, storage or resynthesis. Removal of large chylomicron remnants by adipose and muscle tissues has been demonstrated in humans *in vivo* [16]. This removal was suggested to be mediated by the VLDL receptor [17, 18], which recognises apoE and LPL as ligands [19] and is most abundant in skeletal muscle and adipose tissue.

Metabolism of VLDL and their Remnants

The VLDL particles are synthesized in the liver and contain a single molecule of apoB-100. A model for the assemply/secretion of VLDL has been described by Davis and Hui [20] according to which apoB in the ER has two fates: translocation and formation of lipoproteins in the ER lumen or degradation in the cytoplasm. Translocation of apoB into the ER lumen and assemply into a nascent core-containing particle require the MTP and lipid availability. MTP facilitates the translocation, folding of apoB and the addition of lipids to lipid-binding domains. The nascent particle in the ER lumen can then be "enlarged" to form a mature VLDL. In the absence of sufficient lipid or functional MTP, translocation of apoB becomes blocked and the translocated arrested apoB is rapidly degradated by the ubiquitin-dependent proteasome. In addition to TAG and apoB-100, VLDL contain other apolipoproteins, including apoA-I, A-II, A-IV, the three apoCs and apoE [21]. Newly secreted VLDL particles acquire additional apoE and C from circulating lipoproteins, mainly HDL.

There are at least four sources of fatty acids for TAG synthesis in the liver: plasma non-esterified fatty acids (NEFA), hepatic *de novo* lipogenesis, splanchnic lipid (hepatic and visceral sources) and fatty acids derived from circulating lipoproteins taken up by the liver. It has been shown that in fasted lean subjects, plasma NEFA provide the vast majority (>90%) of the fatty acids secreted in VLDL, whereas *de novo* synthesized fatty acids contribute <5%

[22]. Respective values in individuals with moderate hypetriacylglycerolemia were >80% and <3%, resulting in a greater percentage of VLDL-TAG precursors not accounted for by these two sources [22]. Lipoprotein remnants and splanchnic lipid sources may provide a significant source of VLDL-TG fatty acids in these patients [22].

VLDL catabolism is similar to that of chylomicrons so that LPL hydrolyzes its TAG content and the redundant surface material is passed to other lipoprotein particles, mainly HDL. CETP catalyzes the exchange of lipoprotein core lipids between cholesterol-rich particles (LDL and HDL) and VLDL. As the VLDL particle becomes more delipidated, the remnants can either be cleared by the liver or they can continue through a "cascade" of delipidation to form IDL and finally LDL. The ultimate remnant of VLDL is LDL.

There is evidence that the majority of the largest ($VLDL_1$) particles after hydrolysis are cleared directly from plasma and only a minor fraction (~10%) appears in the LDL pool [23]. An appreciable proportion of $VLDL_1$ does not even appear in the $VLDL_2$ fraction [24]. On the contrary, the smaller, $VLDL_2$, particles which contain both products of $VLDL_1$ delipidation and newly-secreted VLDL particles, are rapidly and substantially (>40%) converted to LDL, suggesting that the major precursor for the latter is the $VLDL_2$ subfraction [23]. Interestingly, substantial metabolic heterogeneity is observed even within the $VLDL_2$ fraction. $VLDL_2$ particles that are derived from $VLDL_1$ catabolism are catabolized slowly within their flotation interval without being significantly transferred to LDL. Conversely, directly synthesized $VLDL_2$ are rapidly converted into LDL [23]. Similar processes to those for chylomicron remnants are likely to mediate the hepatic clearance of $VLDL_1$ and $VLDL_2$, although the LDL receptor pathway seems to be the most important in $VLDL_2$ catabolism [24].

Integration of TRL Metabolism in the Postprandial State

In the postprandial state, chylomicrons and VLDL mix in the peripheral circulation. During this period, VLDL accumulate in plasma and can account for as much as 80% of the postprandial increase in the total apoB-containing TRL particles [25]. This accumulation is probably due to competition between chylomicrons and VLDL for LPL [26], which seems to hydrolyse chylomicron-TAG in preference to VLDL-TAG [27]. A number of studies have supported this speculation [25, 28, 29]. Schneeman *et al* [25] observed a remarkably close correlation between the average concentration, as well as the increment in concentration of TRL apoB-48 and apoB-100 postprandially. Karpe *et al* [28] found that postprandial increases in the concentration of TRL-apoB-48 were accompanied by elevation of $VLDL_1$ and reduced concentration of $VLDL_2$ particles. Additionally, the peak plasma level of the $VLDL_1$ seemed to coincide with that for large chylomicron remnants, arguing for an impeded degradation of VLDL particles. Björkegren *et al* [29], using a short-term intravenous infusion and stable isotope techniques, demonstrated that the TAG-emulsion caused a 75-90% block of the conversion of $VLDL_1$ to $VLDL_2$. Collectively, these findings suggest that VLDL patricles accumulate in the postprandial state most probably because their lipolysis does not "compete" effectively with chylomicron lipolysis.

Heath *et al* [30] recently investigated the appearance of dietary fatty acids in VLDL particles in humans *in vivo* using preparatory immunoaffinity chromatography to separate the intestinally- from the hepatically-derived TRL. As expected, dietary fatty acids were rapidly incorporated into chylomicron remnant-TAG, however, after a 90 min delay there was also a substantial incorporation into the VLDL-TAG pool through hepatic secretion. In addition, docosahexanoic acid was over-incorporated into VLDL-TAG compared with both [1-^{13}C]palmitic and eicosapentanoic acid. This study clearly demonstrated there is efficient recycling of dietary fatty acids into the VLDL-TAG pool and that this recycling can be of different magnitude for different fatty acids.

Regulation of Postprandial TRL Metabolism

Postprandial TRL and TAG metabolism is regulated by a number of factors, more importantly insulin, acylation-stimulating protein (ASP) and the enzyme LPL. The apolipoprotein composition of the particle, such as the apoCs and apoE, is also an important modulator of TRL metabolism. Each of these factors will be discussed in this section.

ApoC-I, II & III and apoE

Each of the individual human ApoCs are important modulators of TRL metabolism and their roles have been extensively studied in *in vitro* and *in vivo* studies (reviewed in [31]). Findings from *in vitro* studies [32] and studies in transgenic mice overexpressing human apoC-I [33] agree that apoC-I inhibits the uptake of TRL remnant particles by hepatic receptors, particularly the LRP. Whether apoC-I exerts a specific inhibitory effect on hepatic particle uptake by conformational changes or displacement of apoE is subject to further investigations. Surprisingly, total apoC-I deficiency also leads to an impaired *in vivo* hepatic uptake of VLDL, which has been speculated to be due to enrichment of the particle with apoA-I [34]. In a recent study, coronary artery disease patients, as compared with control individuals, manifested a postprandial accumulation of large, apoC-I–enriched VLDL. In addition, their small VLDL remnants were enriched with apoC-I and cholesterol [35]. It was suspected that the apoC-I enrichment caused a delay in VLDL clearance contributing to cholesterol enrichment of smaller VLDL. In a subsequent postprandial study in asymptomatic men with early atherosclerosis, the same group demonstrated an exaggerated apoC-I enrichment of large and small TRL remnants and cholesterol enrichment of small TRL remnants [36]. Furthermore, the number of apoC-I molecules per small chylomicron remnant particle was strongly associated with the degree of atherosclerotic lesions. Collectively, the results of these two studies [35, 36] point to a link between apoC-I enrichment of TRL remnants, delayed particle clearance and atherosclerosis in humans.

As discussed previously, apoC-II is the physiological activator of LPL [31]. Surprisingly, transgenic mice overexpressing human apoC-II are hypertriglyceridemic compared to controls in both the fasted and fed states [37] exhibiting delayed VLDL-TAG clearance.

These data suggest a more complex role for apoC-II in plasma TAG metabolism, i.e. apoC-II activates LPL, but its excess on the lipoprotein particle inhibits TAG hydrolysis [31].

Several lines of evidence have implicated apoC-III as possible contributor to the development of hypertriacylglycerolemia. ApoC-III interferes with TRL removal by hepatocytes [38, 39] but its principal effect is to inhibit TRL-TAG hydrolysis by LPL [40, 41]. It is believed that decreased lipolysis due to excess lipoprotein apoC-III relates to decreased binding of lipoproteins to cell-surface glycosaminoglycans. In line with this, Cohn *et al* [42] reported a strong significant relationship between VLDL apoC-III and VLDL-TAG concentrations in humans *in vivo*. Unexpectedly, no significant negative relationship was found between VLDL-apoC-III levels and VLDL-TAG or VLDL-apoB fractional catabolic rates arguing against an association between apoC-III and a disruption in TRL hydrolysis and removal. In contrast, they demonstrated a strong positive relationship between VLDL-apoC-III production rates and VLDL-TAG concentration and production rates. The authors speculated that hepatic apoC-III synthesis and secretion may be important determinants of hepatic VLDL-TAG secretion [42].

ApoE is a key ligand mediating the binding of TRL remnant particles to the LDL receptor and the LRP. In humans, the structural gene locus for apo E is polymorphic: three common alleles (e2,e3,e4) code for three major isoforms E-2, E-3 and E-4. Population studies have shown that the apoE polymorphism has a substantial effect on plasma lipids and lipoproteins [43, 44]. A study in young adults by Dallongeville *et al* [44] showed that postprandial triacyglycerolemia was significantly higher in subjects with an E-2, and to a lesser extent with an E-4, isoform than in subjects homozygous for E-3, independently of baseline TAG. It has been observed that, relative to apoE-3 and E-4, apoE-2 exhibits a defective binding activity to lipoprotein receptors [45]. Bergeron and Havel [46] also found prolonged postprandial increases in TRL apoB-48 and apoB-100 in young men with an apo E4/3 phenotype than in those with an apo E3/3 phenotype. The authors speculated that the apoE on chylomicron and VLDL remnants in humans with the apo E4/3 phenotype may be less accessible to hepatic lipoprotein receptors resulting in slower remnant clearance [46].

Insulin and ASP

Insulin is an important regulator of TAG metabolism. In the postprandial state, it regulates both VLDL production and TRL-TAG hydrolysis. Acute hyperinsulinemia suppresses VLDL-apoB and VLDL-TAG production rates in humans *in vivo* [47-49]. This effect seems to be due to a number of mechanisms. First, insulin decreases NEFA availability for VLDL-TAG synthesis by decreasing intracellular hormone-sensitive lipase (HSL) activity in adipose tissue [50, 51] by dephosphorylation. Elevating plasma NEFA during acute hyperinsulinemia attenuates, but does not completely abolish the suppressive effect of insulin on VLDL-TAG production, indicating that the suppressive effect of insulin is, to some extent, NEFA-independent [47]. VLDL secretion is under complex regulation as insulin acutely suppresses $VLDL_1$-apoB production but has no effect on $VLDL_2$-apoB production by the liver [52]. $VLDL_1$ and $VLDL_2$ production is, therefore, independently regulated. Second, insulin (and ASP, reviewed below) enhances entrapment of LPL-derived fatty acids into the subcutaneous adipose tissue by stimulating their esterification [50, 53]. In this way, insulin exerts a direct effect on the maintenance of a concentration gradient for the flow of fatty acids from the site of LPL action to the adipocytes [50]. Nevertheless, in the postprandial state, a proportion of LPL-derived fatty acids escapes retention into the subcutaneous adipose tissue and enters the plasma NEFA pool [54, 55]. In skeletal muscle, in contrast, all fatty acids released by LPL are taken up by the tissue [54, 55]. A study by Evans *et al* [54] clearly demonstrated that the entrapment of LPL-derived fatty acids by subcutaneous adipose tissue is remarkably regulated, so that it is close to 100% one hour after a mixed meal decreasing to ~10-30% by 6 hours. At the time of peak LPL action (4-5 hours after a mixed meal) approximately 50% of LPL-derived fatty acids are retained in the adipose tissue [50]. The upregulation of fatty acid entrapment by subcutaneous adipose tissue follows a time course similar to that of the increase in plasma insulin concentrations [54]. It has been suggested that this "inefficiency" of fat storage in the subcutaneous adipose tissue may give a high degree of control to the process of net fat storage [56] and play a central role in the distribution of dietary-derived lipid energy to tissues less able to hydrolyze chylomicrons [57].

Insulin directly stimulates LPL in adipose tissue [58, 59], thus enhancing TRL-TAG hydrolysis. The stimulation of adipose tissue LPL by insulin is a complex, not well defined process and seems to involve posttranscriptional (e.g. positive effects on LPL mRNA stability) and post-translational mechanisms [60, 61]. Insulin appears to regulate LPL in a tissue-specific manner [59, 62]. Farese *et al* [62] found that, in normal-weight subjects, insulin infusion, under conditions of euglycaemia, had a stimulatory effect on subcutaneous adipose tissue LPL but an inhibitory effect on skeletal muscle LPL activity. However, a more recent study in normal-weight subjects demonstrated that both skeletal and adipose tissue LPL activity increased significantly from fasted to postprandial state [63], indicating that the postprandial state has an enhancing effect not only on adipose tissue but also on muscle LPL activity.

ASP is a lipogenic hormone synthesized and secreted from the adipocytes by the interaction of three proteins: C3, adipsin and factor B (reviewed in [64]). ASP can provide a powerful drive for adipocyte TAG synthesis, at least in isolated cells. It increases the rate of TAG synthesis by stimulating both fatty acid incorporation (fatty acid trapping) and glucose transport into adipocytes, effects that are additive and independent of those of insulin [64]. A recent study in 3T3-L1 adipocytes has also shown that ASP (as well as insulin) increases in situ LPL activity (i.e. TAG hydrolysis and NEFA incorporation) by increasing the trapping of LPL-derived NEFA within the adipocytes [65]. This study suggested that a major part of the regulatory effect of ASP is to relieve the inhibitory effect of NEFA on LPL activity [65]. Thus, ASP, in combination with insulin, may be important for cellular NEFA uptake and storage in the overall regulation of postprandial TAG clearance. ASP is generated and released *in vivo* by human subcutaneous adipose tissue, and this process is enhanced in the postprandial state [66]. Postprandial production of ASP from subcutaneous adipose tissue bed correlated positively with postprandial net fatty acid trapping across the same bed [66]. Thus, ASP may contribute to coordination of postprandial TAG clearance and storage in humans *in vivo*.

Lipoprotein Lipase

LPL is synthesised in parenchymal cells of several tissues. After processing in the ER and Golgi complex, LPL is translocated, by not well defined mechanisms, to functional heparan sulphate proteoglycan binding sites on the luminal surface of the capillary endothelium, where the TRL-TAG hydrolysis takes place [60]. LPL activity is an indispensable first step for TRL-TAG hydrolysis and disposal. Each particle interacts with several LPL molecules, yielding very rapid catalysis. This is probably achieved by binding of large chylomicrons to the vascular endothelium, i.e. margination [67, 68]. LPL activity of the white adipose tissue and muscular tissues (skeletal muscle and cardiac muscle) accounts for a high proportion of the total LPL activity of the body, and therefore, these tissues are the most important in the bulk removal of TAG from plasma [69].

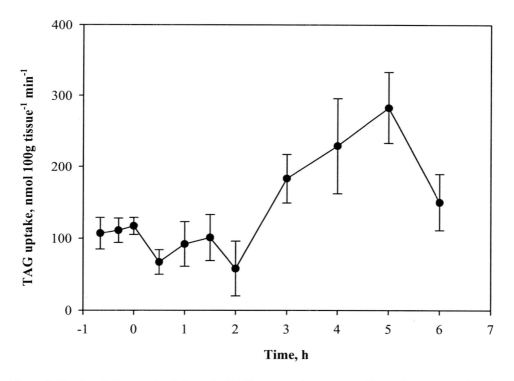

Figure 1. Uptake of plasma triacylglycerols (TAG) across subcutaneous adipose tissue *in vivo* in 13 healthy lean volunteers after overnight fast (-0.7 – 0 h) and after eating a mixed meal. The meal contained 31 g fat, 93 g carbohydrates and 22 g protein. TAG uptake across the tissue was calculated as the TAG arteriovenous difference multiplied by adipose tissue blood flow. Values are means with their standard errors represented by vertical bars. Modified from [56].

LPL activity seems to be altered with nutritional state in a tissue-specific manner directing TRL-TAG disposal according to the metabolic demands of individual tissues. Fasting results in a reduction in LPL activity in adipose tissue but stable or increased levels of LPL in muscle whereas feeding has the opposite effects, at least in the adipose tissue [63,

70-72]. TAG extraction across subcutaneous adipose tissue (a measure of adipose tissue LPL action) is low in the fasted state and rises postprandially to final values 2-3 times those in the fasted state at 4-5 h after the meal [56, 73] (Figure 1). TAG extraction across the leg (representing mainly muscle) also increases postprandially reaching its peak at 3-5 hours after the meal (Figure 2). Interestingly, leg uptake of total and meal-derived TAG has been shown to be higher in women than in men postprandially [74]. Subcutaneous adipose tissue appears to have a predominant role in postprandial clearance of circulating TAG. It has been estimated that TAG clearance by subcutaneous adipose tissue accounts for ~35% of the fat ingested, whereas skeletal muscle's contribution is much less (~14%) [57].

LPL activity is known to be inhibited by NEFA, the main product of TAG hydrolysis [75, 76]. It has been suggested that the local generation and accumulation of fatty acids at the endothelial cell site results in LPL dissociation from the endothelial cells so that fatty acids are not formed more rapidly than they can be taken up by the peripheral tissue [75]. This represents control of endothelial LPL by fatty acids. As discussed above, detachment of LPL from its endothelial binding site and association with the lipoprotein particles may also facilitate TRL removal by the liver [15].

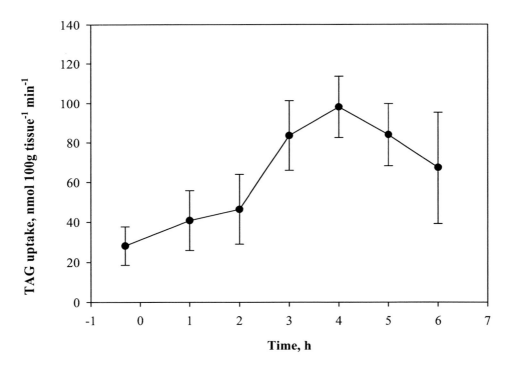

Figure 2. Uptake of plasma triacylglycerols (TAG) across the leg *in vivo* in 8 healthy lean males after an overnight fast (-0.3 h) and after eating a mixed, high-fat meal. The meal contained on average 98 g fat, 98 g carbohydrates and 16 g protein. TAG uptake across the leg was calculated as the TAG arteriovenous difference multiplied by leg blood flow. Values are means with their standard errors represented with vertical bars. Used with permission by the American Physiological Society from [160].

Postprandial TAG Metabolism and Atherosclerosis

Epidemiologic studies have clearly established and independent association between fasting plasma TAG concentration and CHD [77, 78]. Triacylglycerol itself is not a component of atherosclerotic plaques but, as it will be discussed, TRL particles may have both direct and indirect effects on the development of atherosclerosis (reviewed in [79-81]). Postprandial lipemia is transient hypertriacylglycerolemia which, if prolonged and exaggerated, may unfavorably modify plasma lipoproteins generating an atherogenic lipoprotein profile. Unfortunately, there is a complete lack of prospective studies to show that postprandial lipid metabolism is associated with future CHD events or progression of atherosclerosis.

The classic study by Patsch *et al* [82] was one of the first to demonstrate an independent association between increased postprandial TAG levels and CHD in male control and normolipidemic subjects with severe CHD as verified by angiography. CHD patients exhibited a higher and more prolonged postprandial TAG response than the controls. Multivariate logistic-regression analysis, including HDL cholesterol, revealed that postprandial TAG concentrations were independently associated with the disease, whereas fasting TAG was not [82]. Other studies have also reported a pronounced and late postprandial TAG response in normolipidemic patients with severe CHD compared to matched controls [83, 84].

Postprandial TAG concentrations seem to be a potential discriminator not only for the presence of severe CHD but also for early atherosclerosis. In healthy asymptomatic subjects, a commonly used surrogate marker for early atherosclerosis is the intima-media thickness (IMT) of the common carotid artery measured by B-mode ultrasound. Ryu *et al* [85] reported a strong and independent association between peak postprandial TAG concentration and carotid artery IMT in healthy middle-aged men and women. In accordance with these findings, postprandial TAG response [expressed as incremental area under the curve (AUC)] in asymptomatic mildly hyperlipidemic individuals [86] and late (6 h) postprandial TAG concentration in healthy men [87] have been positively associated with early atherosclerosis, independently of both fasting TAG and LDL-cholesterol levels. HDL-cholesterol did not correlate significantly with early atherosclerosis even in univariate analyses [85, 87, 88], implying that this lipid may not be a discriminator of the early phase of CHD.

The way in which postprandial TAG metabolism affects the pathogenesis and progression of CHD is at least partly associated with a constellation of potentially atherogenic lipoprotein changes. These include: i) increase in plasma TRL particles and their remnants; ii) decrease in HDL-cholesterol due to core lipid exchange between HDL and postprandial TRL; and iii) formation of small dense LDL that are potentially atherogenic. Postprandial lipemia may induce an atherogenic state also by impairing endothelial function [89, 90] and exerting clot-promoting and anti-fibrinolytic effects [91, 92] but a detailed discussion is beyond the scope of this review.

Postprandial Increase in TRL Particles and their Remnants

Zilversmit [93] was the first to propose a link between postprandial TRL remnants (principally chylomicron remnants) and atherosclerosis. He proposed that atherogenesis involved the binding of these remnants to the arterial wall, hydrolysis of their TAG by arterial LPL and subsequent internalisation of the remnant by arterial smooth muscle cells. Since then, there has been a wealth of evidence linking TRL remnant particles and risk or progression of atherosclerosis [94, 95].

In vivo measurements of fluxes of various lipoprotein species across the intima of human carotid arteries have shown that elevated plasma concentrations of small remnant lipoproteins (S_f 12-60) shared with LDL the potential for causing lipid accumulation [96]. In accordance with this, small chylomicron remnants (apoB-48-containing TRL in the S_f >20-60 fraction) correlated positively with the rate of progression of coronary artery atherosclerosis, as assessed by coronary angiographies separated by approximately five years in male CHD patients [28]. This relationship was independent of HDL-cholesterol and small dense LDL particle levels [28]. In addition, small cholesteryl-ester rich VLDL particles have been related to CHD severity [97]. Overall, small TRL particles with remnant characteristics may be more atherogenic than large particles, because the latter are less likely to penetrate the arterial endothelium.

Under most circumstances, VLDL particles represent more than 90% of total TRL [79]. Examination of the compositional features of human fasting and postprandial chylomicron and VLDL particles [98, 99] have revealed that VLDL particles attain remnant characteristics in the postprandial state. Specifically, both large and small VLDL become cholesterol, apoE- and apo C-I enriched, but depleted in apoC-II. Large and small chylomicron remnants contain significantly more apoC-II molecules per particle than VLDL in fasted and postprandial states, which helps to explain the reduced efficiency of VLDL, and especially $VLDL_1$, for lipolysis postprandially. The transient increase (by 50%) in cholesterol content [98] and concentration [28] of $VLDL_1$ in the postprandial state could also explain why the postprandial cholesterol accumulation in TRL is mainly accounted for by VLDL particles [25]. An important contribution has been made by Rapp *et al* [100] who used immunoaffinity chromatography to isolate TRL particles from human atherosclerotic plaque removed during surgery. Approximately one-third of the lipoprotein-associated cholesterol was in the IDL/VLDL fraction. This lipoprotein fraction was substantially apo E-enriched, i.e. had remnant characteristics. ApoB-48 was not found.

Remnant lipoproteins are hard to define and even harder to isolate. They exist throughout the Sf <400 density range alongside newly secreted particles. As discussed, remnants are cholesteryl-ester rich and have a high apo E content. A novel immunoaffinity method [101] has been developed to isolate remnant-like particles and measure their cholesterol content as a marker for their accumulation. Increased levels of remnant-like lipoprotein particle (RLP) cholesterol have been found in normolipidemic men with CHD [102]. RLP-cholesterol concentration has been more strongly related with the severity score of coronary atherosclerosis in cases of sudden cardiac death than LDL-cholesterol [103]. Reference values have been published from the Framingham Study [104].

At the moment, there is no evidence that the type of apoB (B-100 or B-48) itself has an effect on atherosclerosis [105, 106]. The study by Veniant *et al* [105] examined the extent of atherosclerosis in apoE knockout mice that synthesize exclusively either apoB-48 or apoB-100. Susceptibility to atherosclerosis was dependent on plasma cholesterol levels. Whether mice synthesized apo-B48 or apo-B100 did not appear to have an independent effect on susceptibility to atherosclerosis.

Low HDL-Cholesterol

HDL particles are the smallest and densest of the lipoprotein classes. HDL mediate the removal and transfer of excess cholesterol from peripheral tissues to the liver, i.e. reverse cholesterol transport [107]. HDL can be separated into mainly two subclasses, the lighter and larger HDL_2 and the denser and smaller HDL_3. HDL_2 contains three to four times more cholesteryl ester and TAG molecules than HDL_3 and is twice as "efficient" as HDL_3 as a vehicle for fat transport [108].

HDL and TRL metabolism is tightly linked so that constituents (free cholesterol and phospholipids) originating from the surface coat of lipolyzed TRL particles constitute a major source of HDL lipids [107]. Fasting HDL-cholesterol concentration shows a strong inverse association with fasting [109] and postprandial [110] plasma TAG levels. It is likely that hypertriacylglycerolemia, either as a metabolic disorder or a transient postprandial phenomenon, results in accelerated exchange of HDL-cholesteryl ester for TRL-TAG mediated by CETP. The TAG-enriched HDL particle is eventually remodeled by the action of hepatic lipase, which hydrolyzes its TAG and phospholipid, leading to the formation of smaller HDL. This remodeling promotes HDL catabolism lowering the concentration of the cardioprotective and metabolically active HDL_2 fraction and thus impairing reverse cholesterol transport [111]. A study by Lamarche *et al* [112] demonstrated that TAG enrichment of HDL particles during an Intralipid infusion enhanced the metabolic clearance of apoA-I (major apolipoprotein component of HDL particle) from the circulation in normolipidemic humans. The authors speculated that increased susceptibility of TAG-rich HDL particles to lipolysis by hepatic lipase compared with fasting HDL could have accounted for the enhanced catabolism of TAG-enriched HDL apoA-I. Large VLDL particles seem to be preferentially involved in the core lipid exchange mediated by CETP [113] and, therefore, the postprandial accumulation of large VLDL [28] could partly explain the inverse relationship between the magnitude of lipemia and fasting HDL_2 or HDL_2-cholesterol levels [114]. In line with this reasoning, it has been suggested that the efficiency of postprandial TRL metabolism determines the plasma level of HDL cholesterol or larger HDL species in the postabsorptive state [82].

An alternative interpretation for the link between HDL-cholesterol levels and postprandial TRL metabolism has been given by Karpe *et al* [115] who investigated men with previous myocardial infarction. These authors observed that if the subjects were arbitrarily divided into two groups according to fasting plasma HDL-cholesterol concentration below and above 1.2 mmol/L, those in the lower HDL-cholesterol range showed strong, negative and linear relation between postprandial TRL responses and HDL-cholesterol. In contrast, only a weak but still negative association was present in subjects in the upper HDL-cholesterol range. The authors speculated that low levels of the larger HDL species or fasting HDL-cholesterol can limit the rate of lipolytic degradation of postprandial TRL, whereas at high levels of HDL, TRL lipolytic degradation depends on factors other than HDL. The potential impact of low HDL levels may be mediated by decreased availability of apoC-II, which would impair TRL-TAG lipolysis by LPL [115]. This hypothesis is in a good agreement with results from a study in endurance-trained men [116] whose HDL-cholesterol levels were well above the distribution in the general population. There was no relationship between fasting HDL-cholesterol and the postprandial TRL response. However, in a subsequent study, Cohen and Grundy [117] demonstrated that normolipidemic men with low (~0.8 mmol/L) or normal (~1.2 mmol/L) HDL-cholesterol concentration exhibited similar postprandial lipemia. Similar results have also been reported by O'Meara et al [109]. These findings argue for a dissociation of postprandial TRL metabolism and fasting HDL-cholesterol, even at a low range of HDL-cholesterol concentration. It may be that high postprandial lipemia is incompatible with high HDL-cholesterol concentrations but that low or normal postprandial TAG metabolic capacity does not automatically confer high HDL-cholesterol. Accordingly, impaired TRL metabolism is not the only cause of low HDL-cholesterol levels.

Small Dense LDL Particles

The role of small dense LDL (defined as pattern B, LDL III or mean diameter of major peak <25.5 nm) as a risk factor for CHD has been well established [118-120]. A number of potential atherogenic mechanisms have been proposed: (i) lower affinity for the LDL receptor which will effectively increase their residence time in circulation for interaction with the arterial wall; (ii) smaller size which allows faster rate of infiltration into the endothelium and subendothelial space than larger LDL; (iii) increased affinity for arterial proteoglycans; and (iv) increased susceptibility to oxidation [121]. All these processes work together in sequence to confer increased risk on small dense LDL.

LDL subclass distribution shows a strong association with fasting plasma TAG levels. In a longitudinal study with a follow up period of approximately three years, McNamara et al [122] showed a significant inverse association between the change in LDL size and the change in plasma TAG. Griffin et al [119] demonstrated a positive association between plasma TAG levels and the concentration of LDL III, when plasma TAG concentration was >1.5 mmol/L. Therefore, it has been suggested that when TAG concentration exceeds this threshold level, formation of small dense LDL is facilitated [123].

The mechanisms of small dense LDL formation in the presence of high plasma TAG concentrations resemble that of HDL particles (discussed in the "Low HDL-cholesterol" section). Briefly, it involves CETP-mediated enrichment of LDL with TAG from TRL particles followed by remodeling of the TAG-enriched LDL particle by hepatic lipase. As the threshold of 1.5 mmol/L for plasma TAG is breached by postprandial lipaemia, the postprandial state could be of great importance in the formation of small dense LDL. Karpe et al [124] showed that the magnitude of postprandial lipemia is positively associated with the fasting levels of small dense LDL particles. Johanson *et al* [125] recently reported a strong inverse correlation between the concentration of TAG in the $VLDL_1$ fraction and LDL size in both healthy controls and first-degree relatives of type 2 diabetic patients. It has been suggested [123] that an increase in large VLDL gives rise to an LDL product that has a prolonged residence time in the circulation (~5 days). This LDL particle can be then converted to small dense LDL by the action of CETP and hepatic lipase [123]. The presence of an increased proportion of small dense LDL has been suggested to represent a fasting marker of impaired postprandial TRL metabolism [126].

Effect of Exercise on Postprandial TAG Metabolism

Exercise has a potent influence on TAG metabolism. Both repeated transitory effects of single, isolated exercise sessions and exercise-training effects may be involved. This section will discuss the effects of exercise on postprandial TAG metabolism and potential mechanisms by which exercise may exert these effects. The scope of this section is not to extensively review all the available literature in the field but, rather, to highlight and discuss recent studies that have contributed substantially to our knowledge and understanding on the impact of exercise on TAG and TRL metabolism (Table 1). It also has to be emphasized that, although this review will focus on the postprandial state, in most studies that will be discussed, exercise reduced both fasting and postprandial TAG concentrations. Since the endogenous TAG pool is an important determinant of the evolution of plasma TAG concentration after fat intake [109, 127], it is obvious that exercise improves postprandial TAG metabolic capacity, to some extent, by decreasing the postabsorptive TAG pool.

Effect of Training and a Single Exercise Session

Several cross-sectional studies have showed that postprandial TAG response to a test meal (40-140 g fat) is consistently lower in endurance-trained men [128, 129] and women [130] than in sedentary individuals. At least in men, this was also observed when the relationship between training and postprandial lipemia was investigated more critically by matching subjects for variables known to influence postprandial TAG metabolism, such as fasting TAG level, body weight and age [128, 129]. However, it is now clear that in the absence of the effects of a recent exercise session, postprandial lipemia is not influenced by habitual physical activity levels [130, 131]. The studies by Tsetsonis *et al* and Herd *et al* [130, 131] compared the postprandial TAG response to a high-fat meal in (endurance- and sprint-) trained and untrained young adults after 2 days' abstistence from exercise. There was no difference in postprandial lipemia between trained and untrained subjects. The effects of the early phase of detraining were specifically examined by Hardman *et al* [132]. Ten

Table 1. Studies that have investigated the impact of exercise on postprandial TAG metabolism

Reference	Subjects	Study design	Test meal fat content	Exercise effect in fasted state	Exercise effect in postprandial state	Comment
[130]	9 F endurance trained 13 F untrained	Control vs 90 min walking at 60% VO_{2max} performed ~15 h prior to test meal	1.7 g/kg FFM	Plasma [TAG]: -27% Ex vs control in trained -16% Ex vs control in untrained	Plasma TAG AUC: -30% Ex vs control in trained -16% Ex vs control in untrained Plasma TAG IAUC: -36% Ex vs control in trained -17% Ex vs control in untrained	1. NS differenceces between groups in the absence of acute exercise 2. Trained group expended more energy during exercise than untrained group
[131]	11 M/9 F endurance trained 10 M sprint/strength trained 11 M/11F untrained	Abstinence from Ex 2 d before test meal	1.2 g/kg BM	NS differences	NS differences	
[132]	9 M/1 F endurance trained	Test meal at 15 h, 60 h, 6.5 d without Ex	1.2 g/kg BM	Plasma [TAG]: +28% at 60h vs control no further increase at 6.5 d	Plasma TAG AUC: +35% at 60 h vs 15 h no further increase at 6.5 d Plasma TAG IAUC: +43% at 60 h vs 15 h no further increase at 6.5 d	Rapid deterioration of TAG metabolic capacity with detraining
[134]	21 M recreationally active	Control vs 60 min Ex at 60% VO_{2max} performed 12 h before (12 h-pre), 1 h before (1 h-pre) or 1h after (1 h-post) the test meal	100 g	NS differences	Plasma TAG IAUC: -51% 12 h-pre vs control -38% 1 h-pre vs control NS 1 h-post vs control	
[136]	5 M/4 F recreationally active	Control vs 180 min walking at 32% VO_{2max} (4.2 MJ) vs 90 min walking at 63% VO_{2max} (4.3 MJ) performed ~15 h prior to test meal	1.3 g/kg BM	Plasma [TAG]: -30% LI & MI walking vs control	Plasma TAG AUC: -33% LI walking vs control -32% MI walking vs control Plasma TAG IAUC: -27% LI & MI walking vs control	NS differences between exercise intensities. Energy expenditure during exercise appears as an important determinant of reduction in lipemic response.

Table 1. Studies that have investigated the impact of exercise on postprandial TAG metabolism (Continued)

Reference	Subjects	Study design	Test meal fat content	Exercise effect in fasted state	Exercise effect in postprandial state	Comment
[137]	12 M physically active	Control vs 90 min running at 60% VO$_{2max}$ (4.8 MJ) performed ~15 h prior to test meal with ingestion of acipimox or placebo	1.2 g/kg BM	NS differences	Plasma TAG AUC: -22% acipimox vs control -21% placebo vs control Plasma TAG IAUC: -33% acipimox vs control -43% placebo vs control	Despite significant differences in the relative contribution of fat and CHO to energy metabolism during exercise, TAG responses were similar between the two exercise conditions.
[138]	3 M/7 F sedentary	Control vs 10 min walking at 60% VO$_{2max}$ before each meal vs 30 min walking at 60% VO$_{2max}$ before breakfast	Breakfast:0.4 g/kg BM Lunch: 0.93 g/kg BM Dinner: 0.56 g/kg BM	NS differences	Day-long plasma [TAG]: -12% short walks vs control -12% long walk vs control	Multiple short exercise sessions achieved a similar effect to this achieved through a long session.
[139]	12 F recreationally active	Control vs 90 min walking at 60% VO$_{2max}$ ~15 h prior to test meal vs an equivalent energy deficit induced by restriction of food intake	1.7 g/kg FFM	Plasma [TAG]: -20% Ex vs control and food intake restriction	Plasma TAG AUC: -20% Ex vs control -7% food intake restriction vs control (NS)	The effect of exercise on postprandial lipemia was greater than that attributable to the energy deficit incurred
[140]	10 M/4 F recreationally weight trained	Control vs aerobic Ex (1.6 MJ) vs resistance Ex (1.7 MJ) performed ~15 h prior to test meal	1.2 g/kg BM	Plasma [TAG]: -21% resistance Ex vs control and aerobic Ex	Plasma TAG AUC: -14% resistance Ex vs control -18% resistance Ex vs aerobic exercise	The first study that investigated the effects of resistance exercise on postprandial lipemia. Aerobic exercise of equal energy expenditure did not have significant effects.

Table 1. Studies that have investigated the impact of exercise on postprandial TAG metabolism (continued)

Reference	Subjects	Study design	Test meal fat content	Exercise effect in fasted state	Exercise effect in postprandial state	Comment
[141]	13 M recreationally active	Control vs 238 min Ex at 25% VO_{2peak} (4.6 MJ) vs 90 min Ex at 65% VO_{2peak} (4.6 MJ) completed 1 h prior to test meal	1.3 g/kg BM	NS differences	Plasma TAG IAUC: -39% MI Ex vs control -34% MI vs LI Ex NS differences between LI Ex and control	LI and MI exercise of equal energy expenditure exerted different effects on lipemic response to a meal consumed 1 h after exercise.
[156]	8 M recreationally active	Control vs 90 min Ex at 60% VO_{2max} (4.5 MJ) performed ~16 h prior the test meal. Muscle biopsy before test meal	1.4 g/kg BM	NS differences	Plasma TAG AUC: -28% Ex vs control Plasma TAG IAUC: -42% Ex vs control NS differences in muscle LPL activity in the fasted state	Exercise reduced postprandial lipemia without significantly affecting muscle LPL activity in the fasted state.
[160]	8 M recreationally active/endurance trained	Control vs 120 min Ex at 60% VO_{2max} (7.2 MJ) performed ~16 h prior the test meal. A-V differences across the leg	1.2 g/kg BM	Plasma and VLDL [TAG] lower in Ex condition than control Similar leg TAG uptake	Plasma, VLDL and chylomicron [TAG] lower in Ex condition. Similar leg TAG uptake	1. Exercise-induced enhancement of fasting and postprandial TAG metabolic capacity could not be explained by higher TAG uptake across the leg. 2. Higher plasma β-hydroxybutyrate levels in the exercise condition suggest higher hepatic fatty acid oxidation.
[159]	8 M recreationally active	Control vs 90 min walking at 60% VO_{2max} performed ~15 h prior the test meal and IVFTT	1.2 g/kg BM IVFTT: 0.5 mL 20% Intralipid per kg BM	Plasma [TAG]: -17% Ex vs control	Plasma TAG AUC after meal: -18% Ex vs control Plasma TAG IAUC after meal: -17% Ex vs control NS differences in TAG clearance during IVFTT between Ex and control	Moderate exercise reduced postprandial lipemia but had no effect on TAG clearance rate of an artificial lipid emulsion given intravenously.

Table 1. Studies that have investigated the impact of exercise on postprandial TAG metabolism (continued)

Reference	Subjects	Study design	Test meal fat content	Exercise effect in fasted state	Exercise effect in postprandial state	Comment
[167]	9 M	Control vs 60 min cycling at 70-75% predicted HR_{max} performed ~15 h prior the test meal	0.66 g/kg BM	NS differences	Plasma TAG AUC: -26% Ex vs control NS differences in plasma TAG IAUC	Exercise ameliorated the plasma TAG response to a moderate-fat mixed meal of a composition closer to that of a typical Western diet.
[164]	8 F recreationally active	Test meal was consumed i) after 3 d on a low-CHO diet; ii) after 3 d on an isoenergetic high-CHO diet, and iii) after 3 d on the same high-CHO with 60 min of walking at 60% VO_{2max} (1.46 MJ) daily	1.0 g/kg BM	Plasma and TRL-TAG, TRL-apoB-48, apoB-100 and apoE and serum RLP-cholesterol concentrations were all higher after the high-CHO diet. Daily exercise significantly attenuated all the above diet-induced increases.	Same effects as in the fasted state.	The first study that directly investigated the effects of exercise on concentrations of TRL particles and serum RLP-cholesterol. Daily exercise opposed the potentially deleterious effects of a short-term high-CHO diet on postprandial lipoprotein metabolism.

FFM, fat-free mass; BM, body mass; [TAG], TAG concentration; AUC, area under the curve; IAUC, incremental area under the curve; Ex, Exercise; NS, non-significant; LI, low intensity; MI, moderate intensity; CHO, carbohydrates; IVFTT, intravenous fat tolerance test.

normolipidemic endurance-trained subjects undertook an oral fat tolerance test 15 h, 60 h and 6.5 d after their last training session, which was ≥30 min in duration. When compared with values at 15 h, postprandial lipemia (expressed as total or incremental AUC) was significantly higher at 60 h and at 6.5 d with most of the increase evident by 60 h. Thus, increased levels of physical activity and improved fitness do not necessarily result in changes in the postprandial lipemic response above those attributable to the residual effects of the last bout of exercise. However, the possibility of a synergistic effect between chronic and acute exercise can not be excluded and has not been investigated.

Although it is known since the early 1960s that a session of exercise diminishes postprandial lipemia [133], it was only recently that the optimal timing to exercise to magnify the effect of exercise was investigated [134]. In the study by Zhang et al. [134], 21 recreationally active male subjects consumed a high-fat meal on 4 occasions, which were in a randomized order: (1), control (no-exercise, fat meal only); (2) exercise at 12 h before the meal; (3) exercise at 1 h before the meal, and (4) exercise at 1 h after the meal. In the 3 exercise conditions, subjects performed a 60 min-exercise session at 60% of their VO_{2max}. Compared with the control condition, the TAG-AUC was 51%, 38% and 5% lower, when the exercise was performed 12 h before, 1 h before and 1h after the meal, respectively. The 5% reduction with the post-meal exercise session was not significant. These findings indicated that exercising 12 h before the meal magnifies the ameliorating effect of exercise on postprandial lipemia, implying a delayed effect of exercise on TAG metabolism.

With some exceptions, the total energy expended during exercise is an important determinant of exercise-induced decreases in postprandial lipemia (reviewed in [135]). Tsetsonis and Hardman [136] were the first to demonstrate that exercise sessions of the same energy expenditure but different intensity elicited similar attenuation in postprandial lipemia. Specifically, they compared the effects of brisk walking, for either 90 min at 63% VO_{2max} or 180 min at 32% $VO_{2\,max}$, with a non-exercise trial. Gross energy expenditure was 4.18 MJ for the low intensity and 4.28 MJ for the moderate intensity exercise session (not significantly different). However, substrate utilization was different between the two intensities, so that oxidized fat represented 40% and 25% of the total energy produced during the low and moderate intensity exercise sessions, respectively ($P <0.05$). On the days after walking, postprandial lipemia was reduced by the low and the moderate intensity walking, the magnitude of these reductions being strikingly similar (~30%). These authors were the first to suggest that acute exercise-induced reduction in postprandial lipemia may be independent of qualitative differences in substrate utilization during exercise [136].

An important contribution to this issue was made by Malkova et al [137]. In this study, subjects underwent three oral fat tolerance tests in a balanced design. On two occasions, subjects ran on the treadmill for 90 minutes at 60% $VO_{2\,max}$ the afternoon prior the fat tolerance test, after having ingested 131 mg acipimox (antilipolytic agent) or placebo. On the third occasion they refrained from exercise (control trial). As acipimox suppresses NEFA supply from adipose tissue, NEFA levels remained suppressed during the exercise session in the acipimox trial. Although gross energy expenditure during exercise was identical in the acipimox (4.83 MJ) and placebo (4.86 MJ) conditions, the relative contributions of fat and carbohydrate were different. The proportion of energy derived from fat during exercise was significantly lower after acipimox (16%) than after placebo (28%) whereas the proportion from carbohydrate was correspondingly greater (placebo 72%, acipimox 84%). Interestingly, even after acipimox administration, fat oxidation contributed 16% of energy expenditure during exercise, implying that intramuscular TAG was the predominant source of fatty acids for oxidation in these circumstances. Despite the significant differences in the relative contribution of fat and carbohydrate to energy metabolism during exercise, postprandial lipemia (total TAG-AUC) was strikingly similar in the two exercise conditions; in both cases, 20% lower than in the control condition.

Different patterns of exercise with equal energy expenditure induce similar reducing effects on postprandial TAG response to meals [138]. Murphy *et al* [138] compared the effects of different patterns of brisk walking on day-long plasma TAG concentrations. Subjects undertook no exercise (control), walked briskly for 10 min before each meal (breakfast, lunch, dinner) or walked briskly for 30 min before breakfast. Average day-long plasma TAG levels were significantly lower during the walking conditions than the control condition but did not differ between the two patterns of walking. Thus, exercise undertaken in one session or accumulated throughout the day is equally effective in ameliorating postprandial TAG concentrations.

Since the reducing effect of exercise on postprandial lipemia is closely related to the energy expended during exercise, it is possible that the attenuation in postprandial lipemia by exercise is attributable to the associated energy deficit rather than to the exercise *per se*. The study by Gill & Hardman [139] compared the effects on postprandial lipemia of a moderate-intensity exercise session (60% of VO_{2max}) and an equivalent energy deficit induced by restriction of food intake. Compared with the control condition (no exercise, consumption of a diet isoenergetic to subjects' habitual diet), 90 minutes of brisk walking reduced postprandial lipemia by 20% ($P < 0.05$), whereas food intake restriction reduced it by 7% (not significantly). Thus, the effect of exercise on postprandial lipemia is greater than that attributable to the energy deficit incurred.

Two recent studies demonstrated that exercise-induced reduction in postprandial lipemia is not always related to the energy expended during exercise [140, 141]. Petitt *et al* [140] were the first to investigate the effects on postprandial lipemia of resistance exercise. The resistance exercise session was completed ~15 h before the test meal and was compared with aerobic exercise of equal energy expenditure (~1.7 MJ) and a non-exercise condition. In agreement with previous reports [142], aerobic exercise of 1.7 MJ energy expenditure did not attenuate the postprandial lipemic response to the meal but the resistance exercise did reduce it by 19% ($P < 0.05$). It was speculated that the lipemic response after resistance exercise may not be related to the energy expended during exercise but to some other factor (e.g. skeletal muscle LPL) linked to the high intensity muscle contraction associated with weight lifting. Katsanos *et al* [141] compared the effects of two exercise sessions of different intensities (25% vs 65 % VO_{2peak}) but equal energy expenditure (~4.6 MJ) on postprandial plasma TAG response to a high-fat meal. Exercise was completed 1 h before the test meal. As compared with a non-exercise condition, the low-intensity exercise did not affect the magnitude of postprandial lipemia but the moderate-intensity exercise significantly attenuated it by 39%. Both these studies [140, 141] point to other physiologic and metabolic factors, in addition to energy expenditure, that regulate the ameliorating effect of exercise on postprandial lipemia.

Mechanisms for Exercise Effects on Postprandial TAG Metabolism

Potential mechanisms for the exercise-induced attenuation of postprandial lipemia include improved capacity for TRL-TAG hydrolysis, suppression of VLDL-TAG secretion and slower rate of chylomicron entry into the systemic circulation.

Effects on TRL-TAG Hydrolysis

Studies that have investigated the hypothesis that exercise reduces plasma TAG concentration by enhancing the TRL-TAG hydrolysis pathway have mostly focused on the key enzyme, LPL. Cross-sectional studies have demonstrated that endurance-trained athletes exhibit higher post-heparin plasma LPL activity than sedentary controls [143, 144]. On a tissue level, Nikkila et al [145] found that LPL activity of both adipose tissue and skeletal muscle was 2.7- and 1.7-times higher, respectively, in male long distance runners than in controls. The authors concluded that endurance training is associated with an adaptive increase in LPL activity not only in skeletal muscle but also in adipose tissue, which aims to increase the body capacity to mobilize and utilize fat as a fuel. Such an increase can allow rapid restoration of TAG stores in both tissues, while increase in adipose tissue LPL activity can also favor release of fatty acids directly from plasma TAG to plasma NEFA pool for oxidation in muscles [145].

Training studies that involved daily, prolonged intense exercise (e.g. sessions of ≥60 minutes at 60-75% of VO_{2max}) have demonstrated a training-induced increase in skeletal muscle LPL activity but no effect on adipose tissue LPL activity [146]. Acute exercise studies showed that 1 h of exhaustive exercise increased adipose tissue (by 44%) but not muscle LPL activity [147], whereas heavy exercise of longer duration (eight-hour (85 km) cross-country skiing race) did increase muscle LPL activity by 240% [148].

Studies that specifically investigated the exercise-induced increase in muscle LPL activity have shown that this increase usually occurs over a period of several hours [148] with a lag time of at least one to two hours [147, 149, 150]. Greiwe et al [151] examined the effect of 60 min cycling at 65% VO_{2peak} on muscle LPL protein content in untrained individuals. LPL mass was increased by 170% at 22 h after exercise compared with baseline. Since LPL protein content usually reflects LPL enzyme activity in skeletal muscle [146], these findings suggest that moderate- to high-intensity exercise induce a delayed increase in LPL activity. Exercise appears to raise muscle LPL activity, at least partly, by pretranslational mechanisms, i.e. by increasing LPL mRNA level [146, 152]. Catecholamines, fatty acids and muscle contraction may be potential regulators of exercise-induced LPL gene expression. Epinephrine has been shown to stimulate human muscle LPL activity *in vivo* [153]. Catecholamines increase intracellular cAMP, and the LPL promoter has a cAMP responsive element [154]. It has also been speculated that both a fall in intramyofibral concentrations of fatty acids (due to increased β-oxidation) and the muscle contractile activity *per se* may signal the induction of LPL gene expression [155].

Does moderate-intensity exercise increase muscle LPL? A study by Herd et al [156] found that 90-min cycling at ~60% VO_{2max} performed 16 h before the test meal did not affect fasting muscle LPL activity but did reduce the postprandial plasma TAG response. Therefore, the findings by Herd *et al* [156] do not directly support muscle LPL as a mechanism for the observed exercise-induced attenuation of postprandial hypertriacylglycerolemia.

Studies that examined the effect of a single exercise session on the rate of clearance of exogenous TAG showed that clearance rate is increased the day after prolonged exercise [157, 158]. Sady *et al* [157] showed that the clearance rate of an intravenous fat emulsion was increased by 76% ($P < 0.01$, range 16-221%) at 18 h after a marathon race, compared to values taken 24 hours before the race. Annuzzi *et al* [158] subsequently showed that the day after 180 min, but not 90 min, of exercise at 77% HR_{max}, clearance rate of an intravenous fat emulsion was significantly increased. Similarly, Gill *et al* [159] found no effect of a 90-min session of moderate-intensity exercise on the clearance rate of an intravenous fat emulsion.

The most convincing evidence that mechanisms other than increased muscle TAG uptake must account for the effects of prior exercise on postprandial lipemia is from the study by Malkova *et al* [160]. These authors compared postprandial plasma TAG extraction across the leg between a control (non-exercise) and an exercise condition. In the exercise condition, subjects ran for 2 h at ~60% VO_{2max} in the evening before the test meal. Postprandial concentrations of total, VLDL- and chylomicron-TAG were all significantly lower in the exercise condition. The majority of the decrease in plasma TAG was attributable to the decrease in VLDL-TAG. TAG uptake by the leg increased significantly from basal to postprandial state in both conditions. There were no significant differences in postprandial TAG uptake, as an absolute measure of extraction. However, postprandial TAG clearance, a measure of fractional extraction, was higher in the exercise condition indicating that leg TAG uptake was maintained despite lower arterial TAG concentrations (Figure 3). Thus, although exercise did not affect the absolute TAG extraction by the leg (muscle), it did enhance the efficiency of muscle to hydrolyze circulating TAG.

Effects on VLDL-TAG Secretion

The evidence on a possible effect of exercise on hepatic VLDL-TAG production is sparse and mostly limited to experimental animals. Using the Triton method, Simoneli and Eaton [161] studied TAG production by the liver. Triton WR-1339 has detergent properties that bind plasma TAG, thereby preventing its clearance from the circulation. Hence, increments in circulating TAG after administration of Triton reflect their secretion by the liver. This study [161] showed that in obese hyperlipidemic Zucker rats, as well as in their thin normolipidaemic littermates, hepatic TAG secretion was reduced by approximately 50% after three weeks of training (running). The study by Mondon *et al* [162] demonstrated similar results. Ten to 12 weeks of training resulted in 50% lower VLDL-TAG secretion rate *in vivo*. TAG secretion by perfused livers of trained and untrained rats were identical in response to given insulin and NEFA levels. This indicated that exercise training did not lead to any intrinsic difference in the ability of liver to esterify NEFA and secrete TAG, when insulin and NEFA were comparable. Rather, the lower TAG secretion rates *in vivo* observed in trained rats seemed to have been due to a reduction in substrate availability during the training period.

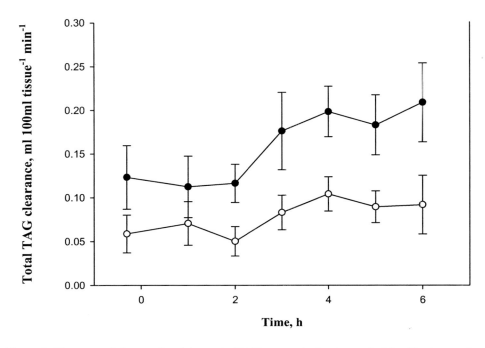

Figure 3. Clearance of plasma triacylglycerols (TAG) across the leg *in vivo* in 8 healthy lean males after overnight fast (-0.3 h) and after eating a mixed, high-fat meal in control (open circles) and exercise (solid circles) conditions. In the control condition, subjects refrained from exercise for 2 d before the test meal. In the exercise condition, subjects ran on the treadmill for 2 h at 60% VO_{2max} the evening before the meal. Clearance of TAG across the leg was calculated as the leg TAG uptake divided by the arterial TAG concentration and represents the "efficiency" of TAG hydrolysis. Values are means with their standard errors represented with vertical bars. Used with permission by the American Physiological Society from [160].

Studies in humans have showed higher fasting and postprandial b-hydroxybutyrate concentrations ~16 h after an exercise session *vs* a control condition possibly indicating higher rates of hepatic fatty acid oxidation [160, 163]. Fasting and postprandial plasma NEFA levels are often elevated in the exercise condition [160, 163] and this may result in higher rates of hepatic fatty acid oxidation due to higher systemic fatty acid delivery to the liver. However, exercise-induced increases in ketone bodies with a concomitant decline in postprandial lipemia have been observed despite similar plasma NEFA levels and, presumably, systemic fatty acid availability to the liver [164]. Evidently, the availability and partition between oxidation and esterification of all sources of fatty acids in the liver and the hepatic VLDL secretory capacity ultimately determine the rate of VLDL-TAG secretion.

Until recently, there was no information on the effect of exercise on VLDL turnover rates in humans. To the best of this investigator's knowledge, two recent studies were the first to investigate VLDL-apoB [165] and VLDL-TAG [166] turnover in humans in response to training or an exercise session. The study by Alam *et al* [165] in type 2 diabetic patients showed that a 6-month exercise training program, involving 20-40 min exercise at 60-85% VO_{2max} 4 times per week, significantly reduced fasting plasma and VLDL-TAG concentrations as well as VLDL apoB secretion rate. VLDL fractional catabolic rate did not change in response to training. These findings were in the absence of the effects of a recent exercise session, because patients had refrained from exercise for 3 d before the study. Thus, the study by Alam *et al* [165] provided evidence that chronic exercise reduces VLDL production, which may explain the beneficial effect of exercise on TAG metabolic capacity. The study by Morio *et al* [166] examined VLDL-TAG turnover during and immediately after a moderate-intensity exercise session in untrained men and women. The authors observed that, whereas VLDL-TAG concentration remained constant throughout the study, VLDL-TAG turnover rate was 70% elevated during exercise and increased to an even greater extent (~90%) in the immediate post-exercise period, i.e. 10-40 min after exercise. VLDL-TAG turnover rate returned to pre-exercise values during the late recovery phase (100-180 min after exercise). The authors speculated that the accelerated VLDL-TAG turnover was due to stimulation of VLDL-TAG synthesis and secretion due to increased delivery of NEFA to the liver [166].

Effects on Intestinal Absorption of Dietary Fat

The potential effect of exercise on gastrointestinal handling of dietary fat has not been specifically investigated. Studies that have looked at gastric emptying using the paracetamol method have found no effect of exercise and by examining the time to peak concentration in the chylomicron-TAG concluded that effects of exercise on the rate of chylomicron appearance into the systemic circulation are unlikely [159, 163]. A study by Kolifa *et al* [167] examined the effects of 1-h exercise performed ~15 h before a meal with a distinct fatty acid composition as compared with fasting plasma TAG-fatty acid composition. They observed that exercise reduced the early postprandial plasma concentrations of dietary fatty acids (as TAG-acyl groups) and speculated it may reflect attenuated release of dietary fat from the intestine but also a more efficient hydrolysis of dietary fat in the exercise condition. The effect of exercise on TAG output from the intestine and its relative contribution, if any, to the post-exercise decline in postprandial lipemia is unknown.

Future Directions

The last two decades significant progress has been made to understand the effects of exercise on postprandial TAG metabolism. However, considering the complexity of the postprandial state and its association with atherosclerosis, a number of unanswered questions remain. The beneficial effects of exercise have been widely documented in healthy individuals and there is a lack of studies to date in individuals with metabolic abnormalities, such as visceral obesity, diabetes, CHD. These conditions are often characterized by postprandial lipoprotein abnormalities [168-170] and so these patients would benefit most from the favorable effects of exercise. Cardiac rehabilitation and exercise training programs have been proven to improve the fasting plasma lipoprotein profile, body composition and other CHD risk factors [171] but information on postprandial lipid metabolism is sparse. The study by Yanes *et al* [172] compared postprandial lipemic response between cardiac patients who had underwent exercise rehabilitation for at least three months and those who had elected not to participate in a regular exercise program. Although fasting lipid profile was improved, no significant differences were observed in the postprandial state. The authors attributed this finding to 1) the large variability in lipemic response within and between the subject groups and 2) the intensity of training which may not have been sufficient to enhance TAG metabolic capacity [172]. Certainly, more studies are needed to examine any favorable effects of exercise on postprandial TRL metabolism in patients with lipoprotein abnormalities.

As discussed, compositional changes of TRL particles in the postprandial state, such as cholesterol-, apoE- and apoC-I enrichment, affect the metabolism and atherogenic potential of these particles. Apo C-II, as LPL activator, and apoC-III also regulate plasma TRL metabolism. It is currently unknown how exercise affects the lipid and apolipoprotein composition of TRL particles. Most of the research for example on the TRL-TAG clearance step in exercise studies has focused on LPL activity, however, it is important to appreciate that several factors other than LPL activity are also critical modulators of the TRL-TAG hydrolysis and clearance process, including the apolipoprotein composition and size of particles. Answers to these questions will increase our understanding on lipoprotein metabolism and its modulation by exercise.

Results from one study that investigated TAG fluxes across leg did not provide direct evidence that increased muscle TAG uptake accounts for the effects of moderate intensity exercise on postprandial lipemia [160]. It is essentially unknown if TRL-TAG clearance by other tissues, such as the splanchnic region and the subcutaneous adipose tissue, is affected by exercise. Under normal conditions, the splanchnic region accounts for as much as 70% of meal-TAG disposal in men [173]. In the case of subcutaneous adipose tissue, which appears to account for ~35% of meal-TAG clearance, it would also be very interesting to know how entrapment of LPL-derived fatty acids is affected and regulated by exercise. The efficiency of entrapment would determine, to some extent, the distribution and availability of TRL-fatty acids to other tissues, such as muscle and liver.

Evidently, exercise may ameliorate fasting and postprandial TAG levels by reducing VLDL-TAG secretion from the liver. Limited information exists in this area in humans. Recent turnover studies [165, 166] showed that chronic exercise reduces VLDL-apoB secretion and that VLDL-TAG turnover is greatly increased during and immediately after moderate-intensity exercise. Whether exercise performed many hours before the meal affects fasting and postprandial TAG secretion rates has never been directly addressed. The mechanisms by which exercise affect TRL metabolism await further investigation. Sex-based exercise effects may also exist considering the distinct sex differences in many aspects of TRL and TAG metabolism [74, 173, 174].

Conclusion

Significant progress has been made in our understanding of postprandial lipoprotein metabolism in health and disease. Postprandial lipemia is transient hypertriacylglycerolemia which, if exaggerated and prolonged, may unfavorably modify plasma lipoproteins generating an atherogenic lipoprotein profile. Regulation of TRL metabolism is complex and TRL particles may have both direct and indirect effects on atherosclerosis. Regular, frequent aerobic exercise may oppose the disturbances to lipoprotein metabolism evident during the postprandial period. Moderate-intensity exercise reduces fasting and postprandial plasma TAG concentrations exerting a delayed and transient effect independent of the energy substrates but dependent on the energy expended during exercise. The impact of exercise on TRL-TAG metabolism is likely to be mediated by enhancement of the TRL-TAG removal pathway as well as reduced hepatic TAG production. Direct evidence for the mechanisms of the exercise effects in humans is scarce. There is much to be learned about the impact of exercise on metabolism and atherogenic potential of TRL particles. As our understanding increases, it will add to the available evidence for the importance of exercise as part of preventive strategies against CHD and other metabolic disorders.

References

[1] Mu, H, Hoy, CE. The digestion of dietary triacylglycerols. *Prog Lipid Res* 2004;43:105-33.

[2] Chen, YD, Reaven, GM. Intestinally-derived lipoproteins: metabolism and clinical significance. *Diabetes Metab Rev* 1991;7:191-208.

[3] Powell, LM, Wallis, SC, Pease, RJ, Edwards, YH, Knott, TJ, Scott, J. A novel form of tissue-specific RNA processing produces apolipoprotein-B48 in intestine. *Cell* 1987;50:831-40.

[4] Green, PH, Glickman, RM. Intestinal lipoprotein metabolism. *J Lipid Res* 1981;22:1153-73.

[5] Hayashi, H, Fujimoto, K, Cardelli, JA, Nutting, DF, Bergstedt, S, Tso, P. Fat feeding increases size, but not number, of chylomicrons produced by small intestine. *Am J Physiol* 1990;259:G709-19.

[6] Hussain, MM. A proposed model for the assembly of chylomicrons. *Atherosclerosis* 2000;148:1-15.

[7] Lundahl, B, Hamsten, A, Karpe, F. Postprandial plasma ApoB-48 levels are influenced by a polymorphism in the promoter of the microsomal triglyceride transfer protein gene. *Arterioscler Thromb Vasc Biol* 2002;22:289-93.

[8] Luchoomun, J, Hussain, MM. Assembly and secretion of chylomicrons by differentiated Caco-2 cells. Nascent triglycerides and preformed phospholipids are preferentially used for lipoprotein assembly. *J Biol Chem* 1999;274:19565-72.

[9] Kayden, HJ, Karmen, A, Dumont, A. Alterations in the Fatty Acid Composition of Human Lymph and Serum Lipoproteins by Single Feedings. *J Clin Invest* 1963;42:1373-81.

[10] Fielding, BA, Callow, J, Owen, RM, Samra, JS, Matthews, DR, Frayn, KN. Postprandial lipemia: the origin of an early peak studied by specific dietary fatty acid intake during sequential meals. *Am J Clin Nutr* 1996;63:36-41.

[11] Jackson, KG, Robertson, MD, Fielding, BA, Frayn, KN, Williams, CM. Olive oil increases the number of triacylglycerol-rich chylomicron particles compared with other oils: an effect retained when a second standard meal is fed. *Am J Clin Nutr* 2002;76:942-9.

[12] Evans, K, Kuusela, PJ, Cruz, ML, Wilhelmova, I, Fielding, BA, Frayn, KN. Rapid chylomicron appearance following sequential meals: effects of second meal composition. *Br J Nutr* 1998;79:425-9.

[13] Mahley, RW, Ji, ZS. Remnant lipoprotein metabolism: key pathways involving cell-surface heparan sulfate proteoglycans and apolipoprotein E. *J Lipid Res* 1999;40:1-16.

[14] Zambon, A, Deeb, SS, Bensadoun, A, Foster, KE, Brunzell, JD. In vivo evidence of a role for hepatic lipase in human apoB-containing lipoprotein metabolism, independent of its lipolytic activity. *J Lipid Res* 2000;41:2094-9.

[15] Heeren, J, Niemeier, A, Merkel, M, Beisiegel, U. Endothelial-derived lipoprotein lipase is bound to postprandial triglyceride-rich lipoproteins and mediates their hepatic clearance in vivo. *J Mol Med* 2002;80:576-84.

[16] Karpe, F, Humphreys, SM, Samra, JS, Summers, LK, Frayn, KN. Clearance of lipoprotein remnant particles in adipose tissue and muscle in humans. *J Lipid Res* 1997;38:2335-43.

[17] Multhaupt, HA, Gafvels, ME, Kariko, K, Jin, H, Arenas-Elliot, C, Goldman, BI, et al. Expression of very low density lipoprotein receptor in the vascular wall. Analysis of human tissues by in situ hybridization and immunohistochemistry. *Am J Pathol* 1996;148:1985-97.

[18] Wyne, KL, Pathak, K, Seabra, MC, Hobbs, HH. Expression of the VLDL receptor in endothelial cells. *Arterioscler Thromb Vasc Biol* 1996;16:407-15.

[19] Niemeier, A, Gafvels, M, Heeren, J, Meyer, N, Angelin, B, Beisiegel, U. VLDL receptor mediates the uptake of human chylomicron remnants in vitro. *J Lipid Res* 1996;37:1733-42.

[20] Davis, RA, Hui, TY. 2000 George Lyman Duff Memorial Lecture: atherosclerosis is a liver disease of the heart. *Arterioscler Thromb Vasc Biol* 2001;21:887-98.

[21] Havel, R. Triglyceride-rich lipoprotein remnants. In: Rifai N, Warnick G, Dominiczak M, editors. Handbook of lipoprotein testing. Washington: AACC Press; 1999.

[22] Parks, EJ, Krauss, RM, Christiansen, MP, Neese, RA, Hellerstein, MK. Effects of a low-fat, high-carbohydrate diet on VLDL-triglyceride assembly, production, and clearance. *J Clin Invest* 1999;104:1087-96.

[23] Packard, CJ, Munro, A, Lorimer, AR, Gotto, AM, Shepherd, J. Metabolism of apolipoprotein B in large triglyceride-rich very low density lipoproteins of normal and hypertriglyceridemic subjects. *J Clin Invest* 1984;74:2178-92.

[24] Packard, CJ, Shepherd, J. Lipoprotein heterogeneity and apolipoprotein B metabolism. *Arterioscler Thromb Vasc Biol* 1997;17:3542-56.

[25] Schneeman, BO, Kotite, L, Todd, KM, Havel, RJ. Relationships between the responses of triglyceride-rich lipoproteins in blood plasma containing apolipoproteins B-48 and B-100 to a fat-containing meal in normolipidemic humans. *Proc Natl Acad Sci U S A* 1993;90:2069-73.

[26] Brunzell, JD, Hazzard, WR, Porte, D, Jr., Bierman, EL. Evidence for a common, saturable, triglyceride removal mechanism for chylomicrons and very low density lipoproteins in man. *J Clin Invest* 1973;52:1578-85.

[27] Potts, JL, Fisher, RM, Humphreys, SM, Coppack, SW, Gibbons, GF, Frayn, KN. Peripheral triacylglycerol extraction in the fasting and post-prandial states. *Clin Sci (Lond)* 1991;81:621-6.

[28] Karpe, F, Steiner, G, Olivecrona, T, Carlson, LA, Hamsten, A. Metabolism of triglyceride-rich lipoproteins during alimentary lipemia. *J Clin Invest* 1993;91:748-58.

[29] Björkegren, J, Packard, CJ, Hamsten, A, Bedford, D, Caslake, M, Foster, L, *et al.* Accumulation of large very low density lipoprotein in plasma during intravenous infusion of a chylomicron-like triglyceride emulsion reflects competition for a common lipolytic pathway. *J Lipid Res* 1996;37:76-86.

[30] Heath, RB, Karpe, F, Milne, RW, Burdge, GC, Wootton, SA, Frayn, KN. Selective partitioning of dietary fatty acids into the VLDL TG pool in the early postprandial period. *J Lipid Res* 2003;44:2065-72.

[31] Jong, MC, Hofker, MH, Havekes, LM. Role of ApoCs in lipoprotein metabolism: functional differences between ApoC1, ApoC2, and ApoC3. *Arterioscler Thromb Vasc Biol* 1999;19:472-84.

[32] Weisgraber, KH, Mahley, RW, Kowal, RC, Herz, J, Goldstein, JL, Brown, MS. Apolipoprotein C-I modulates the interaction of apolipoprotein E with beta-migrating very low density lipoproteins (beta-VLDL) and inhibits binding of beta-VLDL to low density lipoprotein receptor-related protein. *J Biol Chem* 1990;265:22453-9.

[33] Jong, MC, Dahlmans, VE, van Gorp, PJ, van Dijk, KW, Breuer, ML, Hofker, MH, *et al*. In the absence of the low density lipoprotein receptor, human apolipoprotein C1 overexpression in transgenic mice inhibits the hepatic uptake of very low density lipoproteins via a receptor-associated protein-sensitive pathway. *J Clin Invest* 1996;98:2259-67.

[34] Jong, MC, van Ree, JH, Dahlmans, VE, Frants, RR, Hofker, MH, Havekes, LM. Reduced very-low-density lipoprotein fractional catabolic rate in apolipoprotein C1-deficient mice. *Biochem J* 1997;321 (Pt 2):445-50.

[35] Björkegren, J, Boquist, S, Samnegard, A, Lundman, P, Tornvall, P, Ericsson, CG, *et al.* Accumulation of apolipoprotein C-I-rich and cholesterol-rich VLDL remnants during exaggerated postprandial triglyceridemia in normolipidemic patients with coronary artery disease. *Circulation* 2000;101:227-30.

[36] Björkegren, J, Silveira, A, Boquist, S, Tang, R, Karpe, F, Bond, MG, *et al.* Postprandial enrichment of remnant lipoproteins with apoC-I in healthy normolipidemic men with early asymptomatic atherosclerosis. *Arterioscler Thromb Vasc Biol* 2002;22:1470-4.

[37] Shachter, NS, Ebara, T, Ramakrishnan, R, Steiner, G, Breslow, JL, Ginsberg, HN, *et al.* Combined hyperlipidemia in transgenic mice overexpressing human apolipoprotein Cl. *J Clin Invest* 1996;98:846-55.

[38] Windler, E, Havel, RJ. Inhibitory effects of C apolipoproteins from rats and humans on the uptake of triglyceride-rich lipoproteins and their remnants by the perfused rat liver. *J Lipid Res* 1985;26:556-65.

[39] Mann, CJ, Troussard, AA, Yen, FT, Hannouche, N, Najib, J, Fruchart, JC, *et al.* Inhibitory effects of specific apolipoprotein C-III isoforms on the binding of triglyceride-rich lipoproteins to the lipolysis-stimulated receptor. *J Biol Chem* 1997;272:31348-54.

[40] Ginsberg, HN, Le, NA, Goldberg, IJ, Gibson, JC, Rubinstein, A, Wang-Iverson, P, *et al.* Apolipoprotein B metabolism in subjects with deficiency of apolipoproteins CIII and AI. Evidence that apolipoprotein CIII inhibits catabolism of triglyceride-rich lipoproteins by lipoprotein lipase in vivo. *J Clin Invest* 1986;78:1287-95.

[41] Maeda, N, Li, H, Lee, D, Oliver, P, Quarfordt, SH, Osada, J. Targeted disruption of the apolipoprotein C-III gene in mice results in hypotriglyceridemia and protection from postprandial hypertriglyceridemia. *J Biol Chem* 1994;269:23610-6.

[42] Cohn, JS, Patterson, BW, Uffelman, KD, Davignon, J, Steiner, G. Rate of production of plasma and very-low-density lipoprotein (VLDL) apolipoprotein C-III is strongly related to the concentration and level of production of VLDL triglyceride in male subjects with different body weights and levels of insulin sensitivity. *J Clin Endocrinol Metab* 2004;89:3949-55.

[43] Dallongeville, J, Lussier-Cacan, S, Davignon, J. Modulation of plasma triglyceride levels by apoE phenotype: a meta-analysis. *J Lipid Res* 1992;33:447-54.

[44] Dallongeville, J, Tiret, L, Visvikis, S, O'Reilly, DS, Saava, M, Tsitouris, G, *et al.* Effect of apo E phenotype on plasma postprandial triglyceride levels in young male adults with and without a familial history of myocardial infarction: the EARS II study. European Atherosclerosis Research Study. *Atherosclerosis* 1999;145:381-8.

[45] Weisgraber, KH, Innerarity, TL, Mahley, RW. Abnormal lipoprotein receptor-binding activity of the human E apoprotein due to cysteine-arginine interchange at a single site. *J Biol Chem* 1982;257:2518-21.

[46] Bergeron, N, Havel, RJ. Prolonged postprandial responses of lipids and apolipoproteins in triglyceride-rich lipoproteins of individuals expressing an apolipoprotein epsilon 4 allele. *J Clin Invest* 1996;97:65-72.

[47] Lewis, GF, Uffelman, KD, Szeto, LW, Weller, B, Steiner, G. Interaction between free fatty acids and insulin in the acute control of very low density lipoprotein production in humans. *J Clin Invest* 1995;95:158-66.

[48] Lewis, GF, Uffelman, KD, Szeto, LW, Steiner, G. Effects of acute hyperinsulinemia on VLDL triglyceride and VLDL apoB production in normal weight and obese individuals. *Diabetes* 1993;42:833-42.

[49] Mittendorfer, B, Patterson, BW, Klein, S, Sidossis, LS. VLDL-triglyceride kinetics during hyperglycemia-hyperinsulinemia: effects of sex and obesity. *Am J Physiol Endocrinol Metab* 2003;284:E708-15.

[50] Frayn, KN, Shadid, S, Hamlani, R, Humphreys, SM, Clark, ML, Fielding, BA, *et al.* Regulation of fatty acid movement in human adipose tissue in the postabsorptive-to-postprandial transition. *Am J Physiol* 1994;266:E308-17.

[51] Coppack, SW, Jensen, MD, Miles, JM. In vivo regulation of lipolysis in humans. *J Lipid Res* 1994;35:177-93.

[52] Malmstrom, R, Packard, CJ, Watson, TD, Rannikko, S, Caslake, M, Bedford, D, *et al.* Metabolic basis of hypotriglyceridemic effects of insulin in normal men. *Arterioscler Thromb Vasc Biol* 1997;17:1454-64.

[53] Campbell, PJ, Carlson, MG, Hill, JO, Nurjhan, N. Regulation of free fatty acid metabolism by insulin in humans: role of lipolysis and reesterification. *Am J Physiol* 1992;263:E1063-9.

[54] Evans, K, Burdge, GC, Wootton, SA, Clark, ML, Frayn, KN. Regulation of dietary fatty acid entrapment in subcutaneous adipose tissue and skeletal muscle. *Diabetes* 2002;51:2684-90.

[55] Miles, JM, Park, YS, Walewicz, D, Russell-Lopez, C, Windsor, S, Isley, WL, et al. Systemic and forearm triglyceride metabolism: fate of lipoprotein lipase-generated glycerol and free fatty acids. *Diabetes* 2004;53:521-7.

[56] Frayn, KN, Humphreys, SM, Coppack, SW. "Fuel selection in white adipose tissue". *Proc Nutr Soc* 1995;54:177-189.

[57] Coppack, SW, Fisher, RM, Gibbons, GF, Humphreys, SM, McDonough, MJ, Potts, JL, et al. Postprandial substrate deposition in human forearm and adipose tissues in vivo. *Clin Sci (Lond)* 1990;79:339-48.

[58] Sadur, CN, Eckel, RH. Insulin stimulation of adipose tissue lipoprotein lipase. Use of the euglycemic clamp technique. *J Clin Invest* 1982;69:1119-25.

[59] Picard, F, Naimi, N, Richard, D, Deshaies, Y. Response of adipose tissue lipoprotein lipase to the cephalic phase of insulin secretion. *Diabetes* 1999;48:452-9.

[60] Braun, JE, Severson, DL. Regulation of the synthesis, processing and translocation of lipoprotein lipase. *Biochem J* 1992;287 (Pt 2):337-47.

[61] Preiss-Landl, K, Zimmermann, R, Hammerle, G, Zechner, R. Lipoprotein lipase: the regulation of tissue specific expression and its role in lipid and energy metabolism. *Curr Opin Lipidol* 2002;13:471-81.

[62] Farese, RV, Jr., Yost, TJ, Eckel, RH. Tissue-specific regulation of lipoprotein lipase activity by insulin/glucose in normal-weight humans. *Metabolism* 1991;40:214-6.

[63] Yost, TJ, Jensen, DR, Haugen, BR, Eckel, RH. Effect of dietary macronutrient composition on tissue-specific lipoprotein lipase activity and insulin action in normal-weight subjects. *Am J Clin Nutr* 1998;68:296-302.

[64] Cianflone, K, Xia, Z, Chen, LY. Critical review of acylation-stimulating protein physiology in humans and rodents. *Biochim Biophys Acta* 2003;1609:127-43.

[65] Faraj, M, Sniderman, AD, Cianflone, K. ASP enhances in situ lipoprotein lipase activity by increasing fatty acid trapping in adipocytes. *J Lipid Res* 2004;45:657-66.

[66] Saleh, J, Summers, LK, Cianflone, K, Fielding, BA, Sniderman, AD, Frayn, KN. Coordinated release of acylation stimulating protein (ASP) and triacylglycerol clearance by human adipose tissue in vivo in the postprandial period. *J Lipid Res* 1998;39:884-91.

[67] Karpe, F, Olivecrona, T, Hamsten, A, Hultin, M. Chylomicron/chylomicron remnant turnover in humans: evidence for margination of chylomicrons and poor conversion of larger to smaller chylomicron remnants. *J Lipid Res* 1997;38:949-61.

[68] Hultin, M, Olivecrona, T. Conversion of chylomicrons into remnants. *Atherosclerosis* 1998;141 Suppl 1:S25-9.

[69] Cryer, A. Tissue lipoprotein lipase activity and its action in lipoprotein metabolism. *Int J Biochem* 1981;13:525-41.

[70] Eckel, RH. Lipoprotein lipase. A multifunctional enzyme relevant to common metabolic diseases. *N Engl J Med* 1989;320:1060-8.

[71] Ladu, MJ, Kapsas, H, Palmer, WK. Regulation of lipoprotein lipase in adipose and muscle tissues during fasting. *Am J Physiol* 1991;260:R953-9.

[72] Eriksson, JW, Buren, J, Svensson, M, Olivecrona, T, Olivecrona, G. Postprandial regulation of blood lipids and adipose tissue lipoprotein lipase in type 2 diabetes patients and healthy control subjects. *Atherosclerosis* 2003;166:359-67.

[73] Fielding, BA, Frayn, KN. Lipoprotein lipase and the disposition of dietary fatty acids. *Br J Nutr* 1998;80:495-502.

[74] Horton, TJ, Commerford, SR, Pagliassotti, MJ, Bessesen, DH. Postprandial leg uptake of triglyceride is greater in women than in men. *Am J Physiol Endocrinol Metab* 2002;283:E1192-202.

[75] Saxena, U, Witte, LD, Goldberg, IJ. Release of endothelial cell lipoprotein lipase by plasma lipoproteins and free fatty acids. *J Biol Chem* 1989;264:4349-55.

[76] Karpe, F, Olivecrona, T, Walldius, G, Hamsten, A. Lipoprotein lipase in plasma after an oral fat load: relation to free fatty acids. *J Lipid Res* 1992;33:975-84.

[77] Hokanson, JE, Austin, MA. Plasma triglyceride level is a risk factor for cardiovascular disease independent of high-density lipoprotein cholesterol level: a meta-analysis of population-based prospective studies. *J Cardiovasc Risk* 1996;3:213-9.

[78] Jeppesen, J, Hein, HO, Suadicani, P, Gyntelberg, F. Triglyceride concentration and ischemic heart disease: an eight-year follow-up in the Copenhagen Male Study. *Circulation* 1998;97:1029-36.

[79] Karpe, F. Postprandial lipoprotein metabolism and atherosclerosis. *J Intern Med* 1999;246:341-55.

[80] Havel, RJ. Remnant lipoproteins as therapeutic targets. *Curr Opin Lipidol* 2000;11:615-20.

[81] Proctor, SD, Vine, DF, Mamo, JC. Arterial retention of apolipoprotein B(48)- and B(100)-containing lipoproteins in atherogenesis. *Curr Opin Lipidol* 2002;13:461-70.

[82] Patsch, JR, Miesenbock, G, Hopferwieser, T, Muhlberger, V, Knapp, E, Dunn, JK, *et al*. Relation of triglyceride metabolism and coronary artery disease. Studies in the postprandial state. *Arterioscler Thromb* 1992;12:1336-45.

[83] Groot, PH, van Stiphout, WA, Krauss, XH, Jansen, H, van Tol, A, van Ramshorst, E, *et al*. Postprandial lipoprotein metabolism in normolipidemic men with and without coronary artery disease. *Arterioscler Thromb* 1991;11:653-62.

[84] Nikkila, M, Solakivi, T, Lehtimaki, T, Koivula, T, Laippala, P, Astrom, B. Postprandial plasma lipoprotein changes in relation to apolipoprotein E phenotypes and low density lipoprotein size in men with and without coronary artery disease. *Atherosclerosis* 1994;106:149-57.

[85] Ryu, JE, Howard, G, Craven, TE, Bond, MG, Hagaman, AP, Crouse, JR, 3rd. Postprandial triglyceridemia and carotid atherosclerosis in middle-aged subjects. *Stroke* 1992;23:823-8.

[86] Sharrett, AR, Chambless, LE, Heiss, G, Paton, CC, Patsch, W. Association of postprandial triglyceride and retinyl palmitate responses with asymptomatic carotid artery atherosclerosis in middle-aged men and women. The Atherosclerosis Risk in Communities (ARIC) Study. *Arterioscler Thromb Vasc Biol* 1995;15:2122-9.

[87] Karpe, F, de Faire, U, Mercuri, M, Bond, MG, Hellenius, ML, Hamsten, A. Magnitude of alimentary lipemia is related to intima-media thickness of the common carotid artery in middle-aged men. *Atherosclerosis* 1998;141:307-14.

[88] Boquist, S, Ruotolo, G, Tang, R, Björkegren, J, Bond, MG, de Faire, U, *et al.* Alimentary lipemia, postprandial triglyceride-rich lipoproteins, and common carotid intima-media thickness in healthy, middle-aged men. *Circulation* 1999;100:723-8.

[89] Lundman, P, Eriksson, M, Schenck-Gustafsson, K, Karpe, F, Tornvall, P. Transient triglyceridemia decreases vascular reactivity in young, healthy men without risk factors for coronary heart disease. *Circulation* 1997;96:3266-8.

[90] Bae, JH, Bassenge, E, Kim, KB, Kim, YN, Kim, KS, Lee, HJ, *et al.* Postprandial hypertriglyceridemia impairs endothelial function by enhanced oxidant stress. *Atherosclerosis* 2001;155:517-23.

[91] Silveira, A, Karpe, F, Blomback, M, Steiner, G, Walldius, G, Hamsten, A. Activation of coagulation factor VII during alimentary lipemia. *Arterioscler Thromb* 1994;14:60-9.

[92] Byrne, CD, Wareham, NJ, Martensz, ND, Humphries, SE, Metcalfe, JC, Grainger, DJ. Increased PAI activity and PAI-1 antigen occurring with an oral fat load: associations with PAI-1 genotype and plasma active TGF-beta levels. *Atherosclerosis* 1998;140:45-53.

[93] Zilversmit, DB. Atherogenesis: a postprandial phenomenon. *Circulation* 1979;60:473-85.

[94] Hodis, HN, Mack, WJ. Triglyceride-rich lipoproteins and progression of atherosclerosis. *Eur Heart J* 1998;19 Suppl A:A40-4.

[95] Hodis, HN. Triglyceride-rich lipoprotein remnant particles and risk of atherosclerosis. *Circulation* 1999;99:2852-4.

[96] Shaikh, M, Wootton, R, Nordestgaard, BG, Baskerville, P, Lumley, JS, La Ville, AE, *et al.* Quantitative studies of transfer in vivo of low density, Sf 12-60, and Sf 60-400 lipoproteins between plasma and arterial intima in humans. *Arterioscler Thromb* 1991;11:569-77.

[97] Tornvall, P, Bavenholm, P, Landou, C, de Faire, U, Hamsten, A. Relation of plasma levels and composition of apolipoprotein B-containing lipoproteins to angiographically defined coronary artery disease in young patients with myocardial infarction. *Circulation* 1993;88:2180-9.

[98] Björkegren, J, Hamsten, A, Milne, RW, Karpe, F. Alterations of VLDL composition during alimentary lipemia. *J Lipid Res* 1997;38:301-14.

[99] Björkegren, J, Karpe, F, Milne, RW, Hamsten, A. Differences in apolipoprotein and lipid composition between human chylomicron remnants and very low density lipoproteins isolated from fasting and postprandial plasma. *J Lipid Res* 1998;39:1412-20.

[100] Rapp, JH, Lespine, A, Hamilton, RL, Colyvas, N, Chaumeton, AH, Tweedie-Hardman, J, *et al.* Triglyceride-rich lipoproteins isolated by selected-affinity anti-apolipoprotein B immunosorption from human atherosclerotic plaque. *Arterioscler Thromb* 1994;14:1767-74.

[101] Nakajima, K, Saito, T, Tamura, A, Suzuki, M, Nakano, T, Adachi, M, *et al.* Cholesterol in remnant-like lipoproteins in human serum using monoclonal anti apo B-100 and anti apo A-I immunoaffinity mixed gels. *Clin Chim Acta* 1993;223:53-71.

[102] Devaraj, S, Vega, G, Lange, R, Grundy, SM, Jialal, I. Remnant-like particle cholesterol levels in patients with dysbetalipoproteinemia or coronary artery disease. *Am J Med* 1998;104:445-50.

[103] Takeichi, S, Yukawa, N, Nakajima, Y, Osawa, M, Saito, T, Seto, Y, et al. Association of plasma triglyceride-rich lipoprotein remnants with coronary atherosclerosis in cases of sudden cardiac death. *Atherosclerosis* 1999;142:309-15.

[104] McNamara, JR, Shah, PK, Nakajima, K, Cupples, LA, Wilson, PW, Ordovas, JM, et al. Remnant lipoprotein cholesterol and triglyceride reference ranges from the Framingham Heart Study. *Clin Chem* 1998;44:1224-32.

[105] Veniant, MM, Pierotti, V, Newland, D, Cham, CM, Sanan, DA, Walzem, RL, et al. Susceptibility to atherosclerosis in mice expressing exclusively apolipoprotein B48 or apolipoprotein B100. *J Clin Invest* 1997;100:180-8.

[106] Flood, C, Gustafsson, M, Richardson, PE, Harvey, SC, Segrest, JP, Boren, J. Identification of the proteoglycan binding site in apolipoprotein B48. *J Biol Chem* 2002;277:32228-33.

[107] Tall, AR, Jiang, X, Luo, Y, Silver, D. 1999 George Lyman Duff memorial lecture: lipid transfer proteins, HDL metabolism, and atherogenesis. *Arterioscler Thromb Vasc Biol* 2000;20:1185-8.

[108] Eisenberg, S. High density lipoprotein metabolism. *J Lipid Res* 1984;25:1017-58.

[109] O'Meara, NM, Lewis, GF, Cabana, VG, Iverius, PH, Getz, GS, Polonsky, KS. Role of basal triglyceride and high density lipoprotein in determination of postprandial lipid and lipoprotein responses. *J Clin Endocrinol Metab* 1992;75:465-71.

[110] Patsch, JR, Karlin, JB, Scott, LW, Smith, LC, Gotto, AM, Jr. Inverse relationship between blood levels of high density lipoprotein subfraction 2 and magnitude of postprandial lipemia. *Proc Natl Acad Sci U S A* 1983;80:1449-53.

[111] Tall, AR. Metabolic and genetic control of HDL cholesterol levels. *J Intern Med* 1992;231:661-8.

[112] Lamarche, B, Uffelman, KD, Carpentier, A, Cohn, JS, Steiner, G, Barrett, PH, et al. Triglyceride enrichment of HDL enhances in vivo metabolic clearance of HDL apo A-I in healthy men. *J Clin Invest* 1999;103:1191-9.

[113] Eisenberg, S. Preferential enrichment of large-sized very low density lipoprotein populations with transferred cholesteryl esters. *J Lipid Res* 1985;26:487-94.

[114] Patsch, JR, Prasad, S, Gotto, AM, Jr., Patsch, W. High density lipoprotein2. Relationship of the plasma levels of this lipoprotein species to its composition, to the magnitude of postprandial lipemia, and to the activities of lipoprotein lipase and hepatic lipase. *J Clin Invest* 1987;80:341-7.

[115] Karpe, F, Bard, JM, Steiner, G, Carlson, LA, Fruchart, JC, Hamsten, A. HDLs and alimentary lipemia. Studies in men with previous myocardial infarction at a young age. *Arterioscler Thromb* 1993;13:11-22.

[116] Cohen, JC, Stray-Gundersen, J, Grundy, SM. Dissociation between postprandial lipemia and high density lipoprotein cholesterol concentrations in endurance-trained men. *Arterioscler Thromb* 1991;11:838-43.

[117] Cohen, JC, Grundy, SM. Normal postprandial lipemia in men with low plasma HDL concentrations. *Arterioscler Thromb* 1992;12:972-5.

[118] Austin, MA, Breslow, JL, Hennekens, CH, Buring, JE, Willett, WC, Krauss, RM. Low-density lipoprotein subclass patterns and risk of myocardial infarction. *Jama* 1988;260:1917-21.

[119] Griffin, BA, Freeman, DJ, Tait, GW, Thomson, J, Caslake, MJ, Packard, CJ, *et al.* Role of plasma triglyceride in the regulation of plasma low density lipoprotein (LDL) subfractions: relative contribution of small, dense LDL to coronary heart disease risk. *Atherosclerosis* 1994;106:241-53.

[120] Gardner, CD, Fortmann, SP, Krauss, RM. Association of small low-density lipoprotein particles with the incidence of coronary artery disease in men and women. *Jama* 1996;276:875-81.

[121] Griffin, BA. Lipoprotein atherogenicity: an overview of current mechanisms. *Proc Nutr Soc* 1999;58:163-9.

[122] McNamara, JR, Jenner, JL, Li, Z, Wilson, PW, Schaefer, EJ. Change in LDL particle size is associated with change in plasma triglyceride concentration. *Arterioscler Thromb* 1992;12:1284-90.

[123] Packard, CJ. Understanding coronary heart disease as a consequence of defective regulation of apolipoprotein B metabolism. *Curr Opin Lipidol* 1999;10:237-44.

[124] Karpe, F, Tornvall, P, Olivecrona, T, Steiner, G, Carlson, LA, Hamsten, A. Composition of human low density lipoprotein: effects of postprandial triglyceride-rich lipoproteins, lipoprotein lipase, hepatic lipase and cholesteryl ester transfer protein. *Atherosclerosis* 1993;98:33-49.

[125] Johanson, EH, Jansson, PA, Gustafson, B, Lonn, L, Smith, U, Taskinen, MR, *et al.* Early alterations in the postprandial VLDL1 apoB-100 and apoB-48 metabolism in men with strong heredity for type 2 diabetes. *J Intern Med* 2004;255:273-9.

[126] Lemieux, I, Couillard, C, Pascot, A, Bergeron, N, Prud'homme, D, Bergeron, J, *et al.* The small, dense LDL phenotype as a correlate of postprandial lipemia in men. *Atherosclerosis* 2000;153:423-32.

[127] Potts, JL, Humphreys, SM, Coppack, SW, Fisher, RM, Gibbons, GF, Frayn, KN. Fasting plasma triacylglycerol concentrations predict adverse changes in lipoprotein metabolism after a normal meal. *Br J Nutr* 1994;72:101-9.

[128] Cohen, JC, Noakes, TD, Benade, AJ. Postprandial lipemia and chylomicron clearance in athletes and in sedentary men. *Am J Clin Nutr* 1989;49:443-7.

[129] Merrill, JR, Holly, RG, Anderson, RL, Rifai, N, King, ME, DeMeersman, R. Hyperlipemic response of young trained and untrained men after a high fat meal. *Arteriosclerosis* 1989;9:217-23.

[130] Tsetsonis, NV, Hardman, AE, Mastana, SS. Acute effects of exercise on postprandial lipemia: a comparative study in trained and untrained middle-aged women. *Am J Clin Nutr* 1997;65:525-33.

[131] Herd, SL, Lawrence, JE, Malkova, D, Murphy, MH, Mastana, S, Hardman, AE. Postprandial lipemia in young men and women of contrasting training status. *J Appl Physiol* 2000;89:2049-56.

[132] Hardman, AE, Lawrence, JE, Herd, SL. Postprandial lipemia in endurance-trained people during a short interruption to training. *J Appl Physiol* 1998;84:1895-901.

[133] Cohen, H, Goldberg, C. Effect of physical exercise on alimentary lipaemia. *Brookhaven Symp Biol* 1960;5197:509-11.

[134] Zhang, JQ, Thomas, TR, Ball, SD. Effect of exercise timing on postprandial lipemia and HDL cholesterol subfractions. *J Appl Physiol* 1998;85:1516-22.

[135] Petitt, DS, Cureton, KJ. Effects of prior exercise on postprandial lipemia: a quantitative review. *Metabolism* 2003;52:418-24.

[136] Tsetsonis, NV, Hardman, AE. Reduction in postprandial lipemia after walking: influence of exercise intensity. *Med Sci Sports Exerc* 1996;28:1235-42.

[137] Malkova, D, Hardman, AE, Bowness, RJ, Macdonald, IA. The reduction in postprandial lipemia after exercise is independent of the relative contributions of fat and carbohydrate to energy metabolism during exercise. *Metabolism* 1999;48:245-51.

[138] Murphy, MH, Nevill, AM, Hardman, AE. Different patterns of brisk walking are equally effective in decreasing postprandial lipaemia. *Int J Obes Relat Metab Disord* 2000;24:1303-9.

[139] Gill, JM, Hardman, AE. Postprandial lipemia: effects of exercise and restriction of energy intake compared. *Am J Clin Nutr* 2000;71:465-71.

[140] Petitt, DS, Arngrimsson, SA, Cureton, KJ. Effect of resistance exercise on postprandial lipemia. *J Appl Physiol* 2003;94:694-700.

[141] Katsanos, CS, Grandjean, PW, Moffatt, RJ. Effects of low and moderate exercise intensity on postprandial lipemia and postheparin plasma lipoprotein lipase activity in physically active men. *J Appl Physiol* 2004;96:181-8.

[142] Tsetsonis, NV, Hardman, AE. Effects of low and moderate intensity treadmill walking on postprandial lipaemia in healthy young adults. *Eur J Appl Physiol Occup Physiol* 1996;73:419-26.

[143] Kantor, MA, Cullinane, EM, Sady, SP, Herbert, PN, Thompson, PD. Exercise acutely increases high density lipoprotein-cholesterol and lipoprotein lipase activity in trained and untrained men. *Metabolism* 1987;36:188-92.

[144] Podl, TR, Zmuda, JM, Yurgalevitch, SM, Fahrenbach, MC, Bausserman, LL, Terry, RB, *et al.* Lipoprotein lipase activity and plasma triglyceride clearance are elevated in endurance-trained women. *Metabolism* 1994;43:808-13.

[145] Nikkila, EA, Taskinen, MR, Rehunen, S, Harkonen, M. Lipoprotein lipase activity in adipose tissue and skeletal muscle of runners: relation to serum lipoproteins. *Metabolism* 1978;27:1661-7.

[146] Seip, RL, Angelopoulos, TJ, Semenkovich, CF. Exercise induces human lipoprotein lipase gene expression in skeletal muscle but not adipose tissue. *Am J Physiol* 1995;268:E229-36.

[147] Lithell, H, Hellsing, K, Lundqvist, G, Malmberg, P. Lipoprotein-lipase activity of human skeletal-muscle and adipose tissue after intensive physical exercise. *Acta Physiol Scand* 1979;105:312-5.

[148] Lithell, H, Orlander, J, Schele, R, Sjodin, B, Karlsson, J. Changes in lipoprotein-lipase activity and lipid stores in human skeletal muscle with prolonged heavy exercise. *Acta Physiol Scand* 1979;107:257-61.

[149] Kiens, B, Lithell, H, Mikines, KJ, Richter, EA. Effects of insulin and exercise on muscle lipoprotein lipase activity in man and its relation to insulin action. *J Clin Invest* 1989;84:1124-9.

[150] Kiens, B, Lithell, H. Lipoprotein metabolism influenced by training-induced changes in human skeletal muscle. *J Clin Invest* 1989;83:558-64.

[151] Greiwe, JS, Holloszy, JO, Semenkovich, CF. Exercise induces lipoprotein lipase and GLUT-4 protein in muscle independent of adrenergic-receptor signaling. *J Appl Physiol* 2000;89:176-81.

[152] Seip, RL, Mair, K, Cole, TG, Semenkovich, CF. Induction of human skeletal muscle lipoprotein lipase gene expression by short-term exercise is transient. *Am J Physiol* 1997;272:E255-61.

[153] Pedersen, SB, Bak, JF, Holck, P, Schmitz, O, Richelsen, B. Epinephrine stimulates human muscle lipoprotein lipase activity in vivo. *Metabolism* 1999;48:461-4.

[154] Deeb, SS, Peng, RL. Structure of the human lipoprotein lipase gene. *Biochemistry* 1989;28:4131-5.

[155] Seip, RL, Semenkovich, CF. Skeletal muscle lipoprotein lipase: molecular regulation and physiological effects in relation to exercise. *Exerc Sport Sci Rev* 1998;26:191-218.

[156] Herd, SL, Kiens, B, Boobis, LH, Hardman, AE. Moderate exercise, postprandial lipemia, and skeletal muscle lipoprotein lipase activity. *Metabolism* 2001;50:756-62.

[157] Sady, SP, Thompson, PD, Cullinane, EM, Kantor, MA, Domagala, E, Herbert, PN. Prolonged exercise augments plasma triglyceride clearance. *Jama* 1986;256:2552-5.

[158] Annuzzi, G, Jansson, E, Kaijser, L, Holmquist, L, Carlson, LA. Increased removal rate of exogenous triglycerides after prolonged exercise in man: time course and effect of exercise duration. *Metabolism* 1987;36:438-43.

[159] Gill, JM, Mees, GP, Frayn, KN, Hardman, AE. Moderate exercise, postprandial lipaemia and triacylglycerol clearance. *Eur J Clin Invest* 2001;31:201-7.

[160] Malkova, D, Evans, RD, Frayn, KN, Humphreys, SM, Jones, PR, Hardman, AE. Prior exercise and postprandial substrate extraction across the human leg. *Am J Physiol Endocrinol Metab* 2000;279:E1020-8.

[161] Simonelli, C, Eaton, RP. Reduced triglyceride secretion: a metabolic consequence of chronic exercise. *Am J Physiol* 1978;234:E221-7.

[162] Mondon, CE, Dolkas, CB, Tobey, T, Reaven, GM. Causes of the triglyceride-lowering effect of exercise training in rats. *J Appl Physiol* 1984;57:1466-71.

[163] Gill, JM, Frayn, KN, Wootton, SA, Miller, GJ, Hardman, AE. Effects of prior moderate exercise on exogenous and endogenous lipid metabolism and plasma factor VII activity. *Clin Sci (Lond)* 2001;100:517-27.

[164] Koutsari, C, Karpe, F, Humphreys, SM, Frayn, KN, Hardman, AE. Exercise prevents the accumulation of triglyceride-rich lipoproteins and their remnants seen when changing to a high-carbohydrate diet. *Arterioscler Thromb Vasc Biol* 2001;21:1520-5.

[165] Alam, S, Stolinski, M, Pentecost, C, Boroujerdi, MA, Jones, RH, Sonksen, PH, *et al.* The effect of a six-month exercise program on very low-density lipoprotein apolipoprotein B secretion in type 2 diabetes. *J Clin Endocrinol Metab* 2004;89:688-94.

[166] Morio, B, Holmback, U, Gore, D, Wolfe, RR. Increased VLDL-TAG turnover during and after acute moderate-intensity exercise. *Med Sci Sports Exerc* 2004;36:801-6.

[167] Kolifa, M, Petridou, A, Mougios, V. Effect of prior exercise on lipemia after a meal of moderate fat content. *Eur J Clin Nutr* 2004.

[168] Couillard, C, Bergeron, N, Pascot, A, Almeras, N, Bergeron, J, Tremblay, A, *et al*. Evidence for impaired lipolysis in abdominally obese men: postprandial study of apolipoprotein B-48- and B-100-containing lipoproteins. *Am J Clin Nutr* 2002;76:311-8.

[169] Ginsberg, HN, Illingworth, DR. Postprandial dyslipidemia: an atherogenic disorder common in patients with diabetes mellitus. *Am J Cardiol* 2001;88:9H-15H.

[170] Karpe, F, Hellenius, ML, Hamsten, A. Differences in postprandial concentrations of very-low-density lipoprotein and chylomicron remnants between normotriglyceridemic and hypertriglyceridemic men with and without coronary heart disease. *Metabolism* 1999;48:301-7.

[171] Lavie, CJ, Milani, RV. Effects of cardiac rehabilitation and exercise training in obese patients with coronary artery disease. *Chest* 1996;109:52-6.

[172] Yanes, AM, Holly, RG, Schneeman, BO, Amsterdam, EA. Effect of cardiac rehabilitation on postprandial response to a high fat meal in patients with coronary artery disease. *Atherosclerosis* 1989;78:1-8.

[173] Nguyen, TT, Mijares, AH, Johnson, CM, Jensen, MD. Postprandial leg and splanchnic fatty acid metabolism in nonobese men and women. *Am J Physiol* 1996;271:E965-72.

[174] Mittendorfer, B, Patterson, BW, Klein, S. Effect of sex and obesity on basal VLDL-triacylglycerol kinetics. *Am J Clin Nutr* 2003;77:573-9.

Chapter V

Hypothalamo-Pituitary-Adrenal Axis Adaptation to Repeated and Prolonged Exercise-Induced Cortisol Secretion in Endurance Training: Physiology is the First Target

Duclos Martine[*]

Laboratoire Neurogénétique et Stress, INRA-UMR 1243, Institut François Magendie, 146 rue Léo Saignat, Université Bordeaux II, 33077 Bordeaux Cedex, France
Service Sport-Santé, CHU Pellegrin, Pl. A. Raba-Leon, 33077 Bordeaux Cedex, France

Abstract

Exercise represents a potent physiological stimulus upon the hypothalamo-pituitary adrenal (HPA) axis. Glucocorticoids (GC) exert many beneficial actions in exercising humans, increasing availability of metabolic substrates for the need of energy of muscles, maintaining normal vascular integrity and responsiveness and protecting the organism from an overreaction of the immune system in the face of exercise-induced muscle damage. On the other hand, when an acute bout of endurance-exercise is stopped, the hormonal profile is expected to converge towards anabolic processes. However, we have previously demonstrated that after a 2-h run, plasma cortisol levels remain significantly increased during almost two hours after the end of the exercise. When training for a marathon race, subjects run an average of 120-180 km/week. This implies daily sessions of prolonged and/or intense running and consequently prolonged phases of endogenous hypercortisolism (*i.e.* during exercise and during post-immediate exercise recovery). Given the antagonistic action of glucocorticoids on muscle anabolic processes as well as their immunosuppressive effects, this has led us to hypothesize that endurance-trained

---

[*] Mail : duclos@pop.bordeaux.inserm.fr

men might develop adaptive mechanisms in order to protect muscle and other GC sensitive tissues against this increased post-exercise cortisol secretion. Indeed, the response to GC is regulated not only by the concentration of GC but also by the availability of cortisol and the sensitivity to GC of the target tissues. Changes in availability and /or sensitivity to GC may explain the discrepancy between repeated and prolonged exercise-induced HPA axis activation and the lack of metabolic consequences of such increased cortisol secretion.

In this chapter, the data on the effects of endurance training on extra-cellular and intra-cellular cortisol availability are discussed. The results provide supports for the adaptation of the HPA axis to repeated and prolonged exercise-induced increases in cortisol secretion. It is an exciting challenge to understand the differences between the effects of repeated exercise-induced cortisol secretion in well-adapted athletes and the deleterious effects (metabolic, endocrine, cardiovascular) of the subtle hypercortisolism reported in some pathology (visceral obesity, metabolic syndrome, depression) representing, on the other hand, models of disadaptation to subtle hypercortisolism. Limitation of the current litterature and possible direction for future research are discussed.

The activation of the hypothalamo-pituitary-adrenal (HPA) axis represents a physiological response to the energetic, metabolic, vascular and sometimes neuro-physiologic or psychologic needs of exercise. Glucocorticoids (GC), the end-product of the HPA axis, exert many beneficial actions in exercising humans, increasing availability of metabolic substrates for the need of energy of muscles, maintaining normal vascular integrity and responsiveness and protecting the organism from an overreaction of the immune system in the face of repeated exercise-induced muscle damage.

Exercise and Activation of the HPA Axis: Instructions for Use

In humans, the dynamics of the HPA axis activation during exercise associates stimulation of the cosecretion of hypothalamic corticotropin-releasing hormone (CRH) and arginin vasopressin (AVP) (with a major role of CRH) [1;2], production of ACTH from pituitary corticotroph cells preceding the increase of cortisol. This is indirectly confirmed by the study of Cashmore [3] who showed that the variations of plasma cortisol during exercise are linked to variations of the cortisol secretion and not to modifications of its clearance.

To gain insights into the brain activation in response to exercise, Timofeeva *et al.* [4] have realized a full analysis of the brain regions activated by 90 min treadmill running in rats. Brain activation was assessed using the expression of *c-fos* mRNA. The *c-fos* gene is quickly and transiently expressed in response to several stimuli and its expression has been widely used to imprint neuronal activity in laboratory rodents. Their results showed that the expression of *c-fos* was highly enhanced during treadmill running. As expected, the large majority of the CRH-ergics neurons in the paraventricular nucleus (PVN) of the hypothalamus expressed *c-fos* during the treadmill-running session, demonstrating that treadmill running strongly activates the hypophysiotropic CRH system. Moreover, the pattern of *c-fos* mRNA distribution in the brain of rats subjected to treadmill running showed similarities with that exhibited in response to both neurogenic stress and systemic challenges. Finally, *c-fos* mRNA expression returned to control levels after 2 h of recovery.

Two major classic factors modulate the HPA axis response to exercise: intensity and duration of exercise. The training factor do not modify the intensity nor the duration thresholds when exercise is realized at similar percent of VO_2 max between sedentary and trained men [5]. When the intensity of exercise is above a threshold of 60-70% of VO_2 max, the increase in plasma cortisol concentration correlates linearly with the percentage of VO_2 max reached during exercise [6;7]. On the other hand, below this intensity threshold, i.e. during light and prolonged exercise (<60% VO_2 max), ACTH and cortisol concentration may increase, defining a duration threshold (around 90 min of exercise at 40% VO_2 max) [5]. This phenomenon is also independent of training.

Other factors – less frequently taken into account althought very important - can modulate the cortisol response to exercise: meal and time of day. Meals stimulate cortisol release in humans. Exercise performed immediately after food ingestion results in a blunted cortisol response to the exercise stimulus and the postprandial increase in serum cortisol concentrations is attenuated by prior exercise [8].

Kanaley *et al.* [9] investigated whether circadian and diurnal rhythms underlying the secretion of cortisol modulate its reponse to aerobic exercise (30 min treadmill running at ~85% VO_2 max) in moderately trained male subjects. They showed that the cortisol response to exercise was significantly modulated by time of day. Although the duration of the increase in serum cortisol concentrations after exercise was similar (150-155 min) at 0700, 1900, and 2400h, the increase over control day levels was greatest at 2400 h and smallest at 1900h and an intermediate response occurred at 0700h. These differences in serum cortisol concentrations between exercise and control days were transient (~40-130min) and were most apparent when the effects over time were studied, as the 6-h integrated cortisol concentrations did not differ significantly at each time of day. Previous studies have reported discrepant results. Two features of the experimental design in Kanaley's study may account for the differences with the past findings. First, this study controlled for the possible effects of meals (standard last meal 12h before exercise), sleep (no sleep during the 5-h period following the start of exercise) and prior exercise. Second, the pattern of cortisol release overtime under exercise conditions was compared with that observed at rest at the identical time of day for each subject. Early studies did not include a control day and simply compared cortisol concentrations during exercise to the preexercise levels on the same day. Altogether these results reinforce those of Thuma [10] and demonstrate that neglicting the circadian variations may introduce errors into conclusion about the hormone responses to exercise and training and/or overtraining, respectively.

Finally this work of Kanaley *et al.* demonstrated that the effect of time of day on the cortisol response to exercise cannot be completely accounted for by the preexercise baseline cortisol concentrations, as baseline cortisol concentrations were similar at 1900h and 2400h with a greater increase over time occurring in response to exercise at 2400h than at 1900h. Comparing these results to those of pharmacological stimulation emphasizes the complex regulation of the cortisol response to exercise. Indeed, time of day influences the incremental response, but not the peak response, to pharmacological tests of cortisol secretory reserve (insulin-induced hypoglycemia, ACTH test, CRH test). In other words, the regulation of the cortisol response to exercise differs from that observed in response to insulin-induced hypoglycemia, or to CRH or ACTH tests.

In the case of repeated daily bouts of exercise, the study of Ronsen et al. [11] indicated the influence of the recovery time between the sessions. They showed that, in male elite endurance athletes, repeating prolonged strenuous exercise within only a few hours (two bouts of 75min of exercise at 75% VO_2 max each separated by either 3h or 6h of rest) resulted in magnified neuroendocrine stress responses, despite completely normalized plasma concentrations of cortisol and ACTH before the second exercise session (during each trial, the subjects were served four standardized meals). They reported a more pronounced increase in ACTH and cortisol when the previous bout of exercise was performed only 3h as opposed to 6h earlier, supporting the hypothesis that upon a reactivation of the HPA axis by the second bout of exercise, the duration of rest between the first and second exercise becomes a significant determinant for the magnitude of the corresponding stress response. This also suggests that when necessary, the HPA axis is able to respond to a second stimulation in male elite endurance athletes.

Profiling the HPA Axis in Endurance-Trained Men

To define the profile of the HPA axis activity in endurance-training, the effects of an acute exercise and its short-term recovery ($\leq$ 120-150 minutes after the end of exercise) have to be dissociated from long-term exercise recovery (> 3h post exercise recovery), and 24-h cortisol secretion during a day with exercise has to be dissociated from a day without exercise.

HPA Axis of Endurance-Trained Men During a Resting Day

There is a lingering belief in the literature that endurance training implies hypercortisolism [6;12]. With regard to the deleterious effects of prolonged hypercortisolism (impaired microbial killing capacity, muscle catabolism, bone demineralization, antireproductive effects, depression and anxiety), we cannot suscribe to the opinion that chronic mild hypercortisolism could have an adaptative role in endurance training. Support for this opinion comes from the works of our laboratory where we have repeatedly shown that in endurance-trained men, 24 h cortisol secretion under non exercising conditions is normal. Accordingly, 0800 h plasma cortisol and 24 h urinary free cortisol (UFC) in resting endurance-trained men are similar to those of age-matched sedentary subjects [5;13]. Since UFC represents an integrated measure of the 24 h cortisol secretion [14], this is in accordance with the previously reported normal nycthemeral HPA axis rhythm in endurance-trained men [5]. What is very important is that overnight UFC is also non different to sedentary subjects [15]. A reason for pointing out such a result is that the sleeping time represents the period where the hormonal profile is the most anabolic (increased ratio of GH to cortisol and of testosterone to cortisol) [13], and therefore the most favorable phase to exercise recovery and protein synthesis. Moreover, it has been shown that activation of the HPA axis results in more severe metabolic consequences when occuring during the diurnal nadir of circadian activity (i.e. during the night) because physiological elevation of plasma cortisol levels in the evening has more pronounced deleterious effects on glucose regulation than elevation of cortisol levels in the morning [16].

Finally, endurance-trained men maintained the circannual rhythmicity of cortisol excretion. In sedentary men highest concentrations of urinary cortisol [17], morning plasma cortisol [18] and saliva cortisol [19] are evidenced during winter and fall compared with spring and summer. In endurance-trained men such seasonal variations of cortisol secretion have been found in urinary of triathletes [15] and plasma of elite cyclists [20].

The overactivity of the HPA axis reported by others may represent a further step of physical activity strain, leading to overreaching and/or overtraining and pathological adaptations of the HPA axis [6;12]. Moreover, as suggested by Luger [6], their highly trained group presenting with mild evening hypercortisolism may have included subjects whose personalities had anorectic or depressive components, all conditions associated with chronic activation of the HPA axis [21;22]. By contrast, in each of our studies, depression (measured by CES-D scale) and abnormalities of eating behaviour (binge eating, anorexia nervosa) were criteria of exclusion. In women, alterations of the HPA axis in amenorrheic runners have been reported, with urinary free cortisol levels elevated to levels observed in anorexia nervosa [12;23;24]. However, the physiopathology of this increased cortisol secretion has been recently explained by M.J. De Souza and A.B. Loucks [24-27] who successfully and repeatedly demonstrated that this is the stress of chronic energy deficiency (negative energy balance) which induces hypercortisolism and not the stress of exercise by itself which induces this chronic hypercortisolism.

HPA Axis in Endurance-Trained Men During a Day with Exercise

Exercise of sufficient intensity and/or duration increases cortisol secretion. However, whatever the type and the duration of exercise, in non overtrained men, the exercise-induced cortisol increase does not exceed more than 120 to 150 minutes after the end of exercise. This raises the following question: is there a decrease in cortisol production after these 2 hours of exercise recovery in order that average 24h cortisol concentrations remained similar between exercising and non exercising men? Unfortunately, data are lacking to answer with accuracy to this question. Only few studies have dealt whis this important question.

In the study conducted by Kern *et al.* [13], ten trained healthy men participated in an balanced cross over study including three conditions: 1) no exercise, 2) long-duration exercise of low intensity (biking 40 km from 1800 to 2030 h) and 3) long-duration exercise of moderate intensity (biking 120-150 km from 1600 to 2030 h). During the subsequent night, somnopolygraphic sleep recordings were obtained and blood was collected every 15 min for determination of plasma concentrations of cortisol. At the end of long-duration exercise of low intensity, plasma cortisol levels did not differ significantly from baseline value before the exercise (400 nmol/l) whereas cortisol was significantly elevated at the end of the long-duration exercise of moderate intensity (1000 nmol/l) (Fig.1). During the no exercise night, the typical secretory cortisol patterns were present with nadir cortisol concentrations during the first half of sleep but increased cortisol levels during the second part of sleep. Average concentrations of cortisol during the nights did not depend on whether this night was preceded by a period of exercise or not (Fig.2A). Separate analysis of the first and second part of the night indicated that in the long-duration exercise of moderate intensity cortisol levels were increased during the first half of the night whereas the rise in cortisol concentrations during second half of the night was reduced (Fig.2B). Therefore, average cortisol concentrations at night remained unaffected between no exercise and exercise days. Hackney *et al.* [28] also reported that cortisol is suppressed at night after daytime exercise involving two bouts of moderate-intensity exercise (aerobic) or high-intensity exercise (anaerobic). However, in their control condition (no exercise), plasma cortisol levels during the first part of the night (between 2200 and 0200 h) averaged 250 nmol/l. In sleeping subjects, this would be an unusual high cortisol concentrations [29], suggesting that the decrease of cortisol at night may have been overestimated.

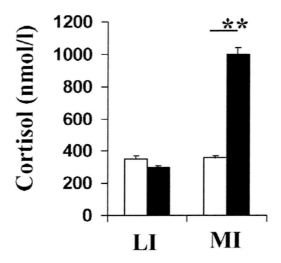

Figure 1. Cortisol concentrations before exercise (white bars) and immediately after exercise (black bars). Exercise was either of long duration low intensity (LI: 40 km biking) or of long duration moderate intensity (MI: 120-150 km biking). Significant differences for pairwise comparisons for corresponding points in time: **$P<0.01$. From [13].

Nindl *et al.* [30] monitored hormone levels during the night after an acute heavy-resistance exercise performed in the late afternoon (from 1500 to 1700 h) on young healthy men. The protocol of exercise was designed to be a high-volume workout (*i.e.*, high total work) that recruited and activated a large amount of muscle tissue. This was accomplished by performing multijoint exercises that required the use of major muscle groups in the lower and upper body. Blood was obtained after the completion of the last set, at a rate of one draw every 10 min from 1700 to 1800 h and one draw every hour thereafter until 0600 h on the following morning. Compared to a control day without any exercise, cortisol levels were significantly increased at the end of exercise (7.1 *vs* 16.9 µg/dl, control *vs* exercise trial), remained elevated two hours after the end of exercise and were restored until control (resting) values thereafter but were not lower than the day without exercise. Therefore whereas on one hand, the influence of the resistance exercise on cortisol concentration do not appear to be long lasting, on the other hand it does not appear to suppress significantly nightime cortisol secretion. But, once again, it remains difficult to conclude on the effects of exercise on 24h cortisol secretion as the sleep patterns have not been studied.

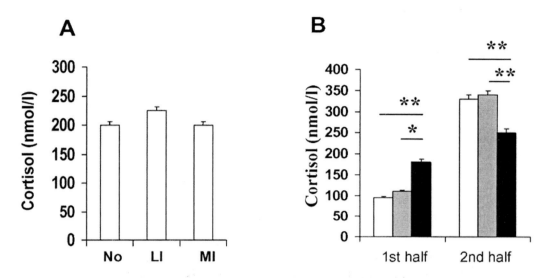

Figure 2. A) Cortisol concentrations averaged across samples collected every 15 min between 2300 and 0700 h during night after no daytime exercise (No), exercise of long duration low intensity (LI) or of long duration moderate intensity (MI). B) Cortisol concentrations separately for first and second half of sleeptime after no daytime exercise (white bar), exercise of long duration low intensity (hatched bar) or of long duration moderate intensity (black bar). Significant differences for pairwise comparisons between experimental conditions: *P<0.05, **P<0.01. From [13].

When instead of repeated plasma samplings, 24h urinary free cortisol (UFC) is used, which is less invasive and allows normal and usual conditions of life, we have shown that in swimmers during a training and/or a competition day, 24h UFC excretion, testimony of 24h cortisol secretion, remained within the normal range of the laboratory [31]. Moreover, in comparison with sedentary men (unpublished results), endurance trained men presented with similar 24h UFC than sedentary men. These findings are in agreement with the absence of difference in the 24h UFC levels between the two hard training days and the two rest days in eumenorrheic women running more than 92.5 km per week for the past 12 months, nor between the two hard training days and the two rest days in the eumenorrheic runners and the two rest days in the eumenorrheic sedentary women [24].

To our knowledge, only one study reported that the increase in 24h UFC coincided very closely with the changes in training volume and intensity in experienced cyclists [32]. However, the results of this study should be interpreted cautiously because after the off-season and before the beguinning of their training program, the cyclists have already higher UFC than sedentary subjects (111.4 ± 8.6 nmol/day *vs* 74.8 ± 10.4 nmol/day, cyclists *vs* sedentary subjects: P<0.05).

Beyond transient exercise-induced increases in cortisol secretion inducing in some cases increased 24h UFC compared to sedentary subjects and sometimes (but not systematically and actually very rarely in non overreached athletes) increased 24h UFC compared to normal values, the question arises whether endurance training induces only transient (the day of exercise) or more sustained changes in the HPA axis physiology and/or set point for 24h cortisol secretion. Indeed, after an endurance exercise at 75% VO_2 max (a 2-h run), cortisol remains significantly increased for almost 2 h after the end of exercise [5;21;33]. This suggests that a 2-h run induces an increase in cortisol concentrations for at least 3 hours (the second hour of exercise and the two hours of post-exercise recovery) [5]. When training for a marathon race, subjects run an average of 120-180 km/week. This implies daily sessions of prolonged and/or intense running and consequently prolonged phases of endogenous hypercortisolism (*i.e.* during exercise and during post-immediate exercise recovery). Given the antagonistic action of glucocorticoids on muscle anabolic processes as well as their immunosuppressive effects, this has led us to hypothesize that endurance-trained men might develop adaptive mechanisms such as decreased sensitivity to cortisol in order to protect muscle and other GC sensitive tissues against this increased post-exercise cortisol secretion.

HPA Axis and Endurance-Training: A Model of Allostasis?

These data raises the intriguing and exciting possibility that endurance-training, i.e. repeated and prolonged exercise-induced HPA axis activation, induces allostatic modifications of the HPA axis physiology. Allostasis is the ability to achieve stability through change [34]. Through allostasis, the HPA axis adapts-copes with repeated stimulations, allowing the ability to respond repeatedly to internal and external stimulations. This is beneficial for the perspective of fuel mobilization. Concurrently, this adaptation also allows protection of the body (at least some tissues) from high cortisol levels.

In lights of our results, we believe that this adaptation exists in endurance-trained men. We have accumulated evidences that when sedentary and healthy endurance-trained men are compared in resting, unchallenged conditions, no difference in HPA axis activity is seen. In other words, our results probe the functional integrity of the HPA axis in healthy endurance-trained men who had been subjected to frequent periods of prolonged HPA axis activation. By contrast, when the HPA axis is challenged, results from endurance-trained men differ from those of sedentary men translating underlying allostatic modifications of the HPA axis due to repeated exercise-induced HPA axis activation.

In a first study, we have monitored plasma cortisol and ACTH concentrations during and 4h after the end of running exercise performed by both endurance trained men and sedentary men [5]. Two parameters, *i.e.* intensity and duration, were changed on 4 consecutive days. The first day (D0) was spent in the laboratory: all blood samples were obtained at rest to determine diurnal variations of each hormone. On the following days (D1 to D4) the subjects exercised: D1 and D2 brief (20 min), light (50% maximal heart rate: HR max, D1) or strenuous (80% HR max, D2), D3 and D4 prolonged (120min), light (D3) or strenuous (D4). In both groups, neither brief (D1, D2) nor prolonged light exercise (D3) induced any significant variation in plasma ACTH or cortisol concentrations. Plasma ACTH and cortisol concentrations increased only if the exercise was intense and prolonged (D4). The training factor did not modify the intensity or duration thresholds for the activation of the pituitary-adrenocortical response to exercise. However, during immediate recovery from the four exercise regimens, the plasma ACTH concentrations of the endurance trained men were constantly above the values of the sedentary subjects, although plasma cortisol concentrations remained similar in both groups. To focus on the relationships between ACTH and cortisol, we compared the areas under the cortisol and ACTH curves (AUC) from 0.5 to 3.5h during recovery from D1 to D4 compared to D0 at the same time (Fig.3). Cortisol AUC were similar in the sedentary subjects and endurance trained men whereas the ACTH AUC were increased in the endurance trained men compared to the sedentary subjects. In other words, during the immediate recovery from exercise whatever its intensity, the magnitude of the ACTH response was increased in the trained subjects but with a reduced effect upon its target, the adrenals glands. Indeed, although plasma cortisol concentration was similar in both populations, in the marathon men, plasma ACTH concentration was significantly increased during immediate exercise recovery when compared to the sedentary subjects.

An increased cortisol clearance in the trained subjects could not explain such results since variations of cortisol concentrations during exercise have been reported to be related to the cortisol secretion rate and not to its clearance [3]. A differential increase in plasma bio-active ACTH-like activity versus immunoreactive ACTH concentations has been reported in human adults subjects after insulin-induced hypoglycemia [35]. Nevertheless, in this study, we did not notice any hypoglycemia, during or after exercise.

Two non-exclusive hypothesis may explain this increased ACTH concentration during exercise immediate recovery: a decreased adrenal sensitivity to ACTH stimulation and/or a decreased HPA axis sensitivity to cortisol negative feed-back.

The hypothesis of a decreased adrenal sensitivity implies that during exercise recovery, there might be a resistance or desensitization of adrenal cells to ACTH. The hypothesis of a decreased hypothalamo-pituitary axis sensitivity to cortisol feedback suggests that the sensitivity of the HPA axis to GC negative feedback is reduced. In the above-cited study [5], this sensitivity had been studied with the cortisol response to food intake. Indeed, in sedentary men, Brandenberger et al. [8] has showed that the daily cortisol pattern results from the interactions between the meal-related peaks, especially the major midday cortisol peak, and the exercise-induced cortisol increases, both of which inhibit the responses to subsequent stimulation. It explains why in conditions of exercise-induced marked cortisol increase (D4), the subsequent stimulation exerted by meal did not elicit a rise of cortisol levels in sedentary men (Fig.4). By contrast, endurance trained men, despite similar increased cortisol concentrations, were able to escape to the blunting effect of the preceeding exercise-induced cortisol increase (GC feedback) and therefore to respond to subsequent stimulation with a significant cortisol increase to noon meal (Fig.4).

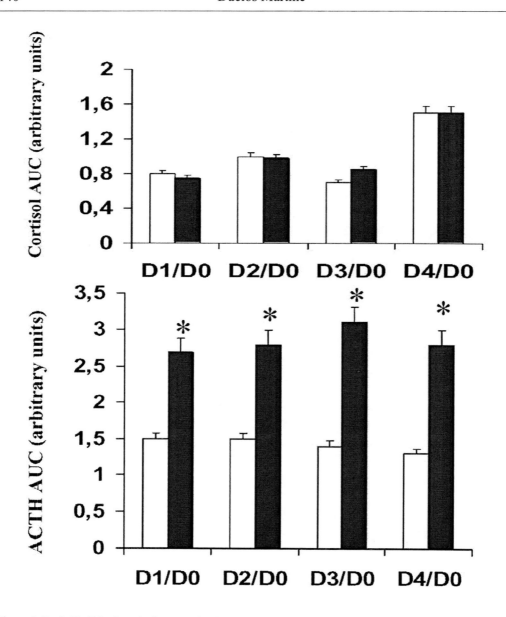

Figure 3. Ratio Dx/D0 of cortisol area under the curve (AUC) (top) and of ACTH AUC (bottom) from day 0 to 4 (D0-D4) during immediate recovery from exercise in the sedentary subjects (white bars) and endurance-trained men (black bars). *: $P<0.05$, sedentary vs endurance-trained subjects. From [5].

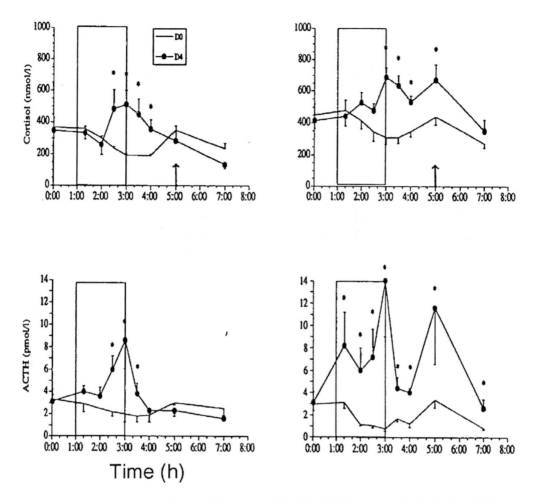

Figure 4. Plasma concentrations of cortisol (upper panels) and ACTH (lower panels) during day 0 (D0: no exercise) and day 4 (D4: running 120 min at 80% HR max) in the sedentary subjects (left panels) and endurance-trained men (right panels). □ Exercise, arrow: meal. * : P<0.05 D0 vs D4. From [5].

To add further insights into the HPA axis sensitivity to an endogenous sustained increase in GC concentrations in endurance-trained men, we next performed pituitary corticotroph stimulation with combined CRH/lysine vasopressin (CRH/LVP) and adrenal stimulation with ACTH [1-24] in endurance trained men both in resting conditions (normal cortisol values) and 2h after the end of strenuous exercise (increased cortisol values). The combined CRH/LVP test is a reliable test to evaluate corticotroph reserve in patients with various pituitary-adrenal diseases or central nervous system disorders [36]. In resting conditions, the combined CRH/LVP test elicited a rise of ACTH and cortisol similar to the values reached during an intense and prolonged exercise [5]. In the exercise session, despite the prolonged increased cortisol secretion (i.e. during exercise and the 2h of exercise recovery [5]) which could impair the ACTH response to CRH/LVP stimulation test, we reported a similar ACTH and cortisol responses after exercise than in resting conditions (Fig.5). The absence of blunted corticotrophin (ACTH) and cortisol responses after pituitary-adrenal stimulation conducted during physiological endogenous "hypercortisolism" suggests an impaired pituitary sensitivity to early GC negative feedback in our endurance-trained athletes. These results are in agreement with the precedent study [5] and with those from Heuser [22] who demonstrated that male endurance athletes running 70 ± 30 km/week have the capacity to overcome dexamethasone suppression during the combined dexamethasone/CRH test. They reported that plasma cortisol and ACTH levels from 1400-1500 h after oral administration of dexamethasone (1.5 mg) the day before at 2300 h were similar in sedentary and endurance-trained men. However, after hCRH infusion, cortisol and ACTH release was markedly increased in endurance-trained men compared to that in the sedentary subjects (Fig.6).

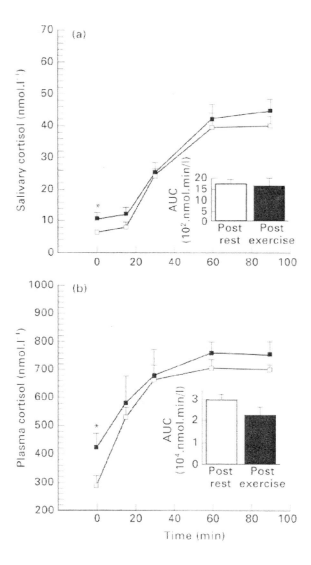

Figure 5. Saliva (a) and plasma cortisol (b) responses to CRH/LVP in post rest (□) and post exercise (■) sessions. Inset panels correspond to AUC responses to CRH/LVP in post rest and post exercise sessions in saliva (upper panel) and plasma (lower panel). * : P<0.05 between post rest and post exercise sessions. From [54].

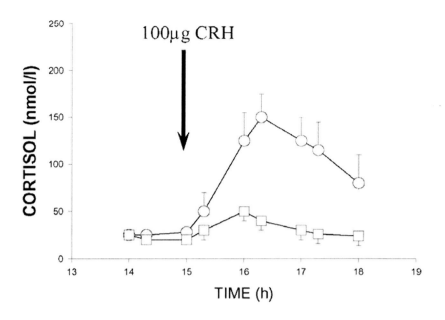

Figure 6. Plasma cortisol response to hCRH challenge after pretreatment with dexamethasone in 10 runners (o) and 13 sedentary subjects (□). From [22].

Finally, in our study the normality of the cortisol reponse after ACTH stimulation both in resting and in exercising conditions discard the second hypothesis of a major decreased adrenal sensitivity to ACTH in endurance-trained men (Fig.7).

Altogether these studies demonstrate that although having a basal-resting functional integrity of their HPA axis, in endurance-trained men, exercise-induced cortisol increase does not impair the ability of the HPA axis to respond to a physiological (food intake) or to a pharmacological challenge.

This impaired sensitivity to early GC negative feedback in endurance-trained men is best explained by the CRH-potentiating effect of vasopressin to release ACTH. According to Hashimoto [37] chronic stimulation of the HPA axis has been found to induce synthesis of vasopressin. As vasopressin-induced ACTH secretion is less sensitive to GC negative feddback than CRH-induced ACTH secretion, vasopressin could limit the relative insensitivity of the pituitary corticotroph cells when an acute stress or stimulation is added to chronic stress. This suggests that a higher vasopressin /CRH ratio may occur in humans under repeated exercise-induced HPA axis activation [2]. We also concur with [38] who hypothetized that a first stress could generate a facilitator priming signal acting on the axis, contributing to an additional positive drive accompanying subsequent stresses sufficient to counterbalance the negative feedback signal from GC. From Akana and Dalmann [39], that facilitation is a dominant effect under conditions of chronic stress in all species. Whether this facilitation represents an adaptive phenomenon or whether this phenomenon exists in sedentary men remains to be determined.

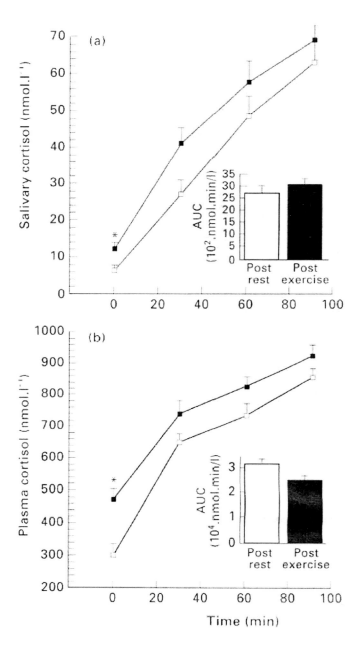

Figure 7. Saliva (a) and plasma cortisol (b) responses to ACTH in post rest (□) and post exercise (■) sessions. Inset panels correspond to AUC responses to ACTH in post rest and post exercise sessions in saliva (upper panel) and plasma (lower panel). * : $p<0.05$ between post rest and post exercise sessions. From [54].

At this point, it is tempting to speculate that enhanced stimulation of the pituitary-adrenal axis due to endurance training induces adrenal hypertrophy, a feature generally associated with increased adrenal sensitivity to ACTH. Nevertheless, this hypothesis of increased adrenal sensitivity to ACTH in endurance-trained men remains unlikely for the following reasons: i) in 1974, Tharp [40] had suggested that the athletes may have reduced adrenal sensitivity to ACTH, a hypothesis which was in keeping with the results of Inder [41] who found elevated basal levels of ACTH without significant elevation in cortisol levels in highly trained male athletes, compared with sedentary subjects; ii) we have previously reported an increased ACTH/cortisol ratio during post-exercise recovery in endurance-trained men compared with matched sedentary subjects, suggesting that, at least in post-exercise recovery, endurance-trained men have a decreased adrenal sensitivity to ACTH [5]. In contrast to the huge literature about the HPA response to acute exercise, no information about adrenal weight in endurance-trained men is presently available.

Allostatic response is devoted to be adaptive and protective. The whole of the data presented in this chapter illustrate the adaptive response of the HPA axis to repeated challenges in endurance-training. With regard to the antagonistic action of cortisol on muscle anabolic processes as well as their immunosuppressive effects, the position set forth in the following discussion to explain the concurrent absence of such clinical findings in healthy endurance-trained men is that they are able to mount protective mechanisms. The question as to what strategy is adopted by the body faced with repeated exercise-induced increased cortisol levels may be answered in terms of tissular sensitivity to GC.

Downstream plasma cortisol concentrations, the biological effects of cortisol on its target tissues are far from being fully known. Indeed, although plasma cortisol concentrations can be measured accurately, studies of plasma cortisol levels are limited because in conditions of normal or subnormal plasma cortisol levels, variations in extracellular and intracellular cortisol availability may occur.

The availability of an accurate measure of the effects of GC on target tissues allows the evaluation of an additional level of GC action. As *in vitro* dexamethasone inhibition of lipopolysaccharide (LPS)-induced interleukine-6 (IL-6) secretion in cultures of peripheral monocytes is an effective means of determining the effects and therefore the sensitivity to GC of one peripheral target of GC *i.e.* the immune tissue [42], we have compared monocytes sensitivity to GC in untrained subjects and in endurance-trained men 24 h after the end of the last session of exercise. Moreover, to evaluate the effect of an exercise-induced increase in GC concentrations in endurance-trained men, sensitivity to GC was further studied at the end of a two-hour run and during exercise recovery [33;43]. We demonstrated an *in vitro* plasticity of sensitivity of monocytes to GC in endurance-trained men, superimposed to changes in systemic cortisol concentrations (plasma and saliva). Compared to sedentary men, similar resting cortisol levels in endurance-trained men are associated with decreased sensitivity of monocytes to GC, 8 h and 24 h after the end of the last training session. Moreover, in these endurance-trained subjects, an acute bout of exercise increased the sensitivity of monocytes to GC to the levels assayed in untrained men (Fig.8).

In other words, compared to sedentary men, similar resting cortisol levels are associated with a decreased sensitivity of monocytes to GC in endurance-trained men. Moreover, an acute bout of endurance exercise increased transiently the sensitivity of monocytes to GC in endurance-trained men.

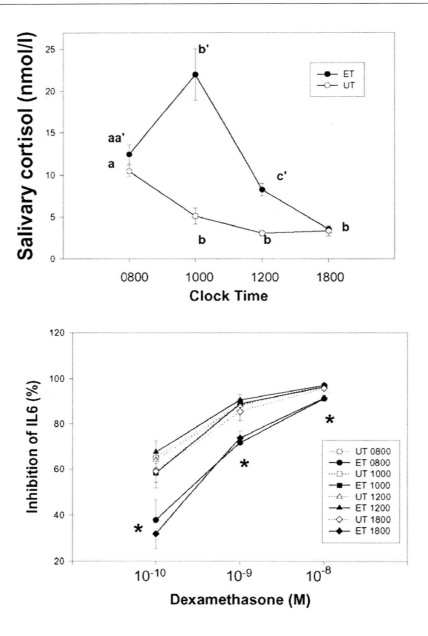

Figure 8. A) Saliva cortisol concentrations across time during the experimental day in endurance-trained men (ET) (exercise and resting sessions) and untrained (UT) men (resting session). ET men realized a two-hour run between 0800 and 1000 h. Bars not sharing a common letter are significantly different from each others. Results are means ± sem. B) Percentage inhibition of lipopolysaccharide (LPS) (0.3 µg/mL) stimulated IL-6 production in ET (solid lines) and UT men (dotted lines). The percent inhibition by dexamethasone was calculated as the percentage of IL-6 produced in the presence of dexamethasone relative to the production of IL-6 in the absence of dexamethasone in the same individual at the dose of 0.3 µg/ml LPS.
*: The percent values of dexamethasone-induced IL-6 inhibition are significantly lower in ET at 0800 h and 1800 h as compared with their values at 1000 h and 1200h, and as compared with the values of UT men at 0800 h, 1000 h, 1200 h and 1800 h ($p<0.05$). From [33].

Results of previous studies are scarce and conflicting. Using a similar *in vitro* technique of dexamethasone suppression of LPS-induced IL-6 production, DeRijk et al. [42] have subjected trained males to a graded exercise of short duration (20 min) and high intensity (70 and 90% VO_2 max) and demonstrated an exercise-induced decrease in sensitivity to GC in peripheral lymphocytes 20 min after the end of exercise. Although the authors stated that the relative amount of monocytes did not change during exercise, it has been previously demonstrated that exercise induces a significant change in specific leukocyte subsets [44]. Since DeRijk et al. [42] used peripheral whole blood cells, it is difficult to discard a role of putative variations in specific lymphocytes subsets. Moreover, in a later study, Smits et al. [45] used an intermittent high intensity exercise (total duration: 15 min at ~ 135% VO_2 max) but specific lymphocyte subsets were studied as well as monocytes. The results showed that exercise differentially affects sensitivity of monocytes and T cells to GC. Nevertheless, when expressed per monocyte, the decrease in IL-6 secretion was significant following exercise. This transient exercise-induced GC resistance contrasts with our demonstration of increased sensitivity to GC after exercise [33;43]. This discrepancy between Smits' study and our studies is likely to be related to the differences in the protocols, the type of exercise and the timing of blood sampling. Comparing the effects of different duration and intensity of exercises and the kinetics of recovery will be necessary to decipher the regulation of sensitivity to GC in trained men.

Taken together, our findings and others support the existence of a plasticity of sensitivity to GC in endurance-trained men. Although changes in sensitivity to GC have mainly been described under pathological conditions [46], this was the first report indicating the kinetics of such rapid and transient changes in healthy subjects. Interestingly, in untrained subjects, a recent paper reported that a psychological stress increased salivary cortisol and sensitivity of monocytes to GC 1 h after stress in men [47]. As running 120 minutes at 65-75% VO_2 max may represent in sedentary subjects an intense psychological stress, among other stress (energetic, metabolic...), we have not submitted our sedentary group to an acute bout of exercise. Although stress has not been evaluated rigorously after exercise, our all six trained men reported increased feelings of well being after exercise. Therefore, the hypothesis of psychological stress-induced increase in GC sensitivity is unlikely. By contrast, these results suggest that different conditions which lead to increased free cortisol concentrations: exercise in endurance-trained men (present study) and psychological stress in sedentary men [47], can be associated with increased sensitivity of monocytes to GC. Therefore, this phenomenon of plasticity of GC sensitivity reported in the present study is not exclusive to endurance-trained men.

The transient exercise-induced increase of sensitivity of monocytes to GC may act to shut off inflammatory reaction and cytokines synthesis [48]. Nevertheless, although such a restrained inflammatory response may, on the one hand, decrease exercise-induced muscle damage or muscle inflammatory reactions, on the other hand, it may lead to increased susceptibility for bacterial and viral infections in immediate post exercise recovery. Inversely, and although hypothetical, the decreased sensitivity of monocytes to GC reported in endurance-trained men 24h after the last bout of exercise, may be related to the process of desensitization which may act to protect the body from prolonged exercise-induced cortisol secretion.

Several mechanisms may explain these transient changes in sensitivity to GC reported in our study: 1) variations in the amount of GC receptors (GR): decreased at rest and increased during exercise, 2) alteration of the ligand binding capacity in peripheral monocytes, 3) changes in direction of GR trafficking, 4) different expression of α and β isoforms of GR receptor [49]. However, upstream these intracellular mechanisms, the extracellular and/or the intracellular cortisol availability could also be modified. Extracellular bioavailability depends on the free fraction of the hormone *i.e.* the free cortisol. Cortisol largely binds to plasma proteins and especially to the cortisol-binding globulin (CBG) [50]. Thus plasma cortisol levels are modulated by variations of CBG and poorly correlates with cortisol production rates unless differences in CBG are corrected [14] (Fig.8). Conversely, saliva cortisol concentrations are independent of CBG concentrations and thus closely reflect the free - active - plasma cortisol [51-53]. In each of our experiments, we have measured both plasma and saliva cortisol concentrations and we did not find differences due to endurance-training (endurance-trained men vs sedentary men, in resting conditions as well as during exercise) [15;21;33;54]. To our knowledge, no human study has dealt with CBG concentrations in endurance-trained men. In rats, Chennaoui *et al.* [55] reported that after treadmill training, despite a certain increase in adrenal weights, no change in CBG capacity occurred, this latter result being consistent with the absence of basal corticosterone changes.

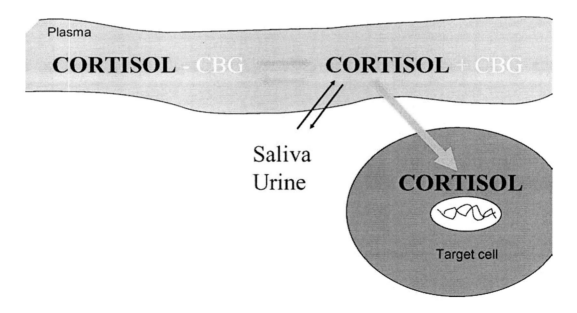

Figure 9. Role of CBG in the extracellular bioavailability of cortisol. Free cortisol (i.e biovailable cortisol) can be easily measured in urine and in saliva.

In addition to CBG which modulates the extracellular availability of cortisol, another recently described level of control of the effect of cortisol on target cells is exerted by pre-receptor metabolism of cortisol by the tissue-specific enzymes 11β hydroxysteroid dehydrogenases (11β-HSD). At the intracellular level, two isoenzyme of 11β-HSD interconvert hormonally active cortisol and inactive cortisone and have been shown to modulate cortisol hormone action in several peripheral tissue [56]. 11β-HSD2 inactivates cortisol to cortisone and is mainly expressed in the kidney, in which it protects the glucocorticoids receptor from cortisol excess [57]. By contrast, 11β-HSD1 is expressed in numerous tissues where it converts the inactive cortisone to active cortisol [56]. The crucial physiological principle illuminated by the action of 11β-HSD is that cortisol action on target cells is determined by enzyme activity within the cells, rather than circulating cortisol levels alone (Fig.10). It has been shown that the peripheral metabolism of cortisol can be assessed accurately from the urinary free cortisol/cortisone ratio, which is a good index of whole body 11β-HSD activity [58]. It should be noted that for determination of urinary free cortisol and urinary free cortisone, the HPLC method showed a better efficiency than the method of competitive binding and must be preferred in the measure of cortisol/cortisone ratio in urine [59].

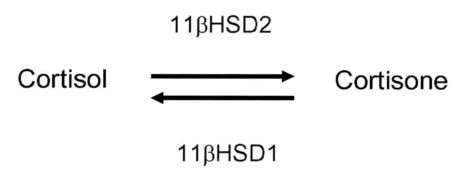

Figure 10. Role of 11βHSD in the intracellular bioavailability of cortisol.

Using this new approach, we have shown that 24-h urinary cortisol/cortisone ratio is positively related to the total training load in a population of swimmers [31]. In a next study, as the nocturnal period is essential for exercise recovery [13], we have focused on overnight glucocorticoids output for monitoring the delicate balance between cumulative fatigue resulting from exercise training and its recovery period over a ten-month season in triathletes. To dissociate the effects of training to those of seasonal hormonal variations, endurance-trained men were compared to sedentary men: nine untrained men and 10 triathletes were followed during a ten-month season, and they reported to the laboratory in November (low training load), March (high training load) and June (moderate training load). Clinical (total score of fatigue, total training load and performances during the competition period) and hormonal parameters (overnight excretion of glucocorticoids and catecholamines, and increment of saliva cortisol response to awakening) were measured [15].

Whereas the measure of overnight excretion of cortisol and cortisone showed a large interindividual variability in response to the different training periods, conversely, overnight urinary cortisol/cortisone ratio showed a good intraindividual and interindividual stability in the untrained men and triathletes group during the follow-up period (Fig.11). More strikingly, the untrained men and triathletes group presented similar ratios without seasonal variation, suggesting that in physiological conditions, any important and prolonged increase in cortisol secretion (seasonal and/or high training load cortisol-induced secretion) is balanced by the parallel increase in its tissular inactivation in cortisone.

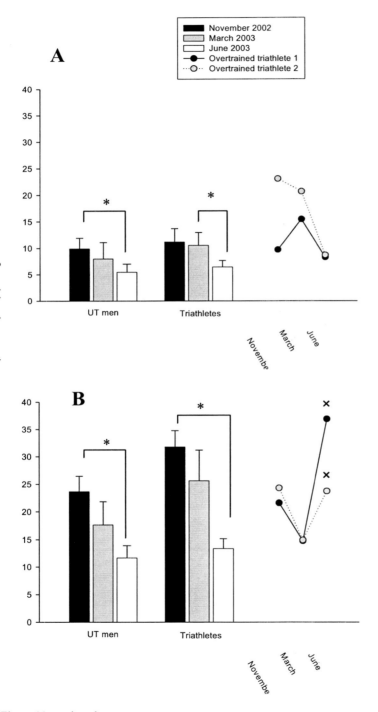

Figure 11 continued on next page

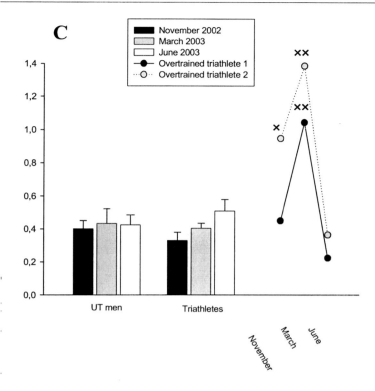

Figure 11. Overnight urinary excretion of cortisol (A) cortisone (B) and cortisol/cortisone ratio (C) in untrained men (UT), trained men (Triathletes) and overtrained men (OT). *p<0.05 compared with June within the same group. No statistical test was used in the comparison between the two overtrained triathletes and the triathletes group. However, for each value of overtrained triathletes, normalized deviation (ND) was calculated by subtracting the value of OT man from the mean values of the group of well trained triathletes and dividing by the standard deviation (SD). Results of the overtrained triathletes were considered as significant, only when ND values were twice less or more than SD values (± 2SD).
× Normalized deviation > 2.0
× × Normalized deviation > 7.0 No significant difference was found between UT men and Triathletes in any sampling. From [15].

Moreover, in this study two triathletes developed an overtraining syndrome (called overtrained triathlete 1 and 2) and were thus removed from the triathletes group and evaluated individually. In November, at the beginning of the training season, overnight urinary cortisol/cortisone ratio of overtrained triathlete 1 was similar those of the untrained men and triathletes group, while the ratio of overtrained triathlete 2 was already higher than the two groups. In March (high training load period), the 2 overtrained men presented the same pattern: their cortisol/cortisone ratios dramatically increased (ratio > 1), whereas the ratio of the triathletes remained stable (Fig.11). During the competition period (June to August), these 2 overtrained triathletes showed severe fatigue and decreased performance. Therefore, our results raise for the first time the possibility that the increase of overnight urinary cortisol/cortisone ratio above 1 might be a predicative marker of overtraining or might translate an important risk for the athlete to develop an overtraining syndrome. The fact that this ratio is not correlated to total score of fatigue excludes it exclusive role as marker of staleness. Assuming the anti-inflammatory action of cortisol, therefore the increase in 24-h cortisol/cortisone ratio reported in athletes with high total training load [31] may be beneficial, acting to stop inflammatory reaction and cytokines synthesis [48]. Inversely, during the night, muscle catabolic process of cortisol is deleterious for the athletes, and the inactivation of cortisol into cortisone protects the glucocorticoids target tissues against the effects of prolonged hypercortisolism due to exercise. Low inactivation of cortisol into cortisone (cortisol/cortisone >1) in overtrained triathletes suggests an inhibition of 11β-HSD2 and translates an increase in cortisol action on the target tissues even if circulating cortisol levels are stable. At present, we can only speculate on the mechanisms that mediate the differences in cortisol metabolism between well trained and overtrained men. It has been proposed that overtraining may be caused by excessive cytokines release during and following exercise [60]. The regulation of 11β-HSD by cytokines has been postulated [61] but remains unknown. This exciting hypothesis of increased intracellular inactivation of cortisol during the night in well-trained men confirms and extends our previous report of the existence of a plasticity of tissular sensitivity to glucocorticoids in endurance-trained men, superimposed to systemic cortisol concentrations (plasma and saliva)[33]. Whatever the mechanisms involved in this plasticity of tissular sensitivity to glucocorticoids in trained men, these new results highlight the diversity of potential mechanisms developed by trained men to protect their tissues against prolonged hypercortisolism.

In summary, the allostatic model of endurance-training includes similar HPA axis activity in resting condition than any (healthy) sedentary men. However, when the HPA axis is challenged, endurance-trained men demonstrate a decreased pituitary (and probably hypothalamic and/or supra-hypothalamic) sensitivity to GC explaining their capacity to achieve successfully a second bout of exercise separated by a short rest period. Their successfull adaptation to exercise-induced repeated and prolonged cortisol secretion also includes decreased peripheral tissue sensitivity to GC in order to protect the body from the severe metabolic and immune consequences of increased cortisol levels. A great diversity of mechanisms are involved in such adaptation, acting at potentially all levels in the cascade leading to the biological effects of cortisol.

Another potentially incisive approach to understand whether subtle modifications in HPA axis function are linked to susceptibility to adaptation or to disadaptation is to compare endurance training and visceral obesity. Although at first approach this may appear counterintuitive, an interesting comparison can be drawn between these two conditions where subtle modifications of the HPA axis profile occur.

Endurance-Training *vs* Visceral Obesity: Adaptation *vs* Disadaptation of HPA axis

The prevalence of obesity increases quickly in developed countries and thus becomes a major problem for public health. Moreover, in addition to total fat mass, the distribution of body fat mass also matters. Using clinical parameters such as waist-to-hip ratio (WHR) or more heavy cost technicals such as resonance magnetic imagery (RMI) or tomodensitometry, two types of obesity have been defined: visceral obesity is characterized by preferential fat deposits at the visceral, central, abdominal level and is opposed to peripheral or gluteofemoral obesity (formerly "android" *vs* "gynoid" obesity).

This visceral obesity, most commonly observed in males and women after menopause has been shown to be an important predictor for increased morbidity and mortality from coronary heart disease [62]. It is therefore a major health question as to what influences this preferential fat distribution. Glucocorticoids have been designed to be potentially important as they promote the differentiation and proliferation of human adipocytes [63], and their receptors are more abundant in visceral adipose tissue than in subcutaneous adipose tissue [64]. This suggests that abdominal body fat distribution and HPA axis activity may be linked but the exact relationship (primary or secondary) still needs more clarifications.

As in premenopausal women the excess in fat mass is less systematically stored in visceral adipose tissue than in men, the factors involved in body fat distribution in premenopausal women should be more discriminant than in men. For these reasons, we have conducted successive studies to assess cortisol secretion, metabolism and tissue sensitivity to glucocorticoids in an homogenous group of premenopausal obese women to determine their HPA axis profile and its relationships with body fat distribution and total fat mass. In all these studies, women with abominal obesity (called A-BFD: (women with) abdominal body fat distribution) were compared to apparied women with peripheral obesity (P-BFD) [29;61;65].

Compared to women with peripheral obesity, women with abdominal obesity have a lower awakening cortisol levels. These differences disappeared in the morning as from 1000 h until 1300 h, similar cortisol concentration were found (Fig.12). Moreover, despite normal and similar 24h UFC, A-BFD women have increased overnight secretion of cortisol (increased nocturnal UFC) [61]. This suggests a flattened diurnal variation in cortisol secretion (decreased in the morning and increased during the night), as reported in subjects submitted to chronic stress (but not in endurance-trained men). Indeed, there is epidemiological evidence that abdominal obesity is associated with various environmental stressors in which frequent or chronic challenges of the HPA axis might be expected.

From a metabolic point of view, this increased overnight cortisol secretion may explain the relatively higher blood glucose levels in A-BFD women (positive relationship between fasting glycemia and overnight UFC levels) suggesting that an enhanced activity of cortisol could contribute to the insulin resistance of women with abdominal obesity.

The dynamic control of the HPA axis in obese women graded by their body fat distribution is also informative of their HPA axis functioning and helps to clarify their HPA axis profile. After stimulation of the adrenals with the low dose ACTH test (1μg), A-BFD women presented a higher cortisol response than P-BFD women suggesting that abdominal obesity is associated with an adrenal hypersensitivity to ACTH. Moreover, and very interestingly in this pathology, in response to food intake, A-BFD women also have a greater food-induced stimulation of cortisol secretion (Fig.12) [29;66;67].

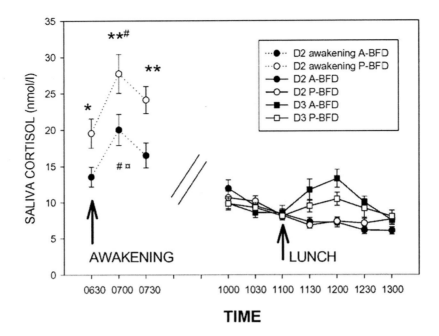

Figure 12. Responses of saliva cortisol to awakening (from 0630 to 0730h in D2: dashed lines) and saliva cortisol concentrations from 1000 to 1300h during the control day (D2) and during D3 where food intake was taken at 1100h (continuous lines). Values are means ± SEM. A-BFD vs P-BFD: * $P<0.05$; ** $P<0.01$; #: $P<0.001$ vs 0630h ; ¤: $P<0.05$ vs 0730h. From [29].

The HPA axis response to a mild negative feed-back has been assessed using the low dose dexamethasone suppression test. Our results showed an increased inhibition of cortisol secretion with low doses of dexamethasone in A-BFD women compared to P-BFD obese women, suggesting an increased pituitary sensitivity to dexamethasone in those with abdominal obesity.

There are many molecular mechanisms potentially involved in the differences in HPA axis activity and reactivity related to body fat distribution in premenopausal obese women. As discussed previously, the bioavailability of cortisol is regulated by the tissular activity of 11βHSD that either activate cortisone to cortisol but can also inactivate cortisol into cortisone. To estimate the whole-body activity of 11βHSD we have measured the urinary ratio of cortisone/cortisol and found an increased urinary cortisone/cortisol ratio in A-BFD women suggesting an increase of the peripheral metabolism of cortisol. Indeed, the plasma metabolic clearance of cortisol is increased in obese subjects [69]. Whatever the mechanism underpinning the pathogenesis of the increased net metabolic clearance of cortisol in abdominal obesity, this would result in decreased cortisol tone on the HPA axis which might explain enhanced positive feedback in abdominal obesity with larger ACTH-induced such as food-induced and/or stress induced cortisol response.

Lastly, the tissular (immune tissue) sensitivity to GC has been assessed using *in vitro* inhibition of lipopolysaccharide-induced IL-6 secretion in cultures of peripheral monocytes: monocytes sensitivity to dexamethasone was significantly decreased in A-BFD women (Fig.13).

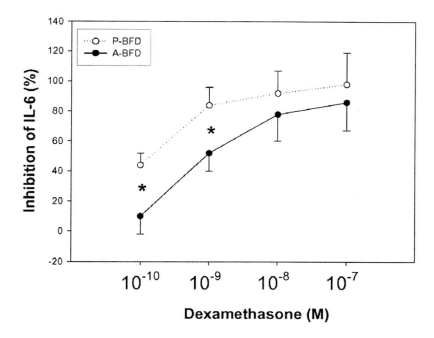

Figure 13. Dexamethasone sensitivity of LPS (0.3 µg/ml) stimulated IL6 production in monocytes in A-BFD (solid lines) and P-BFD obese women (dashed lines). The percent inhibition by dexamethasone was calculated as the percentage of IL-6 produced in the presence of dexamethasone relative to the production of IL-6 in the absence of dexamethasone in the same individual at the dose of 0.3 µg/ml LPS. *: A-BFD vs P-BFD: P<0.05 From [29].

Taken together, the results of these studies indicate that abdominal obesity in women is associated with subtle alterations in the HPA axis activity and reactivity. These differences probably influence metabolic variables. Indeed, greater postprandial hypercortisolism (higher cortisol response to food intake) may worsen insulin sensitivity as GC impair insulin-dependent glucose uptake in the periphery, enhance gluconeogenesis in the liver and inhibit insulin secretion in vitro from pancreatic β-cells {Lambillote 1997}.

Therefore, we are faced with two models where subtle differences in HPA axis activity and reactivity are linked to adaptation (endurance training) or disadaptation and pathology (visceral obesity). In both cases overall 24h cortisol levels are normal (24h UFC). But in visceral obesity overnight UFC is increased and is associated with metabolic disorders such as insulin resistance. On the other hand, whereas 24h UFC may be increased during a day with exercise in endurance training this is associated with decreased tissue sensitivity to GC in resting conditions, allowing the protection of the body from the deleterious effects of prolonged hypercortisolism. This lack of deleterious metabolic effect is evidenced, for example, in the increased insulin sensitivity classically reported in endurance-trained men [68].

Pituitary sensitivity to dexamethasone is increased in visceral obesity but decreased in endurance training leading to facilitated recovery after a strenuous bout of exercise and a capacity to carry on a second session of exercise within few hours.

Finally, the ratio of urinary cortisone to cortisol excretion is increased in visceral obesity. This translates an increased peripheral metabolic clearance of cortisol which induces decreased cortisol tone on the HPA axis and might explain their larger ACTH-induced such as food-induced and/or stress induced cortisol response. By contrast, in endurance trained men, any increase in cortisol concentrations is balanced by the parallel increase in its tissular inactivation into cortisone.

Conclusion

Although women with visceral obesity and endurance-trained men are not very different from healthy sedentary subjects in terms of HPA function, however subtle variations in the HPA axis activity and reactivity are evidenced in women with visceral obesity and in endurance-trained men. This does not imply that, in terms of HPA function, endurance-training should be assimilated to an analogue of visceral obesity nor to two other pathological conditions associated with chronic hypercortisolism: anorexia nervosa and chronic depression, as suggested few years ago. This chapter provides evidence that successfull acclimatation to endurance-training involves allostatic modifications of the HPA axis which are both adaptative to repeated exercise challenges and protective against deleterious effects of increased cortisol levels.

We are far from understanding all the physiology of these adaptative and protective mechanisms reported in endurance-training. This is an exciting future area of research, as endurance training represents an unique model of succesfull adaptation to repeated HPA axis activation.

References

[1] Smoak B, Deuster PA, Rabin D, Chrousos GP. Corticotropin-releasing hormone is not the sole factor mediating exercise-induced adrenocorticotropin release in humans. *Journal of Clinical Endocrinology and Metabolism* 1991; 73:302-306.

[2] Wittert GA, Stewart DE, Graves MP, Ellis MJ, Evans MJ, Wells JE et al. Plasma corticotrophin releasing factor and vasopressin responses to exercise in normal man. *Clinical Endocrinology* 1991; 35:311-317.

[3] Cashmore GC, Davies CTM, Few JD. Relationship between increases in plasma cortisol concentration and rate of cortisol secretion during exercise in man. *Journal of Endocrinology* 1977; 72:109-110.

[4] Timofeeva E, Huang Q, Richard D. Effects of treadmill running on brain activation and the corticotropin-releasing hormone system. *Neuroendocrinology* 2003; 77(6):388-405.

[5] Duclos M, Corcuff J-B, Rashedi M, Fougere V, Manier G. Trained versus untrained men: different immediate post-exercise responses of pituitary-adrenal axis. *European Journal of Applied Physiology* 1997; 75:343-350.

[6] Luger A, Deuster PA, Kyle SB, Gallucci WT, Montgomery LC, Gold PW et al. Acute hypothalamic-pituitary-adrenal responses to the stress of treadmill exercise. *New England Journal of Medicine* 1987; 316:1309-1315.

[7] Kjaer M, Secher NH, Bach FW, Galbo H. Role of motor center activity for hormonal changes and substrate mobilization in humans. *American Journal of Physiology* 1987; 253:R687-R695.

[8] Brandenberger G, Follenius M, Hietter B, Reinhardt B, Simeoni M. Feedback from meal-related peaks determines diurnal changes in cortisol response to exercise. *Journal of Clinical Endocrinology and Metabolism* 1982; 54:592-594.

[9] Kanaley JA, Weltman JY, Pieper KS, Weltman A, Hartman ML. Cortisol and growth hormone responses to exercise at different times of day. *Journal of Clinical Endocrinology and Metabolism* 20011; 86:2881-2889.

[10] Thuma JR, Gilders R, Verdun M, Loucks AB. Circadian rhythm of cortisol confounds cortisol responses to exercise: implications for future research. *Journal of Applied Physiology* 1995; 78:1657-1664.

[11] Ronsen O, Kjeldsen-Kragh J, Haug E, Bahr R, Pedersen BK. Recovery time affects immunoendocrine responses to a second bout of endurance exercise. *American Journal of Physiology* 2002; 283:C1612-C1620.

[12] Villanueva AL, Schlosser C, Hopper B, Liu JH, Hoffman DI, Rebar RW. Increased cortisol production in women runners. *J Clin Endocrinol Metab* 1986; 63(1):133-136.

[13] Kern W, Perras B, Wodick R, Fehm HL, Born J. Hormonal secretion during nighttime sleep indicating stress of daytime exercise. *Journal of Applied Physiology* 1995; 79:1461-1468.

[14] Bright GM. Corticosteroid-binding globulin influences kinetic parameters of plasma cortisol transport and clearance. *J Clin Endocrinol Metab* 1995; 80(3):770-775.

[15] Gouarne C, Groussard C, Gratas-Delamarche A, Delamarche P, Duclos M. Overnight urinary cortisol and cortisone add new insights into adaptation to training. *Medicine & Science in Sports and Exercise* (in press) July 2005

[16] Plat L, Leproult R, L'Hermite-Baleriaux M, Fery F, Mockel J, Polonsky KS et al. Metabolic effects of short-term elevations of plasma cortisol are more pronounced in the evening than in the morning. *Journal of Clinical Endocrinology and Metabolism* 1999; 84:3082-3092.

[17] Hansen AM, Garde AH, Skovgaard LT, Christensen JM. Seasonal and biological variation of urinary epinephrine, norepinephrine, and cortisol in healthy women. *Clinica Chimica Acta* 2001; 309:25-35.

[18] Walker BR, Best R, Noon JP, Watt GCM, Webb DJ. Seasonal variation in glucocorticoid activity in healthy men. *Journal of Clinical Endocrinology and Metabolism* 1997; 82:4015-4019.

[19] King JA, Rosal MC, Ma Y, Reed G, Kelly T-A, Stanek EJ et al. Sequence and seasonal effects of salivary cortisol. *Behavioral Medicine* 2000; 26:67-73.

[20] Guinot M, Duclos M, Idress N, Souberbielle JC, Megret A, Le Bouc Y. Risks of adrenal insufficiency and corticosteroid therapy in elite cyclists. Submitted.

[21] Duclos M, Minkhar M, Sarrieau A, Bonnemaison D, Manier G, Mormede P. Reversibility of endurance training-induced changes on glucocorticoid sensitivity of monocytes by an acute exercise. *Clinical Endocrinology* 1999; 51:749-756.

[22] Heuser IJE, Wark HJ, Keul J, Holsboer F. Hypothalamic-pituitary-adrenal axis function in elderly endurance athletes. *Journal of Clinical Endocrinology and Metabolism* 1991; 73:485-488.

[23] Gold PW, Gwirstman H, Avgerinos PC, Nieman LK, Galluci WT, Kaye W et al. Abnormal hypothalamic-pituitary-adrenal function in anorexia nervosa. Pathophysiologic mechanisms in underweight and weight-corrected patients. *New England Journal of Medicine* 1986; 314:1335-1342.

[24] De Souza MJ, Luciano AA, Arce JC, Demers LM, Loucks AB. Clinical tests explain blunted cortisol responsiveness but not mild hypercortisolism in amenorrheic runners. *J Appl Physiol* 1994; 76(3):1302-1309.

[25] Hilton LK, Loucks AB. Low energy availability, not exercise stress, suppresses the diurnal rhythm of leptin in healthy young women. *American Journal of Physiology* 2000; 278:E43-E49.

[26] De Souza MJ, Van Heest J, Demers LM, Lasley BL. Luteal phase deficiency in recreational runners: evidence for a hypometabolic state. *Journal of Clinical Endocrinology and Metabolism* 2003; 88:337-346.

[27] Loucks AB, Thuma JR. Luteinizing hormone pulsatility is disrupted at a threshold of energy availability in regularly menstruating women. *Journal of Clinical Endocrinology and Metabolism* 2003; 88:297-311.

[28] Hackney AC, Viru A. Twenty-four-hour cortisol response to multiple daily exercise sessions of moderate and high intensity. *Clin Physiol* 1999; 19(2):178-182.

[29] Duclos M, Marquez-Pereira P, Barat P, Gatta B, Roger P. Increased cortisol bioavailability, abdominal obesity and the metabolic syndrome in obese women. *Obesity Research* (in press).

[30] Nindl BC, Kraemer WJ, Deaver DR, Peters JL, Marx JO, Heckman JT et al. LH secretion and testosterone concentrations are blunted after resistance exercise in men. *J Appl Physiol* 2001; 91(3):1251-1258.

[31] Atlaoui D, Duclos M, Gouarne C, Lacoste L, Barale F, Chatard JC. The 24-h urinary cortisol/cortisone ratio for monitoring training in elite swimmers. *Medicine & Science in Sports and Exercise* 36, 218-224. 2004.

[32] Neary JP, Wheeler GD, Maclean I, Cumming DC, Quinney HA. Urinary free cortisol as an indicator of exercise training stress. *Clinical Journal of Sport Medicine* 1994; 4:160-165.

[33] Duclos M, Gouarne C, Bonnemaison D. Acute and chronic effects of exercise on tissue sensitivity to glucocorticoids. *Journal of Applied Physiology* 2003; 94:869-875.

[34] McEwen BS. Protective and damaging effects of stress mediators. *New England Journal of Medicine* 1998; 338(3):171-179.

[35] Goverde HJ, Pesman GJ, Smals AG. The bioactivity of immunoreactive adrenocorticotrophin in human blood is dependent on the secretory state of the pituitary gland. *Clin Endocrinol* (Oxf) 1989; 31(3):255-265.

[36] Favrod-Coune C, Raux-Demay MC, Proeschel MF, Bertagna X, Girard F, Luton JP. Potentiation of the classic ovine corticotrophin releasing hormone stimulation test by the combined administration of small doses of lysine vasopressin. *Clin Endocrinol (Oxf)* 1993; 38(4):405-410.

[37] Hashimoto K, Suemaru S, Takao T, Sugawara M, Makino S, Ota Z. Corticotropin-releasing hormone and pituitary-adrenocortical responses in chronically stressed rats. *Regul Pept* 1988; 23(2):117-126.

[38] Kemppainen RJ, Clark TP. Evidence for a single glucocorticoid regulated pool of adrenocorticotropin in sheep anterior pituitary. *Am J Physiol* 1995; 268:E85-E91.

[39] Akana SF, Dallman MF, Bradbury MJ, Scribner KA, Strack AM, Walker CD. Feedback and facilitation in the adrenocortical system: unmasking facilitation by partial inhibition of the glucocorticoid response to prior stress. *Endocrinology* 1992; 131:57-68.

[40] Tharp GD, Buuck RJ. Adrenal adaptation to chronic exercise. *Journal of Applied Physiology* 1974; 37:720-722.

[41] Inder WJ, Hellemans J, Ellis MJ, Evans MJ, Livesey JH, Donald RA. Elevated basal adrenocorticotropin and evidence for increased central opioid tone in higly trained male athletes. *Journal of Clinical Endocrinology and Metabolism* 1995; 80:244-248.

[42] DeRijk R, Petrides J, Deuster P, Gold PW, Sternberg EM. Changes in corticosteroid sensitivity of peripheral blood lymphocytes after strenuous exercise in humans. *Journal of Clinical Endocrinology and Metabolism* 1996; 81:228-235.

[43] Duclos M, Corcuff J-B, Roger P, Tabarin A. The dexamethasone-suppressed corticotrophin-releasing hormone stimulation test in anorexia nervosa. *Clinical Endocrinology* 1999; 51:725-731.

[44] Moldoveanu AI, Shephard RJ, Shek PN. Exercise elevates plasma levels but not gene expression of IL-1β, IL-6, and TNF-α in blood mononuclear cells. *Journal of Applied Physiology* 2000; 89:1499-1504.

[45] Smits HH, Grünberg K, Derijk RH, Sterk PJ, Hiemstra PS. Cytokine release and its modulation by dexamethasone in whole blood following exercise. *Clinical Experimental Immunology* 1998; 111:463-468.

[46] Walker BR, Phillips DI, Noon JP, Panarelli M, Andrew R, Edwards HV et al. Increased glucocorticoid activity in men with cardiovascular risk factors. *Hypertension* 1998; 31(4):891-895.

[47] Rohleder N, Schommer NC, Hellammer D, Engel R, Kirschbaum C. Sex differences in glucocorticoid sensitivity of proinflammatory cytokine production after psychosocial stress. *Psychosomatic Medicine* 2001; 63:966-972.

[48] Sapolsky RM, Romero M, Munck AU. How do glucocorticoids influence stress responses? Integrating permissive, suppressive, stimulatory, and preparative actions. *Endocrine Reviews* 2000; 21:55-89.

[49] Bamberger CM, Schulte HM, Chrousos GP. Molecular determinants of glucocorticoid receptor function and tissue sensitivity to glucocorticoids. *Endocrine Reviews* 1996; 17:245-261.

[50] Hammond GL. Molecular properties of corticosteroid binding globulin and sex-steroid binding proteins. *Endocrine Review* 1990; 11:65-79.

[51] Laudat MH, Billaud L, Thomopoulos P, Vera O, Yllia A, Luton JP. Evening urinary free corticoids: a screening test in Cushing's syndrome and incidentally discovered adrenal tumours. *Acta Endocrinol* (Copenh) 1988; 119(3):459-464.

[52] Rosner W. The functions of corticosteroid-binding globulin and sex hormone-binding globulin: recent advances. *Endocrine Reviews* 1990; 11:80-91.

[53] Umeda T, Hiramatsu R, Iwaoka T, Shimada T, Miura F, Sato T. Use of saliva for monitoring unbound free cortisol levels in serum. *Clinica Chimica Acta* 1981; 110:245-253.

[54] Duclos M, Corcuff J-B, Arsac L, Moreau-Gaudry F, Rashedi M, Roger P et al. Corticotroph axis sensitivity after exercise in endurance-trained athletes. *Clinical Endocrinology* 1998; 48:493-501.

[55] Chennaoui M, Gomez Merino D, Lesage J, Drogou C, Guezennec CY. Effects of moderate and intensive training on the hypothalamo-pituitary-adrenal axis in rats. *Acta Physiologica Scandinavica* 2002; 175:113-121.

[56] Seckl JR, Walker BR. Minireview: 11β-hydroxysteroid dehydrogenase type 1- A tissue specific amplifier of glucocorticoid action. *Endocrinology* 2001; 142:1371-1376.

[57] Stewart PM, Mason JI. Cortisol to cortisone: glucocorticoid to mineralocorticoid. *Steroids* 1995; 60(1):143-146.

[58] Best R, Walker BR. Additional value of measurement of urinary cortisone and unconjugated cortisol metabolites in assessing the activity of 11 beta-hydroxysteroid dehydrogenase in vivo. *Clin Endocrinol* (Oxf) 1997; 47(2):231-236.

[59] Lin CL, Wu TJ, Machacek DA, Jiang NS, Kao PC. Urinary free cortisol and cortisone determined by high performance liquid chromatography in the diagnosis of Cushing's syndrome. *Journal of Clinical Endocrinology and Metabolism* 82, 151-155. 1997.

[60] Smith LL. Cytokine hypothesis of overtraining: a physiological adaptation to excessive stress? *Med Sci Sports Exerc* 2000; 32(2):317-331.

[61] Duclos M, Corcuff J-B, Etcheverry N, Rashedi M, Tabarin A, Roger P. Abdominal obesity increases overnight cortisol excretion. *Journal of Endocrinological Investigation* 1999; 22:465-471.

[62] Donahue RP, Abott RD, Bloom E, Reed DM, Yano K. Central obesity and coronary heart disease in men. *Lancet* 1987; 1:821-824.

[63] Hauner H, Schmid P, Pfeiffer EF. Glucocorticoids and insulin promote the differentiation of human adipocyte precursor cells into fat cells. *Journal of Clinical Endocrinology and Metabolism* 1987; 64:832-835.

[64] Rebuffe-Scrive M, Walsh VA, McEven BS, Rodin J. Effect of chronic stress and exogenous glucocorticoids on regional fat distribution and metabolism. *Physiology and Behavior* 1992; 52:583-590.

[65] Duclos M, Gatta B, Corcuff JB, Rashedi M, Pehourcq F, Roger P. Fat distribution in obese women is associated with subtle variations of the hypothalamic-pituitary-adrenal axis activity and sensitivity to glucocorticoids. *Clinical Endocrinology* 2001; 55:447-454.

[66] Korbonits M, Trainer PJ, Nelson ML, Howse I, Kopelman PG, Besser GM et al. Differential stimulation of cortisol and dehydroepiandrosterone levels by food in obese

and normal subjects: relation to body fat distribution. *Clinical Endocrinology* 1996; 45:699-706.

[67] Pasquali R, Biscotti D, Spinucci G, Vicennati V, Genazzani AD, Sgarbi L et al. Pulsatile secretion of ACTH and cortisol in premenopausal women: effect of obesity and body fat distribution. *Clinical Endocrinology* 1998; 48:603-612.

[68] Dela F, Mikines KJ, von Linstow M, Secher NH, Galbo H. Effect of training on insulin-mediated glucose uptake in human muscle. *American Journal of Physiology* 1992; 263:E1134-E1143.

[69] Strain GW, Zumoff B, Strain JJ, Levin J, Fukushima DK. Cortisol production in obesity. *Metabolism* 1980; 29:980-984.

In: Focus on Exercise and Health Research
Editor: Thomas B. Selkirk, pp. 163-179

ISBN 1-59454-349-6
© 2006 Nova Science Publishers, Inc.

Chapter VI

The Efficacy of Psyching-Up on Strength Performance

David Tod[1] and Michael McGuigan[2]

[1]Centre for Rehabilitation, Exercise, and Sport Science; Victoria University Melbourne Australia; [2]School of Biomedical and Sports Science; Edith Cowan University; Joondalup, Australia

Abstract

Many people believe that mental preparation influences exercise behaviour and athletic performance. Researchers have examined the effect that a range of cognitive behavioural techniques have on the display of motor skills, and it has been concluded that these interventions may positively influence exercise behaviour and enhance sporting performance. Psyching-up is one type of intervention that has received empirical attention with respect to muscular force production and refers to self-directed cognitive strategies used immediately prior to or during skill execution that are designed to enhance physical performance. In this chapter we review the literature examining the influence of psyching-up on maximal strength, local muscular endurance, and power. The existing research provides evidence that psyching-up may help untrained or neophyte participants improve their maximal strength and local muscular endurance during simple or isolated dynamic contractions. Preliminary evidence also suggests that psyching-up may enhance performance on movements requiring power although more research is needed. Generally, equivocal results have emerged from the few studies in which well-trained samples have been used. Also, the experimental tasks have been restricted to movements such as the handgrip, leg extension, bench press, sit-up, press-up, pull-up, and standing broad jump. Currently, it is unclear why psyching-up may assist novice performers undertaking simple dynamic movements because no explanation has any overwhelming support. To further the understanding of the psyching-up and muscular force production relationship, researchers need to use a wider range of participants, employ complex movements, include multiple control conditions, describe samples on several characteristics, and interpret the meaningfulness of their findings.

Although there is insufficient evidence to indicate that well-trained athletes might profit from psyching-up prior to or during competition, such interventions may be of benefit for novice participants in health and fitness settings.

Many individuals believe that mental preparation influences exercise and sporting behaviour and performance. Within the last thirty years, sport and exercise psychology has become recognised as a separate sport science (Williams & Straub, 2001). Along with this recognition, applied sport and exercise psychologists have increasingly been helping individuals use psychological interventions to influence exercise behaviour and improve sporting performance. Also during this time, exercise and sport psychology researchers have investigated the influence that cognitive behavioural interventions have on sporting performance and exercise behaviour (e.g., Rogerson & Hrycaiko, 2002; Thelwell & Greenlees, 2001; Thelwell & Greenlees, 2003). In the realm of sport, for example, a meta-analysis of 56 studies yielded an effect size of 0.62, with the 95% confidence interval ranging from 0.40 to 0.84 (Meyers, Whelan, & Murphy, 1996). An effect size of 0.62 represents a medium to large effect (Cohen, 1977), suggesting that the use of cognitive behavioural interventions leads to improved performance. In a more recent article, Weinberg and Williams (2001 p. 349) concluded that "a growing body of empirical literature demonstrates the effectiveness of psychological interventions and mental training programs for enhancing athletic performance." Although there is increasing evidence indicating that psychological interventions can influence skill execution, exercise behaviour, and sporting performance, such techniques need to be applied in suitable and creative ways to ensure that exercise and sports participants receive benefits (Tod & Andersen, in press).

One aspect of mental preparation is psyching-up and refers to the use of self-directed cognitive strategies immediately prior to or during skill execution to enhance physical performance (Brody, Hatfield, Spalding, Frazer, & Caherty, 2000; Hardy, Jones, & Gould, 1996). The meta-analysis study cited above reported an effect size of 1.23 (a very large effect, Cohen, 1977), suggesting that psyching-up might have a large influence on performance, although only 5 studies were included (Meyers et al., 1996). In this chapter we will review psyching-up research that has focused on muscular force production. Studies in which other interventions were used such as music, verbal encouragement, and instructor-led guided imagery were not considered to be part of the psyching-up literature. The primary dependent variables that have been measured include maximal strength, local muscular endurance, and power. In this chapter we will review the research under these headings. Strength is considered to be the maximal force generated by a muscle at a particular speed (Harman, Garhammer, & Pandorf, 2000; Kraemer & Fry, 1995), and in this section we have included studies in which force production during a low number of repetitions, such as a 3-repetition maximum (3RM), was measured. Under the local muscular endurance heading we review research in which a high number of repetitions performed at a particular resistance level were assessed, such as the number of bench press repetitions completed until failure. Power refers to the rate at which work can be performed under a given set of circumstances (Abernethy, Wilson, & Logan, 1995; Harman et al., 2000), and in this section we have included research during which the influence of psyching-up on explosive power was investigated.

Maximal Strength

Shelton and Mahoney (1978) were the first investigators to examine the effect of psyching-up on maximal strength. Participants consisted of 30 male competitive weightlifters who had their handgrip strength measured across three trials. No cognitive intervention was used prior to the first trial, and participants counted backwards from a four-digit number in groups of seven prior to the second trial. The purpose of asking participants to count backwards was to assess the effects of a simple distraction task. The weightlifters were randomly assigned to either the experimental ($n = 16$) or control group ($n = 14$) for the final trial. Individuals in the experimental group were asked to psych-up just before their final trial using the mental preparation strategy of their choice, whereas those in the control group counted backwards in groups of six. There was a significant increase in strength from trial two to trial three for the experimental group but not for the control participants. Using trial two as a covariate, there was a significant difference between the groups on the third trial. It would have been interesting to analyse the trial three results using trial one as a covariate to evaluate the effect of psyching-up against a non-intervention condition, but this was not done. A number of other studies have been undertaken since the publication of Shelton and Mahoney's (1978) study, although not all have yielded similar results (Brody et al., 2000; Elko & Ostrow, 1992; Ghiagiarelli, McGuigan, & Tod, 2004; Gould, Weinberg, & Jackson, 1980; Murphy, Woolfolk, & Budney, 1988; Tenenbaum, Bar-Eli, Hoffman, Jablonovski, Sade, & Shitrit, 1995; Theodorakis, Weinberg, Natsis, Douma, & Kazakas, 2000; Tod, Iredale, McGuigan, Strange, & Gill, in press; Tynes & McFatter, 1987; Weinberg, Gould, & Jackson, 1980, 1981; Whelan, Epkins, & Meyers, 1990; Wilkes & Summers, 1984). Across the studies in which psyching-up lead to increased maximal strength, the average increase has been 12% with a range of –1% to 35% (Tod, Iredale, & Gill, 2003). The estimate was obtained by expressing the difference in strength between the intervention and control conditions as a percentage of the control conditions.

Researchers have employed within- and between-participant repeated measure designs and have used different types of control conditions (Brody et al., 2000). The distraction control has been most commonly used where participants have undertaken a cognitive task to prevent them from psyching-up. Other control conditions have included quiet rest, non-intervention, and attention-placebo, which is used to tease out the effects of those factors common to all the interventions (Wilson, 2000). Some researchers have only used the distraction control condition in their studies (e.g., Brody et al., 2000; Elko & Ostrow, 1992; Weinberg et al., 1980; Wilkes & Summers, 1984). In such research designs, if participants performed better in the psych-up condition compared to the distraction control, the results may be difficult to interpret. Although psyching-up might have enhanced performance, it could also be concluded that the distraction task lead to a drop in performance. The only unambiguous conclusion is that psyching-up lead to better performance than distraction. It seems unlikely, however, that many people would actively distract themselves prior to a strength task. One possible solution is for researchers to regularly include more than one control condition in their research designs.

In a number of studies, researchers have allowed participants to use the psych-up strategy of their choice (e.g., Shelton & Mahoney, 1978; Tod et al., in press; Weinberg et al., 1980,

1981; Whelan et al., 1990). The common techniques used have included focussed attention, preparatory arousal, imagery, and self-efficacy statements. Also, a number of participants have used a combination of techniques (Shelton & Mahoney, 1978; Weinberg et al., 1980, 1981). Researchers have also compared the effectiveness of various psych-up strategies by directing participants to use particular techniques, and preparatory arousal, imagery, focussed attention, self-efficacy statements, self-talk, and relaxation have been those methods typically prescribed (Elko & Ostrow, 1992; Gould et al., 1980; Murphy et al., 1988; Theodorakis et al., 2000; Tynes & McFatter, 1987; Whelan et al., 1990; Wilkes & Summers, 1984). Preparatory arousal has been found the most consistently effective strategy, whereas relaxation has been associated with reduced strength performance (Murphy et al., 1988; Tenenbaum et al., 1995).

The types of strength tasks used in the supporting research have been largely limited to simple dynamic movements such as the bench press, handgrip, and leg extension exercises. Strength is defined in part by the task being performed (Blazevich, Gill, & Newton, 2002; Brody et al., 2000; Kraemer & Fry, 1995), and it cannot be assumed that the findings from existing studies are applicable to other movements, particularly compound actions involving a large number of muscle groups. Although a recent study found that psyching-up lead to increased force production during the bench press exercise (Tod et al., in press), researchers need to examine a wider range of complex movements, especially those used in a health, fitness, or sports setting. Also, untrained individuals have been the type of participants predominantly examined and this point will be expanded on later in this chapter.

Preliminary evidence suggests that neither age nor varying the psych-up duration period influences maximal strength, although more research is needed (Elko & Ostrow, 1992; Weinberg et al., 1981). The time intervals used in Weinberg et al.'s (1981) study included (a) 15 seconds, (b) 30 seconds, (c) a self-initiated period where the participants (undergraduate students) determined how long they would prepare themselves, and (d) a yoked condition in which participants were paired with individuals in the self-initiated condition. The leg extension (single joint exercise) was the movement task used and results indicated that the free choice psych-up strategy led to greater strength scores compared with the non-intervention control condition, although there were no differences among the various time intervals. The possible interaction between age and psyching-up was investigated by Elko and Ostrow (1992). Their sample was divided into older males (mean age [M] = 59.9 years, SD = 2.6), older females (M = 60.3 years, SD = 2.3), younger males (M = 22.1 years, SD = 2.8), and younger females (M = 21.0 years, SD = 2.6), and the dependent variable was handgrip strength. Preparatory arousal, imagery, and distraction represented the various intervention conditions. No interactions between psyching-up and age were observed, although imagery was associated with greater strength, and the younger participants were stronger than older individuals.

One study investigated the influence of competitive experience on the psych-up effect, using measured handgrip strength as the dependent variable (Whelan et al., 1990). Individuals classified as having low levels of experience had not played sport or had only participated in recreational exercise. Those people classified as having moderate experience had participated in high school or recreational sport, although they may have also played some college intramural or recreational sport. Individuals classified as having high levels of experience included collegiate or semi-professional athletes or those with a significant history in a number of competitive sports at high school. The various psych-up conditions included preparatory arousal, self-selected psyching-up, attention-placebo, and a distraction task. Preparatory arousal led to greater strength in the moderately experienced participants only, whereas in the highly experienced individuals, self-selected psyching-up was associated with better performance. The authors suggested that mental preparation could be learned through experience or could be quickly trained after moderate amounts of competitive sporting experience.

Not all investigations have yielded positive results, and the non-supportive research has raised a number of questions that are worthy of attention (e.g., Brody et al., 2000; Ghiagiarelli et al., 2004; Murphy et al., 1988; Tenenbaum et al., 1995). In one of the few studies in which well-trained participants were employed, Brody et al. (2000) measured forced produced and electromyogram (EMG) activity during an isometric biceps contraction with a right angle at the elbow. No differences were observed across the psych-up or distraction control conditions. The authors identified two possible reasons why their results were different from the supportive research. Dynamic strength tasks had been used in the previous studies, whereas Brody et al. (2000) examined an isometric contraction. Participants may have had more freedom to vary their movements or posture during the dynamic strength tasks allowing them to gain a biomechanical advantage or recruit more muscle groups. During an isometric contraction participants may not have been able to vary their posture or movement patterns. Psyching-up may not lead to greater force within a single muscle, but may enhance performance because participants can use more of their musculature. It is possible that psyching-up may influence some types of contractions but not others. Alternatively, the type of participants examined may explain Brody et al.'s (2000) results. Most of the supportive research has used untrained participants whereas those used in Brody et al (2000) were well-trained. Brody et al. (2000) suggested that psyching-up may assist untrained rather than well-trained individuals. Trained individuals are likely to have well-developed movement patterns and neural pathways that might not be easily modified via psyching-up, whereas untrained people may have less developed movement patterns and neural pathways that are modifiable. Also, the performance of untrained participants is likely to be characterised by greater variation compared with trained individuals. Empirical evidence, however, regarding the relationships between dynamic and isometric strength is mixed (Murphy & Wilson, 1996; Wilson & Murphy, 1996). It cannot be assumed that the participants were highly trained in an isometric biceps contraction on the basis of their dynamic performance levels. It was not clear if either or both of the explanations accounted for the differences between Brody et al.'s (2000) results and the findings of the supportive investigations, and further research is needed.

In a recent study, the influence of psyching-up on 1RM squat performance was examined in participants with a minimum of one year of weight training experience (Ghiagiarelli et al., 2004). No differences were found between psyching-up and a distraction condition. Ghiagiarelli et al's (2004) investigation is one of the few to have examined a compound strength task that was used by trained participants as part of their regular training and provides evidence that psyching-up may not increase dynamic maximal strength in people who have moved beyond the novice stage. The authors offered a number of reasons why their results may have differed from the supportive research. First, the squat exercise is a compound full body movement, whereas the supportive research has tended to use simpler or single joint strength tasks. Perhaps psyching-up does not assist individuals during compound movements that involve the entire body. Second, the participants had at least one year of weight training experience whereas most of the supportive research has used untrained participants. Some supportive research, however, has used trained participants including Tod et al. (in press) who also used individuals with at least one year of training experience. Psyching-up might be influenced by the interaction between the type of task (e.g., simple versus compound) and participant experience. Third, maybe the participants did not psych-up enough to obtain a benefit. Researchers have not previously considered the possibility that a minimum amount of psyching-up is needed. It is not clear, however, why participants with one year of weight training experience would not be able to psych-up enough, if in the supportive research, novices have been able to mentally prepare themselves sufficiently. It is not possible to determine which, if any, of the proposed explanations accounted for Ghiagiarelli et al.'s (2004) results.

The finding that psyching-up had no effect on strength was also observed by researchers who compared positive self-talk (PS), relaxation-visualisation autogenic training (RVA), and a non-intervention control on peak force and power during an isokinetic bilateral knee extension exercise (Tenenbaum et al., 1995). Although the participants had no prior experience in resistance training, they underwent a three-week weight training programme to become familiar with the strength tests used in the study. In addition, the two intervention groups received four instructional sessions on the use of their respective psych-up strategies. Peak force increased in all groups pre- to post-test, although the control group had a significantly greater improvement. Also, the PS group had a greater improvement than the RVA group. The peak power findings will be discussed later. The non-significant difference between the PS and control groups differs from other research that has used an isokinetic knee extension exercise (e.g., Gould et al., 1980; Theodorakis et al., 2000; Weinberg et al., 1981; Wilkes & Summers, 1984). Participants in the supporting research were not given four sessions of instruction, however, and the authors suggested that as a result of receiving training, their participants might have had to divide their attention across the strength task and a psych-up strategy. In support of the authors' suggestion, evidence does indicate that if attentional demands of a task exceed the available resources then performance levels may decrease (Schmidt & Wrisberg, 2000). Alternatively, if psyching-up is only effective for untrained individuals, as argued by Brody et al. (2000), perhaps the lack of significant differences in Tenenbaum et al.'s (1995) study was because participants were no longer novices at the task after completing a three week training programme. It appears that the knee extension is a simple task to learn. It is not clear which explanation, if either, accounts for Tenenbaum et al.'s (1995) results, but the study illustrates the need to define the differences between novice, untrained, and well-trained individuals.

In another non-supportive study, Murphy et al. (1988) compared fear-, anger-, and relaxation-based imagery with non-intervention pre- and post-tests on handgrip strength using male undergraduate students. Relaxation imagery was associated with lower strength scores compared to the other interventions, and the pre-test led to higher strength scores over the fear-based imagery and post-test trials. The result that fear and anger based imagery were not associated with superior strength conflicts with other investigations that have found imagery to be an effective psych-up strategy (Elko & Ostrow, 1992; Gould et al., 1980; Shelton & Mahoney, 1978). The participants in Murphy et al. (1988) were asked to imagine scenes in which they felt angry, fearful, or relaxed. The images participants produced may have not been related to the handgrip task. In the supportive research, participants have generally been asked to produce images related to the strength task (Elko & Ostrow, 1992; Gould et al., 1980). Perhaps psyching-up leads to improved strength if the strategy is task relevant. Fatigue, however, is a possible rival hypothesis for the Murphy et al. (1988) results. Strength scores decreased between the pre- and post-tests, participants completed multiple trials, and it is not clear how much rest they had between each attempt. Consequently, fatigue may have overshadowed any psych-up effect.

Fitts and Posners' (1967) Stages of Motor Skill Learning

From a motor learning perspective, Fitts and Posner's (1967) classic three phases of learning theory offers one possible way to synthesis the current empirical data on psyching-up and maximal strength. In their early or cognitive phase, the novice lifter attempts to understand the task and its demands. It is usually necessary for participants to focus on the cues, events, and responses associated with the movement. In the squat exercise, for example, individuals need to attend to kinaesthetic information regarding body position, balance, and the effort needed to successfully complete the lift. Novices also often rely on visual feedback via mirrors and directions from instructors as well. According to Fitts' and Posners' (1967) model, a large part of learning a strength task involves cognitive activity and many strength researchers also argue that the initial strength gains novices experience are due to neurological learning (Sale, 1988). Most of the supportive research has used untrained participants and the finding that psyching-up influences maximal strength in novices during simple dynamic tasks seems to be robust.

In the intermediate or associative phase, the movements that must be made have been learned. Although errors still occur, they are gradually eliminated and over time performance becomes more coordinated and efficient. A common observation in a weight-training setting is that novice individuals' movement patterns are initially inefficient and uncoordinated, particularly in complex compound movements. As individuals train over time, their movements become smooth and efficient (Laidlaw, Kornatz, Keen, Suzuki, & Enoka, 1999).

In Fitts' and Posners' (1967) third or autonomous phase, the performance of well-learned skills requires less cognitive processing and becomes automatic. There appears to be some similarities between highly practiced skills and reflexes because both seem to occur without much cognitive activity. Instead, cognitive processing may interfere with movement. Highly trained participants, for example, who are requested to direct to their attention to their muscle movements during a squat may find it difficult to perform the movement in a normal efficient manner.

The support for the psyching-up effect becomes mixed when considering the research in which participants with some degree of training experience have been used (Brody et al., 2000; Ghiagiarelli et al., 2004; Shelton & Mahoney, 1978; Tenenbaum et al., 1995; Tod et al., in press; Tynes & McFatter, 1987; Whelan et al., 1990). A difficulty in synthesising the research has been the variety of criteria used to describe participants and none seem to be without limitations. Criteria have included the number of weight training competitions undertaken (Shelton & Mahoney, 1978), the number of weeks or years of resistance training completed (Ghiagiarelli et al., 2004; Tenenbaum et al., 1995; Tod et al., in press; Tynes & McFatter, 1987), the amount of competitive sporting experience (Whelan et al., 1990), and level of strength (Brody et al., 2000). In two studies, for example, individuals who had at least one years' weight training experience were used, but it isn't certain these participants were highly trained (Ghiagiarelli et al., 2004; Tod et al., in press). The amount of experience on it's own does not indicate individuals' degree of strength. The findings in these two studies were equivocal. Although psyching-up was associated with increased performance in the bench press exercise, there were no differences in the squat (Ghiagiarelli et al., 2004; Tod et al., in press). As another example, participants' 1RM was reported in one study (Brody et al., 2000). Although such data would seem to be a good indicator of training level, the ratio of strength to body weight also needs to be included. One possible solution is for researchers to include a variety of training level indicators when describing participants including performance data, physical characteristics, training experience, and strength to body weight ratio.

Nevertheless, Brody et al.'s (2000) study has perhaps the clearest indication that well-trained participants were used. The sample had an average 1RM unilateral bicep curl of 29.9 kg and body mass of 87.1 kg. The participants' strength to body weight ratio was 0.34. In keeping with Fitts and Posner's (1967) model, there were no differences in maximal force production between the psych-up and distraction conditions. Firm conclusions about the effect that psyching-up may have in trained participants performing strength tasks to which they are accustomed cannot be made until more research has been conducted on well described samples. One reason why well-trained participants have not generally been used could be the relative difficulty in recruiting such individuals compared to undergraduate students, who have often been targeted in psyching-up research.

Conclusions Regarding Maximal Strength

Taken together, the existing research provides evidence that psyching-up may enhance dynamic maximal strength in untrained participants performing simple movements. Also, preliminary evidence suggests that neither age nor the amount of time individuals take to psych-up influences performance. The effectiveness of psyching-up may be influenced by competitive history with more experienced participants benefiting from using self-selected strategies. More investigations, however, are needed to replicate existing studies. Researchers also need to use highly trained participants and a wider range of movements including compound strength tasks. The efficacy of psyching-up for different types of muscular contractions needs to be further explored. Finally, the influence of psychological instruction, specific and non-specific strategies, and intervention familiarity also need to be investigated.

Local Muscular Endurance

Researchers have given limited attention to the influence of psyching-up on local muscular endurance, and more investigations are needed (Caudill & Weinberg, 1983; Lee, 1990; Theodorakis et al., 2000; Weinberg, Jackson, & Seaboune, 1985). Most of the studies conducted provide evidence that psyching-up is associated with increased performance. The average difference between psych-up and control conditions is 11% with a range of –1 to 29% (Caudill & Weinberg, 1983; Lee, 1990; Weinberg et al., 1985) and these figures were calculated in the same way as the corresponding figures for maximum strength (Tod et al., 2003). As an illustration of the muscular endurance research, in Weinberg et al.'s (1985) study 24 males enrolled in weight training classes performed sit-ups, pull-ups, and push-ups for one minute after engaging in a psych-up condition. Participants also completed the standing broad jump, but these results will be discussed in the power section. The psych-up interventions included imagery, preparatory arousal, a free-choice strategy, and a distraction control. The sequencing of the interventions and performance tasks were counterbalanced to avoid any order effects. Across the performance tasks there were no differences among the psych-up conditions, although they all lead to superior performance compared to the distraction control.

Preliminary evidence has indicated that time may not influence the effectiveness of psyching-up on local muscular endurance, but performance may be improved with a task relevant strategy (Caudill & Weinberg, 1983; Lee, 1990). In a study by Caudill and Weinberg (1983), participants were requested to psych-up for 15, 30, or 60 seconds prior to the endurance test. The strategies included preparatory arousal, imagery, and focussed attention, with quiet rest as the control condition. All three psych-up strategies were associated with a greater number of repetitions on the bench press compared with quiet rest. There were no differences among the interventions and there were no interaction effects (Caudill & Weinberg, 1983). Two experiments were reported by Lee (1990) in which male students were randomly assigned to one of three groups. Those participants in the task relevant group were asked to imagine performing their best, whereas those in the irrelevant group were asked to imagine a situation where they were happy and confident. Participants in the control group undertook a distraction task. In both experiments there was an overall improvement in performance between the pre- and post-tests, and the task relevant participants had a greater improvement compared to the others (Lee, 1990).

In one study there were no differences between self-talk and a non-intervention control on the number of sit-ups performed in three minutes (Theodorakis et al., 2000). Participants consisted of high school students who performed a baseline trial before being allocated to a motivational self-talk, instructional self-talk, or control condition. After the baseline measure, participants performed two further trials, with a five-day rest period in between every attempt. All three groups improved across the trials, indicating that a possible learning effect occurred which may have overshadowed any psych-up effect. It may also have been possible that the control participants spontaneously began using self-talk. In a post-experimental manipulation check, 53% of the control group reported thinking about something specific during the trials although the content of their thoughts was not described.

The local muscular endurance research has used both within- and between-participant repeated measures designs, and the control conditions have included non-intervention, quiet rest, and distraction. Samples, however, have consisted of high school and college students with no indication that participants were highly trained lifters. Local muscular endurance has been measured using sit-ups, press-ups, pull-ups, and the bench press exercises. As with the maximum strength research, investigators could examine a variety of compound sport and exercise-specific movements. Participants have typically been allocated a specific psych-up method to employ, although Weinberg et al. (1985) also allowed them to select a preferred method as one of the conditions investigated. The strategies used have typically included imagery, self-talk, preparatory arousal, and attentional focus. There is no evidence suggesting any strategy is better than the others.

Power

Conflicting results have been obtained from the few studies that have examined the influence of psyching-up on performance during power tests (Tenenbaum et al., 1995; Weinberg et al., 1985). In the Tenenbuam et al. (1995) study, described in the maximal strength section, all three groups (control, PS, & RVA) improved their peak power output from pre- to post- test by 9%. Also, the control group had a higher peak power output than the intervention conditions. In contrast, Weinberg et al. (1985) measured power using the standing broad jump and participants consisted of 24 male students enrolled in a weight training class. There were no differences between the psych-up strategies that included imagery, preparatory arousal, and "free choice," although all three yielded significantly greater performances than the distraction control condition by an average of 2%.

More investigations are needed to examine the influence of psyching-up on power, and along with local muscular endurance, such research might be particularly useful. In many movements the development of maximum strength may not lead to enhanced performance. Participants often need to produce strength quickly (power) or maintain their strength over extended periods of time (endurance). Knowledge about the influence of psyching-up on muscular power and endurance may be more widely applicable than the equivalent understanding regarding maximum strength. In addition, researchers need to examine tasks that are relevant to the participants under study. There is some evidence that psyching-up may influence performance in sport specific tasks requiring power. For example, the influence of instructional and motivational self-talk was assessed on the distance achieved by novices when performing a water polo throw (Hatzigeorgiadis, Theodorakis, & Zourbanos, 2004). Motivational, but not instructional, self-talk was associated with increased performance. In another study, Caudill, Weinberg, and Jackson (1983) found psyching-up lead to quicker sprint times in the 100-yard dash and 60-yard hurdles. Caudill et al's (1983) study is one of the few in which experienced participants performed a task with which they were accustomed. The participants were college track athletes who performed the task during training. In replicating Caudill et al.'s (1983) study it would be desirable to evaluate if psyching-up can still influence performance under competitive conditions. In a related study, the combination of psyching-up with music was associated with quicker 60-meter dash performance compared with distraction in intercollegiate male sprinters (Hall & Erickson, 1995). Although not a pure psyching-up study, the result is notable because the runners competed against each other in groups of three.

Researchers who have examined the influence of psyching-up on power, along with local muscular endurance and maximal strength, have seldom interpreted the meaningfulness of their results. It is rare, for example, that effect sizes are reported despite the recommendation that they are included and interpreted in research articles (e.g., Speed & Andersen, 2000). Weinberg et al.'s (1985) study, mentioned above, provides an example. In considering the standing broad jump results, the preparatory arousal condition lead to a 3.9% improvement in performance. If a 3.9% improvement was applicable to trained athletes performing the long jump (an assumption that needs to be tested), then such a result might have large implications. As another example, Tod et al. (in press) used the minimal worthwhile difference method described by Hopkins (2003) to interpret their results. Using 2.5 Kg as the minimal worthwhile difference applicable to the participants (the smallest increment available in many weight training situations), the authors concluded that psyching-up was almost certainly beneficial. It seems useful to recommend that researchers interpret the meaningfulness of their results.

Explanations for the Psych-Up Effect

To examine why psyching-up may influence muscular force production, the selection of suitable variables needs to be based on the factors that influence the display of strength. A number of variables, beginning with input from the higher motor centres and ending with the interaction of actin and myosin, determine strength (Pette & Staron, 2001). The increase in strength resulting from psyching-up might be due to changes in the central nervous system. The cerebral cortex is the first and highest level of muscle contraction control. Psyching-up strategies most likely occur in the cerebral cortex and may stimulate changes that influence motor unit recruitment, synchronisation, or firing rate. Additionally, psyching-up may lead to changes in sympathetic nervous system activity and alterations in peripheral factors such as muscle contractility. Such changes might occur in the primary agonist muscles, antagonist muscles, or other muscles that contribute to the movement (Brody et al., 2000; Tod et al., 2003).

Although there are a number of theoretical reasons why psyching-up might influence muscular force production, there is currently there is no empirical evidence that conclusively supports any explanation (Tod et al., 2003). Some researchers have hypothesised that improved strength performance may result from increased arousal, enhanced self-confidence, or focussed attention (Biddle, 1985; Brody et al., 2000; Hardy et al., 1996). An inconsistent pattern of results, however, has merged from the research and the changes observed in psychological states have often not been in the expected directions. Weinberg et al. (1980) for example, found that higher perceived effort was associated with leg strength when participants psyched-up. In contrast, although Lee (1990) found that task-relevant imagery led to more sit-ups completed in 30 seconds compared with task-irrelevant imagery, higher vigour and lower fatigue was associated with task-irrelevant imagery. In addition, in Brody et al's (2000) investigation there were no differences in performance, whereas participants thought they had higher levels of arousal and attention when they psyched-up. A possible limitation, however, with these investigations could be the reliance on self-reported data (Brody et al., 2000; Caudill & Weinberg, 1983; Elko & Ostrow, 1992; Lee, 1990; Murphy et al., 1988; Weinberg et al., 1980, 1981; Weinberg et al., 1985; Wilkes & Summers, 1984). Perhaps participants may not be capable of accurately reflecting on their relevant cognitive processes (Nisbett & Wilson, 1977). The questionnaire data may have been influenced by participants' beliefs about the extent to which arousal, effort, and attention should have changed with psyching-up. Researchers could advance knowledge in the area by measuring psychological states in a variety of ways, although for some variables, such as confidence, self-report data will probably continue to be collected because other methods are not readily available.

Although some researchers have used physiological measures to evaluate if increased arousal explains the psyching-up effect, the results have not been supportive. Heart rate, for example, was not related to increased strength or psyching-up (Whelan et al., 1990). In addition, related research using instructor-led interventions have produced mixed results (Perkins, Wilson, & Kerr, 2001; Pierce, McGowan, Eastman, Aaron, & Lynn, 1993). In a recent study, cortisol was used as an indicator of physiological stress (Ghiagiarelli et al., 2004). Results revealed a significant elevation in saliva levels of cortisol following 1RM attempts in the squat exercise. There were no significant differences between the self-directed cognitive strategy and distraction control in salivary cortisol responses or performance. The authors suggested the findings could be partially explained by the participants' training experience and because they were not lifting during a competition (Ghiagiarelli et al., 2004). Davis et al (1981) demonstrated that the psychoendocrine response to a novel situation was a major determinant of serum cortisol levels during maximal work. The measurement of physiological variables to assess arousal deserves further attention, although multiple valid measures need to be used. Heart rate, for example, may not be the best variable to measure when examining the effect of psyching-up on strength. Heart rate may increase from enhanced sympathetic nervous system activity and from reduced parasympathetic nervous system activity (Berntson, Cacioppo, & Quigley, 1993; Perkins et al., 2001).

Brody et al. (2000) also assessed physiological measures in an attempt to explain why psyching-up might influence muscular force production. The authors hypothesised that psyching-up might lead to increased motor unit recruitment in the agonist muscles along with a decrease in the antagonist muscles. In their experiment there were no differences in EMG activity in either the biceps or triceps muscles across the psych-up and control groups, although there were also no differences in maximal force production. Taken together the results from the relevant investigations have not helped researchers explain why psyching-up might influence force production. One central reason why there is no substantial support for any explanation is the lack of empirical attention. Researchers need to continue investigating why psyching-up may improve strength performance because such information might underpin practical recommendations.

A Possible Application of the Psyching-Up Effect

To date, the empirical evidence suggests that the group most likely to benefit from psyching-up are novices and those who are not highly trained. Also, most of the research has focussed on simple dynamic strength tasks like the handgrip and leg extension exercises. Tod, Iredale, and Gill (2003) suggested that well-trained sports participants were the individuals most likely to be interested in psyching-up research, but such a suggestion might be inaccurate. Undoubtedly many well-trained sports people would be very interested in the findings from the psyching-up research, but less highly conditioned individuals who also participate in sport may be curious about the possible performance benefits they might receive. There are greater numbers of low to moderately conditioned individuals than those who are highly trained.

The results of the empirical research might also apply to individuals undertaking weight training as part of health and fitness programmes. In addition, Asken and Goodling (1986) published a single case report in which psyching-up enhanced handgrip strength in a female patient with the diagnosis of recurrent CVA with left hemiparesis. It is possible that psyching-up may be applicable in a rehabilitation setting, although more research is needed. Psyching-up may help an individual to train at a higher intensity, providing a greater stimulus for adaptation. Over time psyching-up may be one strategy, among others, that contributes to optimal training gains. In addition, psyching-up may assist in the development of self-efficacy, a variable that has a bi-directional relationship with exercise behaviour (McAuley & Blissmer, 2002). Self-efficacy plays a role in the adoption and maintenance of exercise (Buckworth & Dishman, 2002). Exercise adherence is an important concern because 50% of people who start an exercise programme cease within six months (Buckworth & Dishman, 2002), and many will dropout much earlier. Given that it can take a number of weeks until individuals experience noticeable changes in body shape, weight, and strength, it is possible that some people cease exercising before they have obtained any desired benefits. It would seem that building self-efficacy is a worthy goal. The most influential means of building self-efficacy is performance mastery (Bandura, 1997). If psyching-up helps individuals make optimal training gains then it may indirectly influence self-efficacy. Bandura (1997) has also suggested that self-efficacy may be influenced by cognitive self-modelling and verbal persuasion. It is possible that some specific psych-up strategies such as imagery and self-talk may influence self-efficacy levels. Self-efficacy has not been specifically measured, but there is some evidence that psyching-up may influence self-confidence, a closely related construct (Caudill & Weinberg, 1983; Gould et al., 1980). Although it may be argued that psyching-up could be one strategy, among others, that helps individuals achieve optimal gains and build self-efficacy, thereby leading to the establishment of exercise behaviour, such speculation needs empirical examination. Longitudinal studies may help assess the benefits exercisers receive from including a psyching-up strategy as part of their weight training regimes.

Summary

Psyching-up has been defined as self-directed cognitive strategies used to enhance physical performance. Based on the research reviewed in this chapter, it appears that psyching-up may enhance the performance of novice and sub-elite individuals during simple dynamic tasks requiring maximal strength or muscular endurance. A number of strategies have empirical support, such as imagery, self-talk, and preparatory arousal. It is possible, however, that any technique that leads to suitable activation and attentional states will enhance performance (Hardy et al., 1996). Much remains to be learned about the role of psyching-up on muscular force production and attention needs to be directed to well-trained individuals performing compound strength movements to which they are accustomed. It is also recommended that researchers include a number of control conditions in their designs, provide a variety of details about participants' levels of conditioning, and attempt to interpret their findings. One possible application of the psyching-up literature might be for those individuals who weight train for health and fitness purposes. Given the importance that many individuals place on their mental preparation immediately prior to performance and the potential benefits that sub-elite sports and exercise participants might receive from psyching-up, its seems that further empirical attention is warranted.

References

Abernethy, P., Wilson, G., & Logan, P. (1995). Strength and power assessment: Issues, controversies and challenges. *Sports Medicine, 19*, 401-417.

Asken, M. J., & Goodling, M. D. (1986). The use of sport psychology techniques in rehabilitation medicine. *International Journal of Sport Psychology, 17*, 156-161.

Bandura, A. (1997). *Self-efficacy: The exercise of control.* New York: W. H. Freeman.

Berntson, G. G., Cacioppo, J. T., & Quigley, K. S. (1993). Respiratory sinus arrhythmia: Autonomic origins, physiological mechanisms, and psychophysiological implications. *Psychophysiology, 30*, 183-196.

Biddle, S. J. H. (1985). Mental preparation, mental practice and strength tasks: A need for clarification. *Journal of Sports Sciences, 3*, 67-74.

Blazevich, A. J., Gill, N., & Newton, R. U. (2002). Reliability and validity of two isometric squat tests. *Journal of Strength and Conditioning Research, 16*, 298-304.

Brody, E. B., Hatfield, B. D., Spalding, T. W., Frazer, M. B., & Caherty, F. J. (2000). The effects of a psyching strategy on neuromuscular activation and force production in strength-trained men. *Research Quarterly for Exercise and Sport, 71*, 162-170.

Buckworth, J., & Dishman, R. K. (2002). *Exercise psychology.* Champaign, IL: Human Kinetics.

Caudill, D., Weinberg, R., & Jackson, A. (1983). Psyching-up and track athletes: A preliminary investigation. *Journal of Sport Psychology, 5*, 231-235.

Caudill, D., & Weinberg, R. S. (1983). The effects of varying the length of the psych-up interval on motor performance. *Journal of Sport Behavior, 6*, 86-91.

Cohen, J. (1977). *Statistical power analysis for the behavioural sciences* (Rev. ed.). New York: Academic.

Davis, H. A., Gass, G. C., & Bassett, J. R. (1981). Serum cortisol response to incremental work in experienced and naïve subjects. *Psychosomatic Medicine, 43*, 127-132.

Elko, K., & Ostrow, A. C. (1992). The effects of three mental preparation strategies on strength performance of young and older adults. *Journal of Sport Behavior, 15*, 34-41.

Fitts, P. M., & Posner, M. I. (1967). *Human Performance*. Belmont, Ca.: Brooks/Cole.

Ghiagiarelli, J., McGuigan, M. R., & Tod, D. (2004). *Maximal strength and cortisol responses to psyching up during the squat exercise*. Paper presented at the National Strength and Conditioning Association National Conference, Minneapolis, MN.

Gould, D., Weinberg, R., & Jackson, A. (1980). Mental preparation strategies, cognitions, and strength performance. *Journal of Sport Psychology, 2*, 329-339.

Hall, K. G., & Erickson, B. (1995). The effects of preparatory arousal on sixty-meter dash performance. *Applied Research in Coaching and Athletics Annual*, 70-79.

Hardy, L., Jones, G., & Gould, D. (1996). *Understanding psychological preparation for sport: Theory and practice of elite performers*. Chichester, England: Wiley.

Harman, E., Garhammer, J., & Pandorf, C. (2000). Administration, scoring, and interpretation of selected tests. In T. R. Baechle & R. W. Earle (Eds.), *Essentials of strength training and conditioning* (2 ed., pp. 287-317). Champaign, IL: Human Kinetics.

Hatzigeorgiadis, A., Theodorakis, Y., & Zourbanos, N. (2004). Self-talk in the swimming pool: The effects of self-talk on thought content and performance on water-polo tasks. *Journal of Applied Sport Psychology, 16*, 138-150.

Hopkins, W. G. (2003). *A new view of statistics*. Retrieved 29-May, 2003, from http://www.sportsci.org/resource/stats

Kraemer, W. J., & Fry, A. C. (1995). Strength training: Development and evaluation of methodology. In P. J. Maud & C. Foster (Eds.), *Physiological Assessment of Human Fitness* (pp. 115-138). Champaign, IL: Human Kinetics.

Laidlaw, D. H., Kornatz, K. W., Keen, D. A., Suzuki, S., & Enoka, R. M. (1999). Strength training improves the steadiness of slow lengthening contractions performed by old adults. *Journal of Applied Physiology, 87*, 1786-1795.

Lee, C. (1990). Psyching up for a muscular endurance task: Effects of image content on performance and mood state. *Journal of Sport & Exercise Psychology, 12*, 66-73.

McAuley, E., & Blissmer, B. (2002). Self-efficacy and attributional processes in physical activity. In T. Horn (Ed.), *Advances in sport psychology* (2nd ed., pp. 185-205). Champaign, IL: Human Kinetics.

Meyers, A. W., Whelan, J. P., & Murphy, S. M. (1996). Cognitive behavioral strategies in athletic performance enhancement. In M. Hersen, R. M. Eisler, & P. M. Miller (Eds.), *Handbook of Behavior Modification* (Vol. 30, pp. 137-164). Pacific Grove, CA: Brooks/Cole.

Murphy, A. J., & Wilson, G. J. (1996). Poor correlations between isometric tests and dynamic performance: relationship to muscle activation. *European Journal of Applied Physiology, 73*, 353-357.

Murphy, S. M., Woolfolk, R. L., & Budney, A. J. (1988). The effects of emotive imagery on strength performance. *Journal of Sport & Exercise Psychology, 10*, 334-345.

Nisbett, R. E., & Wilson, T. D. (1977). Telling more than we can know: Verbal reports on mental processes. *Psychological Review, 84*, 231-259.

Perkins, D., Wilson, G. V., & Kerr, J. H. (2001). The effects of elevated arousal and mood on maximal strength performance in athletes. *Journal of Applied Sport Psychology, 13*, 239-259.

Pette, D., & Staron, R. S. (2001). Transitions of muscle fiber phenotypic profiles. *Histochemistry and Cell Biology, 115*, 359-372.

Pierce, E. F., McGowan, R. W., Eastman, N. W., Aaron, J. G., & Lynn, T. D. (1993). Effects of progressive relaxation on maximal muscle strength and power. *Journal of Strength and Conditioning Research, 7*, 216-218.

Rogerson, L. J., & Hrycaiko, D. W. (2002). Enhancing competitive performance of ice hockey goaltenders using centring and self-talk. *Journal of Applied Sport Psychology, 14*, 14-26.

Sale, D. G. (1988). Neural adaptation to resistance training. *Medicine and Science in Sport and Exercise, 20*, S135-S145.

Schmidt, R. A., & Wrisberg, C. A. (2004). *Motor learning and performance* (3rd ed.). Champaign, IL: Human Kinetics.

Shelton, T. O., & Mahoney, M. J. (1978). The content and effect of "psyching-up" strategies in weight lifters. *Cognitive Therapy and Research, 2*, 275-284.

Speed, H. D., & Andersen, M. B. (2000). What exercise and sport scientists don't understand. *Journal of Science and Medicine in Sport, 3*, 84-92.

Tenenbaum, G., Bar-Eli, M., Hoffman, J. R., Jablonovski, R. Sade, S., & Shitrit, D. (1995). The effect of cognitive and somatic psyching-up techniques on isokinetic leg strength performance. *Journal of Strength and Conditioning Research, 9*, 3-7.

Thelwell, R. C., & Greenlees, I. A. (2001). The effects of a mental skills training package on gymnasium triathlon performance. *The Sport Psychologist, 15*, 127-141.

Thelwell, R. C., & Greenlees, I. A. (2003). Developing competitive endurance performance using mental skills training. *The Sport Psychologist, 17*, 318-337.

Theodorakis, Y., Weinberg, R., Natsis, P., Douma, I., & Kazakas, P. (2000). The effects of motivational versus instructional self-talk on improving motor performance. *The Sport Psychologist, 14*, 253-272.

Tod, D., & Andersen, M. B. (in press). Success in sport psych: Effective sport psychologists. In S. Murphy (Ed.), *The sport psych handbook*. Champaign, IL: Human Kinetics.

Tod, D., Iredale, F., & Gill, N. (2003). 'Psyching-up' and muscular force production. *Sport Medicine, 33*, 47-58.

Tod, D., Iredale, F., McGuigan, M., Strange, D., & Gill, N. (in press). "Psyching-up" enhances force production during the bench press. *Journal of Strength and Conditioning Research*.

Tynes, L. L., & McFatter, R. M. (1987). The efficacy of "psyching" strategies on a weight-lifting task. *Cognitive Therapy and Research, 11*, 327-336.

Weinberg, R., Jackson, A., & Seaboune, T. (1985). The effects of specific vs nonspecific mental preparation strategies on strength and endurance performance. *Journal of Sport Behavior, 8*, 175-180.

Weinberg, R. S., Gould, D., & Jackson, A. (1980). Cognition and motor performance: Effect of psyching-up strategies on three motor tasks. *Cognitive Therapy and Research, 4*, 239-245.

Weinberg, R. S., Gould, D., & Jackson, A. (1981). Relationship between the duration of the psych-up interval and strength performance. *Journal of Sport Psychology, 3*, 166-170.

Weinberg, R. S., & Williams, J. M. (2001). Integrating and implementing a psychological skills training program. In J. M. Williams (Ed.), *Applied sport psychology: Personal growth to peak performance* (4th ed., pp. 347-377). Mountain View, CA: Mayfield.

Whelan, J. P., Epkins, C. C., & Meyers, A. W. (1990). Arousal interventions for athletic performance: Influence of mental preparation and competitive experience. *Anxiety Research, 2*, 293-307.

Wilkes, R. L., & Summers, J. J. (1984). Cognitions, mediating variables, and strength performance. *Journal of Sport Psychology, 6*, 351-359.

Williams, J. M., & Straub, W. F. (2001). Sport psychology: past, present, future. In J. M. Williams (Ed.), *Applied sport psychology: Personal growth to peak performance* (pp. 1-12). Mountain View, CA: Mayfield.

Wilson, G. J., & Murphy, A. J. (1996). The use of isometric tests of muscular function in athletic assessment. *Sports Medicine, 22*, 19-37.

Wilson, G. T. (2000). Behavior therapy. In R. J. Corsini & D. Wedding (Eds.), *Current psychotherapies* (6 ed., pp. 205-240). Itasca, Il: F. E. Peacock.

Chapter VII

Exercise-Induced Cardiovascular Adjustments by Muscle Receptors Stimulation

Antonio Crisafulli* and Alberto Concu

From: Department of Sciences applied to Biological Systems, section of Human Physiology, School of Sports Medicine, University of Cagliari, Italy

Abstract

During exercise cardiovascular apparatus operates some adjustments which aim at meeting the metabolic needs of exercising muscle. Both mechanical (skeletal-muscle and respiratory pumps) and nervous (centrally and peripherally originating) mechanisms contribute to regulate blood pressure and flow to the metabolic demand.

Concerning the nervous component of this regulation, there are several inputs of both central/cortical and peripheral/intravascular origin that converge to the brain-stem neurons controlling cardiovascular activity and regulate the hemodynamic responses to exercise on the basis of the motor strategy. Furthermore, evidences support the concept that also nervous signals of extravascular origin, i.e. arising from muscle mechano- and/or metabo- receptors, activate the same control areas on the basis of the muscle mechanical and metabolic involvement.

This review focuses on inputs arising from exercising muscles which modulate cardiovascular system in order to connect blood pressure and flow with the actual muscle mechanical status (muscle length and strain, and tissue deformation due to muscle movements) and metabolic condition (concentration of catabolites in the extra-cellular compartment produced by muscle activity).

It was reported that the stimulation of type I afferent nervous fibers from muscle receptors increases blood pressure through a mechanism of peripheral origin. Among sub-groups of type I afferents, indirect findings suggest that type Ib from Golgi tendon

---

* Via Porcell 4, 09124 Cagliari (Italy); Phone: +390706758918; Fax: +390706758917; e-mail: crisaful@unica.it / concu@unica.it

organs may contribute to the muscle-induced cardiovascular reflex. On the contrary, it appears that group Ia from muscle spindle primary ending and group II afferents are not involved in this reflex. Opposite, it seems ascertained that type III and IV afferent nervous fibers can be activated by exercise-induced mechanical and chemical changes in the extracellular environment into they are scattered. It is believed that type III afferents act mainly as "mechanoreceptors", as they respond to muscle stretch and compression occurring during muscle contraction, while type IV fibres act as "metaboreceptors", since they are stimulated by end-products of muscle metabolism. The activity of both type III and IV afferents can reflexely increase heart rate and systemic vascular resistance which, in turn, lead blood pressure to raise. Moreover, there are several growing evidences that also myocardial contractility, stroke volume and cardiac pre-load can be modulated by the activity of these reflexes of muscular origin.

These findings suggest that signals arising from exercising muscle act to regulate cardiovascular adjustments during exercise so that blood flow can be set to meet the muscle metabolic request.

Introduction

The main task of the cardiovascular apparatus is to provide the blood flow needed to serve the contracting skeletal muscles. This activity is particularly emphasized during strenuous physical exertions such as running or cycling, when heart rate, cardiac contractility, and sympathetic nerve activity increase and cardiac output can reach and even exceed values of 30 liters•min^{-1}, which is about six folds higher than the normal resting value of human beings [Mitchell et al. 1983(a), Lewis et al. 1983, Nishiyasu et al. 2000, Ichinose et al. 2004]. At the same time, vasodilatory substances released by working muscles greatly decrease peripheral vascular resistance and counteract the effect of the elevated cardiac output upon blood pressure. Inasmuch as arterial blood pressure is the product of cardiac output by peripheral vascular resistance, the resulting effect is that mean arterial pressure is kept stable or slightly increased with respect to rest. This fact indicates that mechanisms controlling the circulatory system can defend blood pressure homeostasis in spite of the cardiovascular stress caused by exercise and that some adjustments must be made to achieve a balance between cardiac output and peripheral vascular resistance, i.e. working muscles must be supplied of blood flow without inducing great changes in arterial blood pressure.

Several mechanisms are believed to be responsible for this cardiovascular regulation: mechanical mechanisms, which include the muscle pump and the respiratory pump activity [Higginbotham et al.1986, Laughlin 1987, Carter et al. 1999, Crisafulli et al. 2003(b)], and neural mechanisms. Mechanical mechanisms act as facilitator of cardiac filling and their activity is testified by the increase in stroke volume that takes place at the beginning of muscle activity, i.e. when muscle and respiratory pump start working. Clearly, the isolated effect of muscle and respiratory pumps would be to raise blood pressure through a flow-increased mechanism if vasodilation did not contemporary lower systemic vascular resistance.

Concerning the neural component, its action is essential for a normal blood pressure regulation during exercise, as testified by subjects with spinal cord injuries who develop a marked hypotension in response to muscle vasodilation during electrically-induced exercise because of the absence of neural feedback [Dela et al. 2003]. There are strong evidences that both central and peripheral control mechanisms operate the cardiovascular adjustments of neural origin occurring during exercise [Mitchell et al. 1983(a)]. In the central mechanism, commonly known as "central command", the activation of regions of the brain responsible for motor unit recruitment also activates the cardiovascular control areas located in the medulla [Goodwin et al. 1972, Strange et al. 1993]. It is thought that the central command establishes at the onset of exercise a basal level of sympathetic and parasympathetic efferent activity tightly linked to the intensity of the effort. This basic pattern of autonomic activity is then modulated by peripheral signals which reflexly activate the cardiovascular control centers. The peripheral reflexogenic areas considered important for the cardiovascular regulation during exercise are the arterial baroreceptors and the receptors within muscle. In particular, baroreceptors operate in order to maintain blood pressure and counteract any mismatch between vascular resistance and cardiac output by controlling muscle vasodilation and cardiac chronotropism through sympathetic modulation. On the other hand, receptors within muscle can activate afferent nerves and, in turn, induce sympathetic-mediated cardiovascular adjustments in response to the mechanical and the metabolic condition of the contracting muscle [Mitchell et al. 1983(b), Stebbins et al. 1988, Rowell et al. 1990, Shi et al. 1995, Iellamo et al. 1997]. Thus, the balance between cardiac output and peripheral resistance is governed by an interplay between influence on the heart, released vasodilatory substances, and sympathetic vasoconstriction.

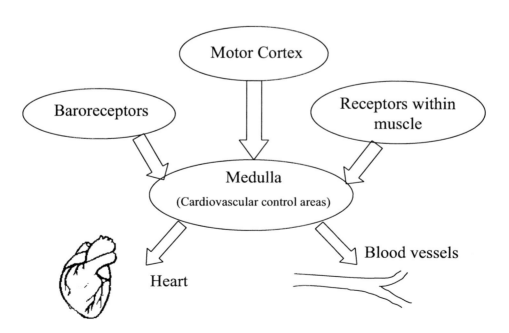

Figure 1. schematic representation of nervous inputs and outputs to the cardiovascular control areas of the Medulla.

In short, the autonomic nervous outputs to the cardiovascular system depend on the inputs to the cardiovascular control areas from cerebral motor cortex and from the peripheral reflexogenic areas (figure 1). Central and peripheral neural mechanisms probably work together and are not mutually exclusive in the regulation of cardiovascular response to exercise. Moreover, it would exist some redundancy between the two mechanisms and neural occlusion may be operative [Rybicky et al. 1989]. The system manages to regulate cardiac output and vascular conductance in order to defend blood pressure against changes in arterial resistance induced by vasodilatory substances produced during muscle contraction and to provide sufficient blood flow to working muscle.

This article focuses on the role played by the nervous peripheral inputs arising from exercising muscle; in the first part, the effects of mechanical stimulation of muscle receptors and nerve fibers are discussed, while in the second part we analyze reflexes of chemical origin and their possible involvement in the regulation of cardiovascular apparatus during exercise.

Cardiovascular Reflexes Arising from Mechanical Stimuli within Muscle

Afferent fibers from skeletal muscle are classically subdivided in four groups (I to IV) on the basis of their anatomical and electro-physiological characteristics [Mathews 1972]. Group I fibers have diameters of 12-20 µm and conduct impulses at 72-120 m sec^{-1}; group II have diameter of 2-16 µm and conduct impulses at 12-72 m sec^{-1}; group III have diameter of 1-6 µm and conduct impulses at 3-30 m sec^{-1}; finally, group IV, which, opposite to the first three groups are unmyelinated fibers, have diameters of 1µm or less and conduct impulses at 2.5 m sec^{-1} or less.

Almost all these fibers are susceptible of changing their firing rates towards the spinal cord when mechanical stimuli are applied to their endings and, in this way, they may contribute to the modulation related to muscle mechanical status made by the autonomic nervous system upon cardiovascular apparatus during exercise.

Type I Nervous Fibers and the Proprioceptive Cardiovascular Reflex

Decandia et al. [1991] found that electrically-stimulated group I afferent fibers of anaesthetized cats induced and increase in both systolic left ventricle pressure and systolic arterial pressure. Propanolol did not eliminate this reflex, thus excluding sympathetic heart activation as a cause of the phenomenon. Opposite, Phentolamine, which is a sympathetic alfa-receptor antagonist, blocked this blood pressure response, indicating that this muscle reflex acts by vasoconstricting blood vessels and by increasing peripheral vascular resistance to which follows a Starling-mediated increase in systolic left ventricular pressure and in systolic arterial pressure [Orani and Decandia 1994].

The above results followed a very accurate experiment, made by Orani et al. [1990] on anaesthetized cats, in which the effect of group I afferents stimulation on cardiovascular activity was clearly elucidated. After lumbo-sacral laminectomy the ventral roots were cut on both sides from L_5 to S_2 to avoid either spontaneous or reflex movements of both hind limbs. Thus, the nerves of the lateral gastrocnemius-soleus and medial gastrocnemius muscles were isolated on the left side and placed on a pair of silver stimulating electrodes. All other sciatic trunk nerves on the same side were also cut and gastrocnemius nerve endings were stimulated by connecting electrodes to a constant current stimulation unit. During two consecutive respiratory cycles continuous trains of electrical stimuli of 0.1 ms were applied with a frequency ranging from 200 to 300 Hz. Stimuli intensity was set at a value which ranged from 1 x to 2 x threshold (T) for the most excitable afferent fibers which, as it is known, are those comprised in the I group of the Matthews classification [Mathews 1972]. From the distal end of a small rootlet disconnected from the spinal cord, the afferent volleys were assessed during the gastrocnemius stimulation, in order to individuate the T stimuli intensity for group I fibers. It was also individuated the maximal intensity to excite group I fibers, which ranged from 1.8 to 2.0 x T. At near-maximal intensities stimulation, also small volleys attributable to group II afferents appeared after the first rapid volley due to group I firing. Increasing the intensity of stimuli up to 4 x T a third volleys appeared after those corresponding to group I and II afferents. These volleys were attributable to the most excitable group III afferent fibers. In brief, thanks to this technique, cardiovascular effects of different mechanoreceptor afferent fibers could be distinguished on the basis of the intensity of electrical stimulation. Inasmuch as in this experiment the stimuli intensity did not overcame 2.0 x T for group I fibers, it was unlikely that group III and IV afferents were stimulated.

Results showed that, at the start of the gastrocnemius stimulation, mean arterial blood pressure suddenly increased and, within two respiratory cycles which lasted the stimulation, it reached a value significantly higher (+6%) with respect to a control condition. Mean arterial pressure control values were reached between the first and the second breath following the stimuli cessation.

Subsequently, stimulation tests were repeated during anodal block of the most excitable afferent fibers (i.e. group I fibers) by applying a continuous electrical current at the site of stimulation. During a 50 ηA anodal block the volleys from gastrocnemius terminations to spinal cord of group I afferents were selectively blocked without having any effect on the amplitude and duration in the volleys of the group II fibers. Stimulation of gastrocnemius during anodal block was ineffective in eliciting the arterial pressure increase previously observed. When anodal block was removed, group I volleys reappeared and arterial pressure increased as it did during the test before the block. These results clearly indicate that excitation of group I afferents from muscle proprioceptors (i.e. anulospiral endings of Ia fibers in the muscle spindles and Ib endings in the Golgi tendon organs) and not of group II fibers from other mechanoreceptors were capable to evoke an arterial pressure response.

Inasmuch as the raise in systolic arterial pressure could be also explained by the fact that gastrocnemius stimulation induced an increase in pulmonary ventilation which in turn, through enhanced ventricle pre-load, caused a Starling-mediated increase in left ventricular systolic pressure and, consequently, in systolic arterial pressure, the muscle stimulation was repeated after curarisation while animals breathed at a constant artificial ventilation. In this setting, gastrocnemius stimulation during controlled ventilation produced the same arterial pressure response as in non-curarised animals, thus demonstrating that the raise in ventilation could not be responsible for the evoked pressor response. The results of the aforementioned experiment were interpreted by the authors through a sudden cardiovascular modulation of nervous origin (i.e. a reflex) at the start of physical exercise which preceded the chemically-mediated vasodilatation due to end-products of muscle metabolism.

However, it should be noticed that these results did not agree with those of some other experiments in which the effect on cardiovascular function of stimulation of group I fibers was investigated [Sato et al. 1981, Mitchell et al. 1983(a), Terui and Koizumi 1984]. In particular, McCloskey and Mitchell [1972] reported arterial pressure increases during the contraction of the hind limb muscles in cats and during simultaneous anodal block of group I afferents. From these results they deduced that these fibers were not involved in the evocation of the pressor reflex. However, the possibility that group I fibers may be effective cannot be excluded since their inefficacy would be definitely proved only if their selective stimulation did not produce excitatory effects. But Decandia et al. [1990] experiments, in which group I fibers were selectively stimulated, strongly support the effectiveness of these afferents in eliciting a pressor reflex, even if the specific importance of their involvement in the overall blood pressure response to exercise may be small and deserves to be better investigated.

Nevertheless, it must be considered that group I fibers contain both Ia and Ib contingents, the former of which concern afferent volleys from muscle spindle primary endings while the second concern the afferent volleys from Golgi tendon organ endings. Selective stimulation of muscle spindles, as it does the muscle vibration or the succinylcholine administration (a drug which specific excites muscle spindle primary endings) were utilized to elucidate possible effects of these proprioceptors on cardiovascular apparatus. McCloskey et al. [1972] applied mechanical vibration of 100-300 Hz (amplitude of vibration of 100-200 µ) along the length of the muscles of both hind limbs of anaesthetized cats and they did not discover any appreciable change in arterial pressure. On the other hand, Gautier et al. [1969] showed a very slight increase in heart rate after succinylcholine administration to anaesthetized cats. However, Kidd and Kucera [1969] demonstrated that this drug can also excite the endings of smaller myelinated fibers, so that cardiovascular responses to succinylcholine does not need to be necessarily attributed to Ia volleys.

Stimuli which are considered putative for muscle spindle excitation are also the passive muscle stretches. In conscious men, by means of a calf ergometer, Baum et al. [1995] produced a passive stretch of plantar flexor muscles. The stretch lasted 10 min and the increase reached in the angle joint of the ankle was of about 20 degrees. During the test electromiograms (EMG) of both the stretched soleus and gastrocnemius muscles were assessed to ensure that no active or reflex contractions did occur in these muscles. A Borg scale was also utilized to evaluate subjective ratings of pain sensations during the muscle stretching (values from 6 = painless to 20 = extremely painful). It was found that, during the stretching, no EMG changes took place, thus indicating that in the stretched muscles no active or reflex contraction occurred. This meant that, among the I group fibers, only the group Ia from primary ending of muscle spindles and not Ib from Golgi tendon organs were excited. On the other and, the Borg scale subjective ratings of pain at the end of the test gave a maximum value of 9. This fact indicated a very low pain sensation due to the ankle stretch and, consequently, not significant excitation of slow conducting nerve fibers of groups III and IV. Therefore, this muscle stretching protocol reasonably excited only group Ia fibers from primary endings of muscle spindles. No changes in arterial pressure were detectable during the test, thus the authors concluded that volleys in group Ia fibers were ineffective in eliciting any cardiovascular effect when muscles were stretched.

Similar conclusions can be deduced from the experiments made by Concu [1988] in which a passive sequence of alternative plantar and dorsal flexion of both ankles were applied in seated conscious men by an oscillating foot-board driven by an electromechanical apparatus. Heart rate, cardiac output, and stroke volume did not change when passive ankle oxillations were applied along the time corresponding to 3 respiratory cycles.

It is suggestive to consider that, in anaesthetized cats in which group I fibers were electrically stimulated, Carcassi et al. [1983] individuated Ib contingent as the hyperventilation eliciting fibers, whereas Ia contingent were ineffective in eliciting any ventilatory response. Considering that in almost all the experiments concerning the effects on pressor reflex from nervous muscle fibers, both respiratory and cardiovascular apparata were excited when these fibers were stimulated, it may be speculated that Golgi tendon organs rather than muscle spindles are responsible for the arterial blood pressure increase shown during the group I afferents stimulation. Indeed, active muscle contraction, which excites Golgi tendon organs, rather than passive muscle stretch, which excites muscle spindles, is probably more effective in reflecting the increased demand of blood from exercising muscles. It is our speculation that Ib fiber group should be suitable for sending this kind of information to nervous controllers of the cardiovascular system in order to correct any mismatch between cardiac output and vascular conductance, i.e. the blood pressure error that activates the arterial blood pressure response.

In any case, even if some cardiovascular effect can be produced by stimulation of group I fibers, the role played by these afferents on the arterial pressure adjustments during muscle activity appears the least if compared with that played by slow conducting nerve fibers of groups III and IV.

Type II Nervous Fibers Effect on Cardiovascular Activity

Group II afferent fibers effects on cardiovascular activity are scarcely investigated. However, Waldrop et al. [1984] failed to demonstrate any effectiveness of these afferents in eliciting heart rate and arterial blood pressure responses when they were selectively stimulated by succinylcholine injected into aorta of anaesthetized cats. After succinylcholine injection, these authors recorded the afferent impulse activity of fibers filaments dissected from either the L_7 and S_1 dorsal roots, among which afferent fibers arising from hind limb muscles, joints, and skin are comprised. They found that this drug induced high frequency volleys in group II but not in group III and IV fibers, both in paralyzed and non paralyzed condition. They also found that, when muscle fasciculation due to succinylcholine injection was abolished by paralysis induced with gallamine, succinylcholine-induced increase in firing activity of group II fibers did not produce any increase in heart rate and/or arterial pressure. Moreover, passive sequence of alternative plantar and dorsal flexion of both ankles, applied by Concu [1988] in conscious men, which along with group I afferents also produced group II fibers excitation from joint mechanoreceptor, did not produce any detectable cardiovascular effect. The fact that group II fibers excitation had no effect on cardiovascular apparatus has been demonstrated also by Decandia et al. in anaesthetized cats [1990]. When group I fibers volleys were selectively eliminated by anodal block, the remaining volleys from the group II fibers did not elicit any cardiovascular response.

It may be concluded that the secondary endings of muscle spindles or the corpuscolate endings inserted in muscles, joints, and skin, most of which send mechanocetive informations to spinal cord by means of group II afferent fibers, seem not to be involved in inducing cardiocirculatory changes when their respective receptive fields are stimulated.

Type III and IV Nervous Fibers and their Respective Influence on Cardiovascular Activity on the Basis O their Specific Sensibility to Mechanical Stimuli

Slow conducting nerve fibers of groups III and IV are thought to be excitable by mechanical stimulation. However, group III rather than group IV seems to be more sensible to this kind of stimulation [Kaufman et al. 1984, Leshnower et al. 2001]. Difficulties do exist in discriminating purely ergoreceptor from nociceptor function among group III and IV muscle afferents. Classically, ergoreceptors are considered those fibers in which muscle contraction induces an almost instantaneous increase in the firing rate of the corresponding afferents proportional to the intensity of the contraction. Moreover, often ergoreceptors transduce the touch sensation. On the contrary, nociceptors are considered those fibers that are stimulated by vigorous pinching of the muscle and transduce pain sensation. These latter fibers may be stimulated also by algesic chemicals such as bradykinin, serotonin, potassium, capsaicin, and hyperosmolar lactate an phosphate [Mitchell et al. 1983(b)].

In anaesthetized cats, Kaufman et al. [1983] induced gastrocnemious muscle static contraction by electrical stimulation of the cut peripheral end of L_7 ventral root which lasted 30-45 s, and selectively recorded group III and IV volleys from L_7-S_1 dorsal roots. During muscle contraction, an increase in arterial pressure was found which started on average about 6 s after the onset of the ventral root stimulation and reached a value 13% greater than control. These findings suggest that mechanical stimulation of skeletal muscle associated with contraction may stimulate afferents nerve endings and evoke cardiovascular reflexes. The discharge pattern of the most of the group III fibers excited during the muscle contraction (53%) was characterized by a sudden increase, with a short onset latency (about 0.8 s), in the firing frequency, which was proportional to the developed muscle tension. However, almost all of these fibers adapted their discharge rates to low values before the end of the muscle stimulation. On the contrary, muscle static contraction induced in 63% of excited group IV fibers a firing rate increase with an average onset latency of about 3.8 s. In the half of these fibers this firing rate was maintained throughout the contraction and they continued to fire for 10-12 s after the end of the contraction. The rapid response to contraction shown by many of the group III afferents suggest that they contribute to the initiation of the exercise pressor reflex [Matsukawa et al. 1994]. On the contrary, the firing behavior found in several fibers of group IV appeared especially well suited to function as the metabolic receptors, which are believed to signal a mismatch between blood supply and demand in contracting skeletal muscle [Haouzi et al. 1999, Gallagher et al. 2001]. In fact, their onset latency is a period of time compatible to allow the metabolic product of contraction to accumulate in a muscle undergoing static contraction. Moreover, the firing rate of these group IV fibers gradually increased as the contraction lasted, due to buildup of metabolites in the contracting muscles. However, it has been reported that a sub-population of group III/IV afferent fibers are polymodal, i.e. they respond to both mechanical and chemical stimuli [Kaufman et al. 1983, Matsukawa et al. 1994].

From the above results it seems clear that receptors within muscles gather information concerning the mass and the mechanical condition (muscle length and strain as well as tissue compression and deformation due to contractions) of the muscles involved in the exercise being performed. Mechanical information is then provided to the cardiovascular controlling areas which operate the hemodynamic adjustments in order to regulate blood flow on the basis of muscle status.

Type III and IV Nervous Fibers and the "Metaboreflex"

In this section we focus on the reflex cardiovascular response generated by nerve fibers which can be activated by the accumulation of end-products of muscle metabolism, i.e. the "metaboreceptors". As stated in the previous chapter, group III and IV are small slow-conducting nerves which are thought to be nociceptors [Mense 1993] and to be sensitive to mechanical distortion [Kaufman et al. 1983, Kaufman et al. 1987] as well as to end-products of muscle metabolism such as lactic acid, potassium, bradykinin, arachidonic acid products, and adenosine [Kniffki et al. 1978, Mense et al. 1983]. Both are composed of fine nerve fibers with either a myelin sheath (group III) or without myelin sheath (group IV). All group IV and most group III fibers terminate as free endings within muscle. The majority of group III fibers are mechano-sensitive and respond to mechanical events during muscle contraction such as stretch and compression, whereas group IV afferents are probably insensitive to mechanical stimuli but are activated by muscle metabolite accumulation [Kniffki et al. 1978, Mense et al. 1983, Leshnower et al. 2001]. Indeed, group III afferent fibers discharge at the onset of contraction and their firing rates tend to adapt if the muscle tension is maintained, which is coherent with the behavior of mechano-receptors; differently, group IV afferents discharge with latency after the beginning of muscle contraction and this pattern has been related with muscle metabolite production [Kaufman et al. 1983, Mense et al. 1983]. However, as previously stated, it has been reported that a sub-population of groups III/IV fibers responds to both mechanical and chemical stimuli [Kaufman et al. 1983, Mense et al. 1983]. Thus, group IV and at least in part group III afferents act as "metaboreceptors" and are involved in the cardiovascular chemoreflex originating in working muscle.

The presence of a controlling neural signal linked to metabolic events occurring within active muscle has been several times postulated and its contribution to the hemodynamic and autonomic response to exercise is now accepted [Rowell et al. 1990, O'Leary 1993, Strange et al. 1993, Piepoli et al. 1995]. The current thinking is that, when O_2 delivery does not suffice to meet the metabolic needs of contracting muscle, by-products accumulate because of a mismatch between metabolism and blood flow. This in turn causes activation of muscle metaboreceptors (free endings of group IV and perhaps III afferents) which leads to a reflex-increase in arterial blood pressure. Since this blood pressure response is abolished when group III and IV affernts are blockade, it could be stated that it is a nervous reflex, which is commonly called "metaboreflex" [Rowell et al. 1990, Piepoli et al. 1995, O'Leary et al. 1998]. It is believed that the metaboreflex-induced increase in blood pressure aims at restoring blood flow to the hypoperfused muscle. Nevertheless, it should be noted that this restoring effect has been demonstrated in dogs [Sheriff et al. 1987, O'Leary et al. 1995, O'Leary et al. 1999] whereas controversy exists whether or not it exists also in humans [Joyner 1991, Rowell et al. 1991]. In any case, the stimulation of group III and/or IV afferents appears to be essential for the normal hemodynamic response to exercise, since its absence abolishes the normal increase in blood pressure [Strange et al. 1993].

Little is known about the central projection of the afferent arms and the central pathways of integration of metaboreflex response. Most group III and IV fibers enter the spinal cord via the dorsal root and distribute in the dorsal horn of the segment of entry and for several segments up and down the spinal cord. Inputs from these fibers may have several levels of integration. The reflex seems not to require the rostral brain even if it a supraspinal level of integration may exist. In particular, the lateral reticular nucleus may be important for its expression and integration. It was proposed that the medulla is the area controlling the cardiovascular response during metaboreflex activation, while the spinal cord seems not to be operative in the intact animal [Mitchell et al. 1983 (a)]. Figure 2 is a schematic simplified picture of the putative mechanism of how metaboreflex works. Briefly, free endings of group IV and possibly III afferents are activated by end-products of muscle metabolism generated within muscle during contraction. These afferents, in turn, activate the cardiovascular control areas (probably located in the medulla) which operate the reflex response consisting in an increase in arterial blood pressure.

It is not clear whether or not a threshold for metaboreceptors stimulation by muscle end-products exists, i.e. whether metaboreflex operates only at moderate-high exercise intensities, when metabolites accumulate within working muscle, or even at mild muscle strain, when probably there is not a mismatch between muscle blood supply and demand and metabolites do not accumulate. It was reported in humans that the muscle metaboreflex has a threshold around a pH of 6.9 units and that mean arterial pressure increases linearly with decreasing muscle pH [Nishiyasu et al. 1994(b)]. Besides, studies employing ^{31}P nuclear magnetic resonance spectroscopy found that decrements in intramuscular pH were coupled to the rise of sympathetic nerve activity, thus suggesting that an event associated with glycolysis and lactate production may be important in activating the reflex [Victor et al. 1988, Sinoway et al. 1989, Cornett et al. 2000].These findings are consistent with the concept that the metaboreflex is activated whenever blood flow to contracting muscle is insufficient to warrant both oxygen delivery and metabolite washout [Rowell et al. 1990, Piepoli et al. 1995, Cornett et al. 2000]. According to this viewpoint, the metaboreflex acts to correct any mismatch between muscle blood flow and metabolism by superimposing to the central command activity.

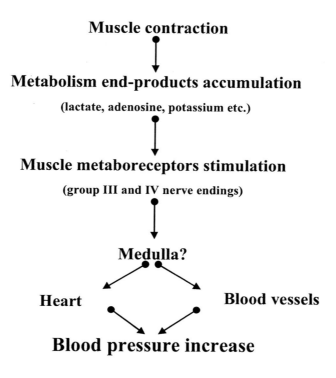

Figure 2. putative mechanisms of metaboreflex working.

However, it was also demonstrated that group IV fibers of cat muscle were responsive to a low level of exercise, i.e. when there was not a mismatch between blood delivery and metabolic needs of working muscle [Andreani et al. 1997]. The response at low level stimulation was interpreted with the fact that the metaboreflex plays a role in the cardiovascular regulation even when there is not an insufficient O_2 delivery to muscle and a mismatch between muscle flow and metabolism is not yet detectable. This is in accordance with the findings of Strange and co-workers [1993] who demonstrated in humans the essential role of the metaboreflex for reaching a normal blood pressure response even for mild exercise eliciting heart rate below 100 bpm. Therefore, it is possible that the metaboreflex is evoked even at low workloads, without any apparent accumulation of end-products of metabolism. According to this viewpoint, metaboreflex is responsible for a tonically active feedback to the cardiovascular control areas that starts working whenever the metabolism is activated by muscle contraction.

Hemodynamic Effects of Metaboreflex Activation

The typical hemodynamic feature of metaboreflex activation is the raise in arterial blood pressure [Mitchell et al. 1983 (a), Rowell et al. 1990, Piepoli et al. 1995]. With regard to the mechanisms responsible for the blood pressure response, it is commonly believed that it is achieved primarily by an increase in systemic vascular resistance caused by peripheral sympathetic vasoconstriction [Rowell et al. 1990, Piepoli et al. 1995]. The reflex effect on heart rate is supposed to be small or absent, and this fact led some authors to speculate that metaboreflex has little or no effect on cardiac output. However, it should be noticed that the effect on heart rate strongly depends on the setting of metaboreflex activation. In fact, two approaches have been used to study the relationship between hemodynamics and metaboreflex: 1) reducing muscle blood flow during effort, or 2) reducing blood flow at the cessation of effort by post-exercise ischemia in order to trap metabolites produced during previous muscle contraction [O'Leary 1993, Clark et al. 1995, Piepoli et al. 1995]. This latter study protocol is used in order to isolate central command and muscle mechanoreflexes from metaboreflex. While the activation of muscle metaboreflex during exercise can elicit some heart rate response through an increase in sympathetic activity towards sinus node, during post-exercise ischemia the rise of sympathetic activity is masked by the concomitantly enhanced parasympathetic outflow due to the loss of central command. The parasympathetic tone during post-exercise ischemia can be further increased by the arterial baroreflex, which responds to the metaboreflex-induced increase in blood pressure by buffering the elevated sympathetic drive to the heart and arteriolar vessels [Iellamo et al. 1999]. Thus, if metaboreflex is activated by post-exercise ischemia, the elevated sympathetic activity to sinus node is counteracted by enhanced parasympathetic tone due to the withdraw of central command and to the sympathetic-buffering effect of baroreflex activation. The resulting effect is that heart rate decreases despite the sympathetic tone to the heart is kept high [O'Leary 1993, Nishiyasu et al. 1994(a)]. Furthermore, it should be also considered that acetylcholine and norepinephrine have complex interaction at the pre-synaptic and post-synaptic level of sinus node [Levy 1971] and that the heart rate behavior may become remarkably unstable during situations resulting in accentuated sympatho-vagal antagonism. A characteristic aspect of sympathetic-parasympathetic interaction is represented by the "accentuated antagonism", which consists in a more pronounced bradycardia in response to vagal stimulation when sympathetic activity is elevated, as it occurs when metaboreflex is evoked [Stramba-Badiale et al. 1991, Tullpo et al. 1998]. Therefore, the lack of heart rate response to metaboreflex during post-exercise ischemia reported by several papers is not unexpected and can be explained through the elevated parasympathetic tone that takes place in this setting which accompanies the metaboreflex-induced increase in sympathetic drive [O'Leary 1993, Piepoli et al. 1995, Crisafulli et al. 2003(a)].

While the effect of metaboreflex upon systemic vascular resistance and heart rate is well established and accepted, less is known about its action upon central hemodynamics, i.e. cardiac output, stroke volume, myocardial contractility, and cardiac pre-load. As stated above, metaboreflex is considered to raise blood pressure primarily through an increase in systemic vascular resistance rather than through a flow-increase mechanism. This concept is based upon the fact that metaboreflex is supposed to induce little changes in cardiac output since it exerts little effects upon heart rate. However, as cardiac output is the product of heart rate and stroke volume, the lack of heart rate response to metaboreflex engagement does not necessary rule out a response in cardiac output, i.e. to detect any flow response the knowledge of both heart rate and stroke volume is necessary. In fact, several lines of evidence suggest that the activation of metaboreflex can actually affect also central hemodynamics. In particular, it was found in dogs that the muscle metaboreflex was capable to increase ventricular performance which, in turn, kept stroke volume constant despite the concomitant increase in heart rate and the consequent reduction in diastolic time and cardiac filling [O'Leary et al. 1998]. Similarly, it was reported in humans that myocardial contractility and stroke volume can be increased during metaboreflex activation caused by post-exercise ischemia [Bonde-Petersen et al. 1978, Bonde Petersen et al. 1982, Crisafulli et al. 2003(a)]. This hemodynamic responses aim at maintaining cardiac output despite the raise in after-load that takes place in this condition as a consequence of vasoconstriction. Indeed, stroke volume and consequently cardiac output would drop in response to any raise in after-load if myocardial contractility did not increase. Clearly, this occurrence could be detrimental since would reduce blood flow to contracting muscle and further impair the mismatch between metabolic demand and need. The importance of increasing cardiac contractility and stroke volume appears particularly when the metaboreflex is evoked during post-exercise ischemia, i.e. when bradycardia occurs, since in this circumstance the cardiovascular apparatus can rely only on the enhanced myocardial contractility to keep stroke volume and cardiac output constant in response to vasoconstriction [Crisafulli et al. 2003(a)].

It was also proposed that the muscle metaboreflex is capable of increasing cardiac filling pressure through splanchnic vasoconstriction and venoconstriction which expel blood volume into the central circulation [Sheriff et al. 1998, Gouvêa Bastos et al. 2000]. The rationale behind this blood volume "centralization" relies on the fact that any increase in cardiac output produced by improvement in heart rate and/or cardiac performance increases also pressure in the peripheral vascular bed and, as blood vessels are distensible, blood volume tends to accumulate in the periphery. Actually, there is a reciprocal relationship between cardiac output and ventricular filling pressure and increases in cardiac output will decrease central venous pressure and cardiac pre-load and this fact, in turn, will produce a drop in cardiac output, especially if muscle pump is not operating [Sheriff et al. 1993]. Thus, any increase in cardiac output must be accompanied by blood flow redistribution towards the central circulation to be effective since increases in heart rate or contractility, either alone or together, cannot effectively induce any flow improvement if they are not supported by an enhanced pre-load. It was speculated that the modulation of central venous pressure and cardiac filling are important mechanisms which accompany the rise in heart rate and cardiac contractility in order to increase cardiac output during metaboreflex response [Sheriff et al. 1998].

Therefore, from the above results it appears that metaboreflex can induce peripheral vasoconstriction as well as affect central hemodynamics by modulating cardiac contractility and pre-load. So, at least in the normal heart, the blood pressure response elicited by metaboreflex can be reached by adjusting both peripheral and central hemodynamics. Figure 3 shows the putative mechanisms through metaboreflex acts to increase blood pressure.

It is noteworthy that the strategy chosen to achieve the blood pressure response appears to depend on the intensity of exercise. It was reported both in humans and in animals that the cardiovascular response to metaboreflex relies mainly on cardiac output during mild exercise, whereas peripheral vasoconstriction becomes more important as exercise intensity rises [Augustyniak et al. 2001, Crisafulli et al. 2003(a)]. This behavior was attributed to the fact that the ability of increasing cardiac output depends on the presence of a cardiac reserve, which represents the heart possibility of increasing contractility and in turn stroke volume. If the cardiac reserve can be still used (i.e. if the contractility was not fully used during exercise), then the metaboreflex-induced pressure response relies mainly on cardiac output; differently, if there is not cardiac reserve further available for increasing stroke volume and cardiac output, as it is during and/or after strenuous efforts, then the response relies on peripheral vasoconstriction and systemic vascular resistance increase. These findings suggest that the intensity of exercise possibly dictates the mechanism by which the blood pressure response is elicited by metaboreflex [Fadel 2003]. If this concept was correct, then it would be no surprising that some human studies, which employed moderate and/or heavy rather than mild exercise, did not provide any changes in stroke volume during metaboreflex response [Bonde-Petersen et al. 1978, Gouvêa Bastos et al. 2000]. Moreover, these results indicate that the hemodynamic response to metaboreflex is complex and not merely constituted by a peripheral vasoconstriction. Further studies are needed to better clarify the role played by stroke volume and contractility responses in achieving the metaboreflex-induced raise in blood pressure.

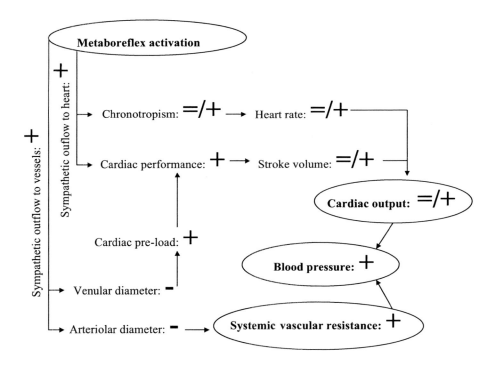

Figure 3. hemodynamic mechanisms of metaboreflex-induced blood pressure response.

In summarizing, it would seem that the cardiovascular apparatus operates with plasticity in order to regulate cardiovascular response to exercise and that the metaboreflex-induced increase in blood pressure can be reached even through the contractility reserve of myocardium.

Metaboreflex and its Possible Involvement in the Genesis of Heart Failure Exercise Intolerance

The hallmark symptom of congestive heart failure is exercise intolerance, which can severely limit the normal daily activities of patients such as working, going up a stair, or simply walking. In this disease a reduction in cardiac function induces a condition where the cardiovascular apparatus fails to meet the flow demand of exercising muscle and, in response to this situation, changes in sympathetic activity and alterations of mechanisms controlling the cardiovascular system also develop [Wilson et al. 1986, Van Der Borne et al. 1997, Shoemaker et al. 1999, Smith et al. 2003]. It was reported that an excessive vasocontriction in the splanchnic beds occurs and even active skeletal muscle may become vasoconstricted due to overactive sympathetic activity [Leimbach et al. 1986, Wilson et al. 1986, Sullivan et al. 1990, Floras 1993]. Yet, blood pressure response to exercise is more elevated than in normal individuals and this occurrence further worsens the myocardium performance, although what causes this altered cardiovascular response is not completely understood yet.

There are several clues that also the metaboreflex is involved in this abnormal blood flow dynamic. In particular, it is thought that one possible explanation of sympathetic overdrive is an exaggerated metaboreflex activity that takes place in response to under-perfusion of contracting muscle. This phenomenon, in turn, leads to vasoconstriction and exaggerated blood pressure response and, at least in part, this situation is responsible for the exercise intolerance shown by these patients [Piepoli et al. 1996, Shoemaker et al. 1998, Notarius et al. 2001]. Thus, according to this hypothesis, in chronic heart failure the metaboreflex activation does not effectively improve blood flow to exercising muscle; rather it would appear that metaboreflex engagement contributes to vasoconstrict the active muscle.

The origin of the overactive metaboreflex may be related to the progressive atrophy of skeletal muscle probably due to the chronic physical de-conditioning often observed in heart failure patients. Such condition increases the accumulation of end product of metabolism during effort because of the reduced oxidative capacity of muscle cells [Wilson et al. 1985, Massie et al. 1987, Drexler et al. 1992]. This causes over-activation of muscle metaboreceptors which, in turn, induces sympathetic vasocostriction and elevated blood pressure response to exertion. Moreover, inasmuch as physical training has been associated to attenuated blood pressure responses to metaboreflex [Mostoufi-Moab et al. 1998], it is possible to speculate that the chronic inactivity of subjects suffering from heart failure exerts an opposite effect, i.e. leads to a more pronounced blood pressure response during metaboreflex engagement. However, this scenario is not universally accepted and some authors reported blunted metaboreflex response in heart failure [Sterns et al. 1991, Negrão et al. 2001].

Moreover, it is conceivable to hypothesize that, together with the over-activation of the reflex, also the inability of increasing myocardial contractility and, consequently, stroke volume in response to metaboreflex may be in part responsible for the exaggerated vasoconstriction during exercise that occurs in heart failure. In fact, these patients can not rely on cardiac reserve to achieve the blood pressure response and, in absence of this mechanism, they can only utilize reflex vasoconstriction. Thus, heart failure causes a functional shift from cardiac output to vasoconstriction in order to achieve the blood pressure response to metaboreflex. This scenario has been demonstrated in an animal model, where the raise in blood pressure during metaboreflex activation was reached by reflex vasoconstriction rather than by a flow increase [Hammond et al. 2000, O'Leary et al. 2004], thus demonstrating that when the cardiac reserve can not be further utilized, then the vasoconstriction becomes the main mechanism through which a blood pressure raise can be reached. Nevertheless, the accentuated vasoconstriction that occurs in this setting leads to detrimental hemodynamic consequence. Indeed, vasoconstriction, by inducing an after-load increase, can further impair the myocardial performance of the already failing heart and this, in turn, may further worsen the skeletal muscle perfusion. Therefore, heart failure may be considered as a disease which disrupts the normal plasticity of cardiovascular response to exercise; in this condition the metaboreflex engagement may be responsible for accentuated vasoconstriction in the active muscle, which is opposite to the flow restoring effect supposed to be in the normal individuals.

Conclusion

The regulation of circulation during exercise implies various levels of control which include central and peripheral mechanisms. There are growing evidences that a peripheral signal of muscular origin acts as regulator of the cardiovascular response to exercise by modulating the basic pattern of autonomic activity established by central command. This mechanism works in response to the mechanical and the metabolic condition of the contracting muscle and it appears to be essential for the normal blood pressure response to muscular work. However, there is still the need to expand our understanding of the mechanisms through which the mechano-metaboreflexes operate. The effects upon central hemodynamics in normal humans are not completely understood yet, and further studies are needed to better elucidate the role of reflex-mediated myocardial contractility and stroke volume response. Moreover, research focusing on central hemodynamics during metaboreflex engagement in heart failure would help to further clarify the origin of exercise intolerance in this cardiac disease.

References

Andreani CM, Hill JM, Kaufman MP (1997). Responses of group III and IV afferents to dynamic exercise. *J. Appl. Physiol.* 82: 1811-1817.

Augustyniak RA, Collins HL, Ansorge EJ, Rossi NF, O'Leary DS (2001). Severe exercise alters the strength and mechanisms of the muscle metaboreflex. *Am. J. Physiol.* 280 *(Heart Circ. Physiol):* H1645-H1652.

Baum K, Selle K, Leyk D, Essfeld D (1995). Comparison of blood pressure and heart rate responses to isometric exercise and passive muscle stretch in humans. *Eur. J. Appl. Physiol.* 70 : 240-245.

Bonde-Petersen F, Rowell LB, Murray RG, GG Blomqvist, R White, E Karlsson, W Campbell, JH Mitchell (1978). Role of cardiac output in the pressor responses to graded muscle ischemia in man. *J. Appl. Physiol.* 45: 574-580.

Bonde-Petersen F, Suzuki Y (1982). Heart contractility at pressure loads induced by ischemia of exercised muscle in humans. *J. Appl. Physiol.* 52: 340-345.

Carcassi AM, Concu A, Decandia M, Onnis M, Orani GP, Piras MB (1983). Respiratory responses to stimulation of large fibers afferent from muscle receptors in cats. *Pflugers Arch.* 399: 309-314.

Carter III R, Watenpaugh DE, Wasmund WL, Wasmund SL, Smith ML (1999). Muscle pump and central command during recovery from exercise in humans. *J. Appl. Physiol.* 87: 1463-1469.

Clark AL, Piepoli M, Coats AJS (1995). Skeletal muscle and the control of ventilation on exercise: evidence for metabolic receptors. *Eur. J. Clin. Invest.* 25: 299-305.

Concu A (1988). Respiratory and cardiac effects of passive limb movements in man. *Pflugers Arch.* 412: 548-550.

Cornett JA, Herr MD, Gray KS, Smith MB, Yang QX, Sinoway LI (2000). Ischemic exercise and the muscle metaboreflex. *J. Appl. Physiol.* 89: 1432-1436.

Crisafulli A, Scott AC, Wensel R, Davos CH, Francis DP, Pagliaro P, Coats AJS, Concu A, Piepoli MF (2003a). Muscle metaboreflex-induced increases in stroke volume. *Med. Sci. Sports Exerc.* 35: 221-228.

Crisafulli A, Orrù V, Melis F, Tocco F, Concu A (2003b) Hemodynamics during active and passive recovery from a single bout of supramaximal exercise. *Eur. J. Appl. Physiol.* 89: 209-216.

Decandia GF, Decandia M, Orani GP (1991). Group I fibers: pressor reflex and cardiac activity. *Cardioscience* 2: 189-192.

Dela F, Mohr T, Jensen CMR, Haahr HL, Secher NH, Biering-Sørensen F, Kjær M (2003). Cardiovascular control during exercise. Insight from spinal cord-injured humans. *Circulation* 107: 2127-2133.

Drexler H, Riede U, Munzel T, Konig H, Funke E, Just H (1992). Alterations of skeletal muscle in chronic heart failure. *Circulation* 85: 1751-1759.

Fadel PJ (2003). Muscle metaboreflex-induced increases in stroke volume. Commentary to accompany. *Med. Sci. Sports Exerc.* 35: 229.

Floras JS (1993). Clinical aspects of sympathetic activation and parasympathetic withdrawal in heart failure. *J. Am, Coll. Cardiol.* 4 (suppl. A): 72A-84A.

Gallagher KM, Fader PJ, Smith SA, Norton KH, Querry RG, Olivencia-Yurvati A, Raven PB (2001). Increases in pressure raise arterial blood pressure during dynamic exercise. *J. Appl. Physiol.* 91: 2351-2358.

Gautier H, Lacaisse A, Djours P (1969). Ventilatory response to muscle spindle stimulation by succinylcholine in cats. *Respiration Physiol.* 7: 383-88.

Goodwin GM, McCloskey DI, Eckberg DL (1972). Cardiovascular and respiratory responses to changes in central command during isometric exercise at constant muscle tension. *J. Physiol. (Lond.)* 226: 173-190.

Gouvêa Bastos B, Williamson JW, Harrelson T, Nôbrega ACL (2000). Left ventricular volumes and hemodynamic responses to postexercise ischemia in healthy humans. *Med. Sci. Sports Exerc.* 32: 1114-1118.

Hammond RL, Augustyniak RA, Rossi NF, Churchill PC, Lapanowsky K, O'Leary DS (2000). Heart failure alters the strength and mechanisms of the muscle metaboreflex. *Am. J. Physiol. 278 (Heart Circ. Physiol)*: H818-H828.

Haouzi P, Hill JM, Lewis BK, Kaufman MP (1999). Responses of group III and IV muscle afferents to distension of the peripheral vascular bed. *J. Appl. Physiol.* 87: 545-553.

Higginbotham MB, Morris KG, Williams RS, McHale PA, Coleman RE, Cobb FR (1986). Regulation of stroke volume during submaximal and maximal upright exercise in normal man. *Circ. Res.* 58: 281-291.

Ichinose M, Saito M, Wada H, Kitano A, Kondo N, Nishiyasu T (2004). Modulation of arterial baroreflex control of muscle sympathetic nerve activity by muscle metaboreflex in humans. *Am. J. Physiol. 286 (Heart Circ. Physiol.)*: H701-H707.

Iellamo F, Legramante JM, Raimondi G, Peruzzi G (1997). Baroreflex control of sinus node during dynamic exercise: effect of central command and muscle reflexes. *Am. J. Physiol. 272 (Heart Circ. Physiol.)* : H1157-H1164.

Iellamo F, Pizzinelli P, Massaro M, Raimondi G, Peruzzi G, Legramante JM (1999). Muscle metaboreflex contribution to sinus node regulation during static exercise. *Circulation* 100: 27-32.

Joyner MJ (1991). Does the pressor response to ischemic exercise improve blood flow to contracting muscles in humans? *J. Appl. Physiol.* 71: 1496-1501.

Kaufman MP, Longhurst JC, Rybicki KJ, Wallach JH, Mitchell JH (1983). Effect of static muscular contraction on impulse activity of group III and IV afferents in cats. *J. Appl. Physiol.* 55: 105-112.

Kaufman MP, Waldrop TG, Rybicki KJ, Ordway GA, Mitchell JH (1984). Effects of static and rhytmic twitch contractions on the discharge of group III and IV muscle afferents. *Cardiovasc. Res.* 18: 663-668.

Kaufman MP, Rybicki KJ (1987). Discharge properties of group III and IV muscle afferents: their responses to mechanical and metabolic stimuli. *Circ. Res.* 61 *suppl.*: 160-165.

Kidd GL, Kucera J (1969). The excitation by suxamethonium of non proprioceptive afferents from caudal muscles of the rat. *Experientia* 25: 158-160.

Kniffki KD, Mense S, Schmidt RF (1978). Responses of group IV afferent units from skeletal muscle to stretch, contraction, and chemical stimulation. *Exp. Brain Res.* 31: 511-522.

Laughlin MH (1987). Skeletal muscle blood flow capacity: role of muscle pump in exercise hyperemia. *Am. J. Physiol. 253 (Heart Circ. Physiol.)*: H993-H1004.

Leimbach WN, Wallin BG, Victor RG, Aylward PE, Sundlof G, Mark AL (1986). *Circulation* 73: 913-919.

Leshnower BG, Potts JT, Garry MG, Mitchell JH (2001). Reflex cardiovascular responses evoked by selective activation of skeletal muscle ergoreceptors. *J. Appl. Physiol.* 90: 308-316.

Levy MN (1971). Sympathetic-parasympathetic interactions in the heart. *Circ. Res.* 29: 437-445.

Lewis SF, Taylor RM, Graham RM, Pettinger WA, Schutte JE, Blomqvist CG (1983). Cardiovascular responses to exercise as functions of absolute and relative work load. *J. Appl. Physiol.* 54: 1314-1323.

Massie BM, Conway M, Yonge R, Frostick S, Sleight P, Ledingham J, Radda G, Raiagopalan B (1987). $_{31}$P nuclear magnetic resonance evidence of abnormal skeletal muscle metabolism in patients with congestive heart failure. *Am. J. Cardiol.* 60: 309-315.

Mathews PB (1972). *Muscle receptors and their central actions.* London; Arnold.

Matsukawa K, Wall PT, Wilson LB, Mitchell JH (1994). Reflex stimulation of cardiac sympathetic nerve activity during static muscle contraction in cats. *Am. J. Physiol. 267 (Heart Circ. Physiol.):* H821-H827.

McCloskey DI, Matthews PBC, Mitchell JH (1972). Absence of appreciable cadiovascular and respiratory responses to muscle vibration. *J. Appl. Physiol.* 33: 623-626.

McCloskey DI, Mitchell JH (1972). Reflex cardiovascular and respiratory responses originating in exercising muscle. *J. Physiol. London* 224: 173-186.

Mense S, Stahnke M (1983). Responses in muscle afferent fibers of slow conduction velocity to contractions and ischemia in cat. *J. Physiol. (Lond.)* 342: 383-397.

Mense S. Nociception from skeletal muscle in relation to clinical muscle pain (1993). *Pain* 54: 241-289.

Mitchell JH, Kaufman MP, Iwamoto GA (1983a). The exercise pressor reflex: its cardiovascular effects, afferent mechanisms, and central pathways. *Ann. Rev. Physiol.* 45: 229-242.

Mitchell JH, Schmidt RF (1983b). Cardiovascular reflex control by afferent fibers from skeletal muscle receptors. In *Handbook of Physiology* vol. III, part 2, ed. Shepherd JT & Abboud FM, pp. 626-658. American Physiological Society, Bethesda USA.

Mostoufi-Moab S, Widmaier EJ, Cornett JA, Gray K, Sinoway LI (1998). Forearm training reduces the exercise pressor reflex during rhythmic handgrip. *J. Appl. Physiol.* 84: 277-283.

Negrão CE, Brandão Rondon MUP, Tinucci T, Alves MJN, Roveda F, Brage AMW, Reis SF, Nastari L, Barretto ACP, Krieger EMK, Middlekauff HR (2001). Abnormal neurovascular control during exercise is linked to heart failure severity. *Am. J. Physiol. 280 (Heart Circ. Physiol.)*: H1286-H1292.

Nishiyasu T, Nobusuke T, Morimoto K, Nishiyasu M, Yamaguchi Y, Murakami N (1994a). Enhancement of parasympathetic cardiac activity during activation of muscle metaboreflex in humans. *J. Appl. Physiol.* 77: 2778-2783.

Nishiyasu T, Ueno H, Nishiyasu M, Tan N, Morimoto K, Morimoto A, Deguchi T, Murakami N (1994b). Relationship between mean arterial pressure and muscle pH during forearm ischemia after sustained handgrip. *Acta Physiol. Scand.* 151: 143-148.

Nishiyasu T, Nagashima K, Nadel ER, Mack GW (2000). Human cardiovascular and humoral responses to moderate muscle activation during dynamic exercise. *J. Appl. Physiol.* 88: 300-307.

Notarius CF, Atchinson DA, Floras JS (2001). Impact of heart failure and exercise capacity on sympathetic response to handgrip exercise. *Am. J. Physiol. 280 (Heart Circ. Physiol.)*: H969-H976.

O'Leary DS (1993). Autonomic mechanisms of muscle metaboreflex control of heart rate. *J. Appl. Physiol.* 74: 1748-1754.

O'Leary DS, Sheriff DD (1995). Is the muscle metaboreflex important in control of blood flow to ischemic active skeletal muscle in dogs? *Am. J. Physiol. 268 (Heart Circ. Physiol. 37)* H980-H986.

O'Leary DS, Augustyniak RA (1998). Muscle metaboreflex increases ventricular performance in conscious dogs. *Am. J. Physiol. 275 (Heart Circ. Physiol. 44)*: H220-H224.

O'Leary DS, Augustyniak RA, Ansorge EJ, Collins H (1999). Muscle metaboreflex improves O_2 delivery to ischemic active skeletal muscle. *Am. J. Physiol. 276 (Heart Circ. Physiol.45)*: H1399-H1403.

O'Leary DS, Sala-Mercado JA, Augustyniak RA, Hammond RL, Rossi NF, Ansorge EJ (2004). Impaired muscle metaboreflex-induced increases in ventricular function in heart failure. *Am. J. Physiol 287 (Heart Circ. Physiol.)*: H2612-H2618.

Orani GP, Decandia M (1990). Group I afferent fibers: effects on cardiorespiratory system. *J. Appl. Physiol.* 68: 932-937.

Orani GP, Decandia M (1994). Role of the heart and peripheral resistance in the reflex effect of group I afferent fibers on blood pressure. *Cardioscience* 5: 25-30.

Piepoli M, Clark AL, Coats AJS (1995). Muscle metaboreceptors in hemodynamic, autonomic, and ventilatory responses to exercise in men. *Am. J. Physiol. 269 (Heart Circ. Physiol. 38)*: H1428-H1436.

Piepoli M, Clark AL, Volterrani M, Adamopoulos S, Sleight P, Coats AJS (1996). Contribution of muscle afferents to hemodynamic, autonomic, and ventilatory responses to exercise in patients with chronic heart failure. *Circulation* 93: 940-952.

Rowell LB, O'Leary DS (1990). Reflex control of the circulation during exercise: chemoreflexes and mechanoreflexes. *J. Appl. Physiol.* 69: 407-418.

Rowell LB, Savage MV, Chambers J, Blackmon JR (1991). Cardiovascular responses to graded reductions in leg perfusion in exercising humans. *Am.. J. Physiol. 261 (Heart Circ. Physiol. 30)* H1545-H1553.

Rybicki KJ, Stremel RW, Iwamoto GA, Mitchell JH, Kaufman MP (1989). Occlusion of pressor responses to posterior diencephalic stimulation and static muscular contraction. *Brain Res. Bull.* 22: 305-312.

Sato A, Sato Y, Schmidt RF (1981). Heart rate changes reflecting modifications of afferent crdiac sympathetic outflow by cutaneous and muscle afferent volleys. *J. Auton. Nerv. Syst.* 4: 231-247.

Sheriff DD, Wyss C, Rowell L, Scher A (1987). Does inadequate oxygen delivery trigger pressor response to muscle hypoperfusion during exercise? *Am. J. Physiol. 253 (Heart Circ. Physiol.)*: H1199-H1207.

Sheriff DD, Zhou XP, Scher AM, Rowell LB (1993). Dependence of cardiac filling pressure on cardiac output during rest and dynamic exercise in dogs. *Am. J. Physiol. 265 (Heart Circ. Physiol. 34)* H316-H322.

Sheriff DD, Augstyniak RA, O'Leary DS (1998). Muscle chemoreflex-induced increases in right atrial pressure. *Am. J. Physiol. 275 (Heart Circ. Physiol. 44)*: H767-H775.

Shi X, Potts JT, Raven PB, Foresman BH (1995). Aortic-cardiac reflex during dynamic exercise. *J. Appl. Physiol.* 78: 1569-1574.

Shoemaker JK, Kunselman AR, Silber DH, Sinoway LI (1998). Maintained exercise pressor response in heart failure. *J. Appl. Physiol.* 85: 1793-1799.

Shoemaker JK, Naylor HL, Hogeman CS, Sinoway LI (1999). Blood flow dynamics in heart failure. *Circulation* 99: 3002-3008.

Sinoway L, Prophet S, Gorman I, Mosher T, Shenberger J, Dolecki M, Briggs R, Zelis R (1989). Muscle acidosis during static exercise is associated with calf vasoconstriction. *J. Appl. Physiol.* 66: 429-436.

Smith SA, Mammen PPA, Mitchell JH, Garry MG (2003). Role of the exercise pressor reflex in rats with dilated cardiomyopathy. *Circulation* 108: 1126-1132.

Stebbins CL, Brown B, Levin D, Longhurst JC (1988). Reflex effect of skeletal muscle mechanoreceptor stimulation on the cardiovascular system. *J. Appl. Physiol.* 65: 1539-1547.

Sterns DA, Ettinger SM, Gray KS, Whisler SK, Mosher TJ, Smith MB, Sinoway LI (1991). Skeletal muscle metaboreceptors exercise responses are attenuated in heart failure. *Circulation* 84: 2034-2039.

Stramba-Badiale M, Vavoli E, DE Ferrari GM, Cerati D, Foreman RD, Schwartz PJ (1991). Sympathetic-parasympathetic interaction and accentuated antagonism in conscious dogs. *Am. J. Physiol. 260 (Heart Circ. Physiol.)*: H335-H340.

Strange S, Secher NH, Pawelczyk JA, Karpakka J, Christensen NJ, Mitchell JH, Saltin B (1993). Neural control of cardiovascular responses and of ventilation during dynamic exercise in man. *J. Physiol. (Lond.)* 470: 693-704.

Sullivan MJ, Green HJ, Cobb FR (1990). Skeletal muscle biochemistry and hystology in ambulatory patients with chronic heart failure. *Circulation* 81: 518-527.

Terui N, Koizumi K (1994). Responses of cardiacvagus and sympathetic nerves to excitation of somatic and visceral nerves. *J. Auton. Nerv. Invest.* 10: 73-91.

Tulppo MP, Makikallio TH, Sepanen T, Airaksinen JKE, Huikuri H (1998). Heart rate dynamics during accentuated sympathovagal interaction. *Am. J. Physiol. 274 (Heart Circ. Physiol.)*: H810-H816.

Van Der Borne P, Montano N, Pagani M, Oren R, Somers VK (1997). Absence of low-frequency variability of sympathetic nerve activity in severe heart failure. *Circulation* 95: 1449-1454.

Victor RG, Bertocci LA, Pryor SL, Nunnally RL (1988). Sympathetic nerve discharge is coupled to muscle cell pH during exercise in humans. *J. Clin. Invest.* 82: 1301-1305.

Waldrop TG, Rybicki KJ, Kaufman MP (1984). Chemical activation of group I and II muscle afferents has no cardiocirculatory effects. *J. Appl. Physiol.* 56: 1223-1228.

Wilson JR, Fink L, Maris J, Ferraro N, Power-Vanwart J, Eleff S, Chance B (1985). Evaluation of energy metabolism in skeletal muscle of patients with heart failure with gated phosphorus-3 I nuclear magnetic resonance. *Circulation* 71: 57-62.

Wilson JR, Falcone R, Ferraro N, Egler J (1986). Mechanisms of skeletal muscle underperfusion in a dog model of low-output heart failure. *Am. J. Physiol. 251 (Heart Circ. Physiol.)*: H227-H235.

Chapter VIII

Thermoregulatory Responses of Athletes with a Spinal Cord Injury to Prolonged Wheelchair Exercise in Cool and Warm Conditions

M. J. Price[*,1] and I. G. Campbell[2]

[1] School of Science and the Environment, Coventry University, Coventry UK.
[2] Lane 4 Management Group Ltd, Bourne End, Buckinghamshire UK

Abstract

This chapter examined the thermoregulatory responses of athletes with a spinal cord injury (T3/4-L1) at rest, during exercise and recovery in cool (21.5 ±1.3°C; 54.2 ±6.3% relative humidity) and warm conditions (31.3 ±0.4°C; 42.3 ±6.3% relative humidity).

Subjects exercised on a wheelchair ergometer at 60% of peak oxygen uptake ($\dot{V}O_2$ peak) for 60 minutes in both conditions. Aural and skin temperatures were continually monitored. Aural temperature increased from rest by 0.6 ±0.3°C (P<0.05) during exercise in cool conditions with relatively steady state aural temperature values from 20 minutes of exercise. During exercise in warm conditions aural temperature increased continually to 1.2 ±0.5°C above resting levels (P<0.05). Differences between conditions were observed from 10 minutes of exercise (P<0.05). Skin temperatures demonstrated differences between conditions from rest in the environmental chamber until the end of recovery (P<0.05). Sensate upper body skin sites demonstrated a balance between heat gain and heat loss in both conditions. Insensate lower body skin temperatures increased by greater amounts, particularly during warm conditions, suggesting an imbalance in thermoregulation and indicating the lower body to be a potent site for heat storage. Whole body heat storage was much greater at the end of exercise in warm (5.44 ±1.8 J.g-

---

[*] School of Science and the Environment, Coventry University, Priory Street, Coventry, CV1 5FB. Tel.no.: 02476 888163; Fax no.: 02476 888702; E-Mail.: m.price@coventry.ac.uk

1) when compared to cool conditions (0.99 ±1.58 J.g-1; P<0.05). Fluid consumption and changes in plasma volume and body mass were similar during exercise in both trials. During the initial 5 minutes recovery, heart rate was greater during warm conditions. The results of this study suggest that trained athletes with a spinal cord injury are able to tolerate prolonged wheelchair exercise in the conditions studied, although greater physiological strain was evident during exercise and the initial stages of recovery in warm when compared to cool conditions. The influence of regional heat storage, voluntary fluid intake and sweat rates in relation to limitations to exercise are discussed.

Introduction

Wheelchair athletes with predominantly low level spinal cord injuries (SCI; T3/4 – L1) have been reported to be able maintain thermal balance during prolonged exercise in cool conditions (Price and Campbell, 1997, 1999a). However, due to the well known loss of blood redistribution and sweating capacity below the level of spinal cord lesion (Randall *et al.*, 1966; Hopman, 1994) the insensate lower body has been considered a potent site for heat storage (Price and Campbell, 1997, 1999a). Considering that increases in body temperature during prolonged upper body exercise in warm conditions for able bodied athletes are twice those observed in cool conditions (Price and Campbell, 2002), the thermoregulatory responses of athletes with SCI may become compromised in such conditions due to the reduced thermoregulatory capacity and heat storage within the lower body. However, there is relatively little known regarding the thermoregulatory responses of this population during exercise and recovery in warm conditions.

Studies examining the thermoregulatory responses of athletes with SCI during exercise in warm conditions have generally employed arm crank ergometry (Hopman *et al.*, 1993; Petrofsky, 1992; Dawson *et al.*, 1994). However, this exercise mode results in greater physiological and thermoregulatory strain when compared to wheelchair ergometry and may overestimate the thermal strain that wheelchair athletes would habitually experience (Price and Campbell, 1999b). The thermoregulatory differences between exercise modes were considered to be due to differences in the application of force to the ergometer flywheel, and consequently propulsion technique. A further contribution was considered to be from local cooling of the arm during wheelchair propulsion. Based on this information it would seem appropriate to examine the thermoregulatory responses of athletes with a SCI to prolonged exercise in warm conditions using specific wheelchair exercise. Only one study has reported the thermoregulatory responses of wheelchair athletes during wheelchair ergometry in a warm environment (~33°C; Armstrong *et al.*, 1995). This study was primarily concerned with evaluating the effectiveness of two cooling strategies during a 30 min bout of exercise at an intensity relating to 10 km race pace. Consequently, the exercise duration employed was short and the exercise intensity was not directly measured and due to the nature of the study no control environment was employed.

The importance of a control environment is evident when considering avenues of heat loss other than sweating i.e. dry heat exchange, in the region below the level of spinal cord lesion. For example, Fitzgerald *et al.* (1990) observed an elevated mean skin temperature in wheelchair dependent women during wheelchair ergometry in 24 – 25°C conditions suggesting an increased contribution to heat loss from dry heat exchange. Furthermore, even with much cooler local skin temperatures below the level of spinal cord injury when compared to those above the lesion prior to exercise, lower body skin temperatures still increased to 30 – 31°C for SCI individuals during arm crank ergometry in 21.5°C conditions (Price and Campbell, 1997). Consequently, both at rest and during exercise in relatively cool conditions a significant thermal gradient does exist for dry heat exchange in the area below the level of spinal cord lesion. However, during exercise in the heat, the thermal gradient may be reduced or even reversed contributing to gains in heat within the lower body that would normally be dissipated by sweating. Such gains in heat may therefore occur early during exercise and contribute to total heat storage. The possible contribution of dry heat exchange from the area below the lesion has not yet been fully considered in this population. Examining this aspect of heat exchange in a cool environment will provide a solid baseline to which heat exchange in other conditions can be compared.

Therefore the aim of this study was to compare the thermoregulatory responses of wheelchair athletes at rest, during prolonged wheelchair exercise and recovery in cool and warm conditions. It is hypothesized that exercise in a warm environment will result in greater increases in body temperature than in a cool environment primarily due to heat storage within the lower body.

Subjects and Methods

Eight trained wheelchair athletes, all with complete spinal cord injury (T3/T4-L1), volunteered to participate in this study. All athletes trained regularly and competed in a variety of wheelchair sports, predominantly athletics and basketball, at a national and international level. The mean age, body mass and sum of four skinfolds were, 29.0 ±4.5 yrs, 64.2 ±11.8 kg and 42.9 ±19.4 mm, respectively. All subjects attended the laboratory on three separate occasions. Further information regarding the subjects is shown in Table 1.

Table 1. Characteristics of the paraplegic athletes (all athletes were complete lesions)

Subject	Lesion level	Aetiology of spinal cord injury	Time since injury (yrs)	Sport
1	L1	Spina Bifida	21.0	Athletics
2	T3/T4	Traumatic	10.0	Athletics
3	T12	Traumatic	16.0	Basketball
4	T8	Traumatic	35.0	Basketball
5	T12	Spina Bifida	22.0	Basketball
6	T8	Traumatic	11.5	Athletics
7	T6/T7	Traumatic	26.0	Weight Training
8	T10	Spina Bifida	22.0	Swimming

Preliminary Tests

Following familiarisation, subjects performed four stages of submaximal wheelchair exercise followed by an incremental test for peak oxygen uptake ($\dot{V}O_2$ peak). The submaximal stages enabled steady state metabolic responses to be measured and the accurate determination of the power output eliciting 60% $\dot{V}O_2$ peak for the prolonged exercise trials. Athletes exercised in their own sports specific wheelchair on a wheelchair ergometer (Bromking Turbo Trainer, Loughborough, England). Athletes exercising in track wheelchairs performed exercise stages at workloads of 30, 40, 50 and 60W. Subjects then undertook an incremental test for $\dot{V}O_2$ peak. This involved subjects propelling their wheelchairs at an increment of 5W.min^{-1} from an initial workload of 30W until volitional exhaustion. As the basketball players were unable to push their sports chairs at these power outputs and to maintain exercise specificity a protocol employing push rate, developed by Wicks et al. (1983), was used. This involved submaximal exercise stages of 30, 40, 50 and 60 pushes per minute with the test for $\dot{V}O_2$ peak involving increases in push rate of 10 pushes per minute until volitional exhaustion. These push rates were equivalent to power outputs of 8, 10, 12 and 14 Watts, respectively, and a ramp of 2 Watts.min^{-1} (Price and Campbell, 2003).

Prolonged Exercise Tests

On subsequent visits to the laboratory subjects performed 60 minutes of wheelchair ergometry (WCE) at a workload set to elicit 60% $\dot{V}O_2$ peak. The prolonged exercise tests were undertaken in either a normal laboratory environment ('cool' environment; 21.5 ±1.3°C; 54.2 ±6.3% relative humidity) or a warm environment (31.3 ±0.4°C, 42.3 ±6.3 % relative humidity). The order of testing was randomised.

On arrival at the laboratory for the 60 minute test, subjects rested quietly for 15 minutes. At the end of this period resting heart rate (HR) was recorded (Polar Sports Tester PE4000, Kempele, Finland) along with resting thermoregulatory data. Subjects then entered the environmental chamber where a resting expired air sample was obtained. A small 20 µl capillary blood sample was obtained from the earlobe and analysed for blood lactate concentration (BLa; YSI 2000 Sport lactate analyser, Yellow Springs, USA). A 5 ml venous blood sample was obtained from the antecubital vein from which haemoglobin (Clandon HemoCue, HemoCue Ltd, Sheffield, England) and haematocrit (Hawksley Reader, Hawksley & Sons, Sussex, England) were subsequently analysed to determine plasma volume (Dill and Costill, 1974). Body mass was then recorded (Seca 710, seated scales, Hamburg, Germany) after individuals had evacuated their bladders. Skinfold measurements were taken from the biceps, triceps, subscapular and suprailiac sites (Durnin and Wormersley, 1974) using Harpenden skinfold callipers (British Indicators Ltd, Luton, England).

Thermisitors were positioned for measures of aural and skin temperatures. Aural temperature was measured by an aural thermistor inserted into the subjects' auditory canal (Benzinger and Taylor, 1963) and securely plugged and taped in position. The external ear was then insulated with cotton wool. Aural temperature was employed in the present study as subject discomfort is often reported from the use of rectal and oesophageal probes (Armstrong et al., 1994; Sato et al., 1996) and rectal temperature has been considered inappropriate for use with the spinal cord injured (Gass et al., 1988). Skin thermistors were placed at the forehead, forearm, upper arm, back, chest, abdomen, thigh and calf in order to establish the whole body thermoregulatory response. Thermistors were attached to the skin using narrow strips of water permeable surgical tape (3M Transpore, Loughborough, England) in a criss-cross pattern. The ends of the strips were anchored with surgical tape. This technique maintained an appropriate skin-to-thermistor interface while minimising the area of skin covered by the surgical tape (Goss et al., 1989). Subjects then undertook a standardised five minute warm up on the wheelchair ergometer. Once completed subjects were allowed to undergo their usual stretching routine. Subjects then exercised at an intensity of 60% $\dot{V}O_2$ peak for 60 minutes and were allowed to drink plain water *ad libitum*. On completion of the exercise test, subjects remained in the seated position and a second 5 ml venous blood sample was obtained. Post-exercise haemoglobin concentration and haematocrit were subsequently analysed. Subjects then rested quietly for 30 minutes and were re-weighed.

Aural and skin temperatures were recorded at rest, post warm-up and every 5 minutes during the exercise period and during the first 30 minutes of recovery. Values were recorded by a Grant Squirrel meter logger (1250 Series, Grant Instruments, Cambridge, England) via Edale thermistors (Edale Instruments, Cambridge, England). Heat storage was calculated from the following formula employed by Havenith et al. (1995) where;

$$\text{Heat Storage} = (0.8\, \Delta T_{core} + 0.2\, \Delta T_{MST}) \cdot C_b,$$

and C_b is the specific heat capacity of the body tissue (3.49 $J \cdot g^{-1} \cdot °C^{-1}$). Values were calculated from changes in aural (ΔT_{core}) and mean skin temperature (ΔT_{MST}; Ramanathan, 1964) from resting values at 5, 15, 30, 45 and 60 minutes of exercise and 15 and 30 minutes of recovery. Small 20 µl capillary blood samples were obtained from the earlobe at 5, 15, 30, 45 and 60 minutes during the exercise period and 5 minutes post-exercise. One minute expired air samples were collected via the Douglas bag technique at 5, 15, 30, 45 and 60 minutes during the exercise period. Ratings of perceived exertion (RPE; Borg Scale) were also obtained after each expired air collection.

Statistical Analysis

Thermoregulatory and physiological data of the group during prolonged WCE in both cool and warm conditions were compared by two-way Analysis of Variance with repeated measures. Significance was accepted at the $P<0.05$ level. Where significance was obtained Tukey post-hoc analysis was undertaken.

Results

Peak Physiological Responses

The peak physiological responses to incremental wheelchair ergometry are shown in Table 2. $\dot{V}O_2$ peak and heart rate peak values for the group were 2.00 ±0.40 $l.min^{-1}$ and 183

±14 beats.min^{-1}, respectively. The subject with the spinal cord lesion at T3 demonstrated no adverse cardiovascular responses during any of the exercise tests. Furthermore, the inclusion of this subjects' thermoregulatory data did not affect mean values and was therefore included in the group data analysis.

Table 2. Peak physiological characteristics for group (Mean ± S.D.)

$\dot{V}O_2$ peak l.min.$^{-1}$	2.00 ±0.40
$\dot{V}O_2$ peak ml.kg.min.$^{-1}$	32.3 ±8.8
Ventilation rate l.min.$^{-1}$	75.5 ±16.0
Heart rate peak bts.min^{-1}	183 ±14
Blood lactate peak mmol.l.$^{-1}$	5.77 ±1.74
RER	1.05 ±0.13

Physiological Responses During Prolonged Exercise

During the prolonged exercise test oxygen uptake ($\dot{V}O_2$) at 5 minutes of exercise was similar between trials (1.19 ±0.33 l.min^{-1} and 1.09 ±0.30 l.min^{-1} in cool and warm conditions, respectively) representing 59.5 ±7.9% and 54.5 ±10.1% $\dot{V}O_2$ peak. Heart rate increased from 5 minutes of exercise until the end of exercise in both conditions (152 ±30 bts.min^{-1} and 164 ±29 bts.min^{-1} for cool and warm conditions, respectively, $P<0.05$). After 5 minutes of recovery from exercise in the warm environment HR was greater than when compared to cool conditions ($P<0.05$). No differences were observed between BLa or RPE during exercise in either condition. However, RPE was elevated earlier during exercise in the warm (10.9 ±1.9 at 15 minutes vs. 9.4 ±1.7 at 5 minutes of exercise, $P<0.05$) when compared to the cool environment (12.9 ±1.7 at 45 minutes vs. 11.4 ±1.1 at 5 minutes; $P<0.05$).

Aural Temperature During Prolonged Exercise and Recovery

Aural temperature for the group at rest, during exercise and recovery in the cool and warm conditions is shown in Figure 1. Aural temperature increased by 0.6 ±0.3 and 1.2 ±0.5°C during exercise in cool and warm conditions, respectively ($P<0.05$). During exercise in cool conditions aural temperature was elevated from rest after 15 minutes of exercise ($P<0.05$), whereas during exercise in warm conditions aural temperature was elevated from rest after 10 minutes of exercise (P<0.05). Differences between trials were observed from 10 minutes of exercise until the end of the recovery period (P<0.05).

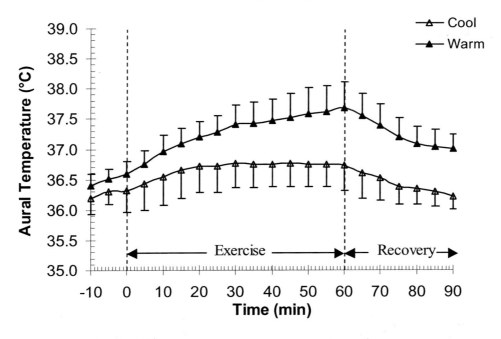

Figure 1. Aural temperature for athletes with a spinal cord injury at rest, during prolonged wheelchair exercise and recovery in cool (21.5 ±1.3°C; 54.2 ±6.3% relative humidity) and warm (31.3 ±0.4°C; 42.3 ±6.3% relative humidity) conditions.

Skin Temperature During Prolonged Exercise and Recovery

During exercise in cool conditions skin temperatures for the group, with the exception of the upper arm, remained unchanged from resting values. Upper arm skin temperature was cooler throughout exercise when compared to resting values (P<0.05; Figure 2) returning to pre-exercise levels on the cessation of exercise. During exercise in warm conditions upper body skin temperatures for the group were elevated above resting values throughout exercise and until the end of the recovery period (P<0.05) being warmer at all time points when compared to the cool condition (P<0.05). Thigh skin temperature was elevated from 55 minutes of exercise in warm conditions until the end of recovery (P<0.05), whereas calf skin temperature was elevated during the final 15 minutes of the recovery period only (P<0.05; Figure 3). Individual skin temperatures at rest in cool conditions, prior to exercise in both conditions and local thermal gradients with the environment are shown in Table 3 and 4.

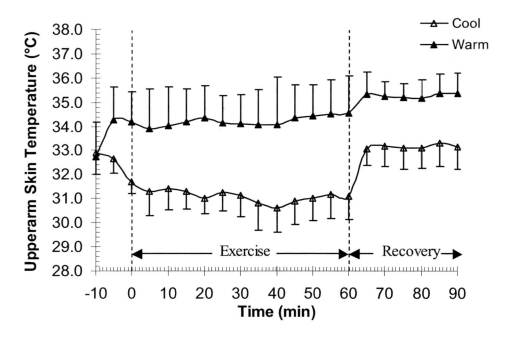

Figure 2. Upper arm skin temperature for athletes with a spinal cord injury at rest, during prolonged wheelchair exercise and recovery in cool (21.5 ±1.3°C; 54.2 ±6.3% relative humidity) and warm (31.3 ±0.4°C; 42.3 ±6.3% relative humidity) conditions.

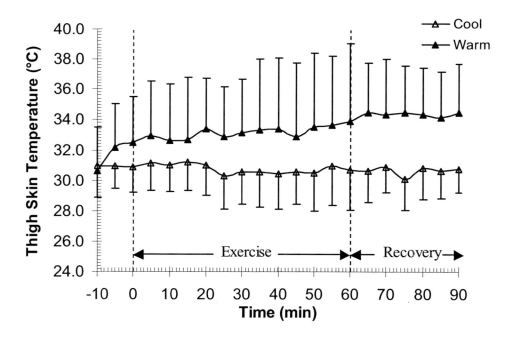

Figure 3 continued on next page

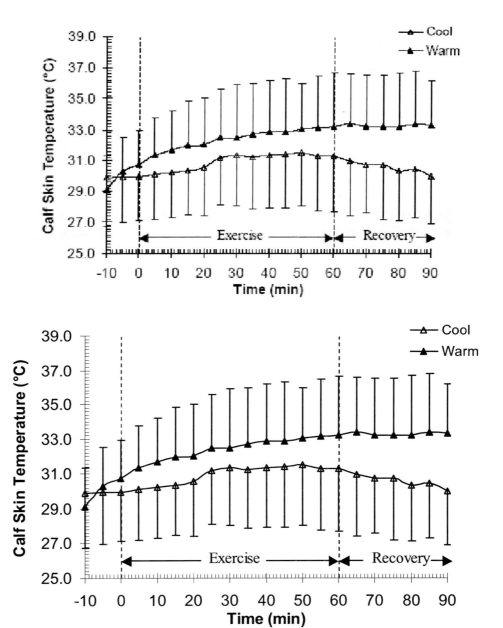

Figure 3. Thigh and calf skin temperature for athletes with a spinal cord injury at rest, during prolonged wheelchair exercise and recovery in cool (21.5 ±1.3°C; 54.2 ±6.3% relative humidity) and warm (31.3 ±0.4°C; 42.3 ±6.3% relative humidity) conditions.

Table 3. Change in skin temperatures (Δ°t) during exercise and local thermal gradients (ambient – skin temperature) at rest and during exercise in cool conditions (End Ex. = end of exercise)

Site	Skin Temperature (Rest)	Skin Temperature (End Ex.)	Δ°t	Thermal Gradient (Rest)	Thermal Gradient (End Ex.)
Forehead	33.5	34.0	0.5	-12.0	-12.5
Forearm	32.1	32.0	-0.1	-10.6	-10.5
Upperarm	32.9	31.1	-1.8	-11.4	-9.6
Back	32.6	32.4	-0.2	-11.1.	-10.9
Chest	32.6	32.7	0.1	-11.1	-11.2
Abdomen	32.8	32.8	0.0	-11.3	-11.3
Thigh	31.0	30.7	-0.3	-9.5	-9.2
Calf	29.1	31.3	2.2	-7.6	-9.8

Table 4. Change in skin temperatures (Δ°t) during exercise and local thermal gradients (ambient – skin temperature) at rest and during exercise in warm conditions (End Ex. = end of exercise)

Site	Skin Temperature (Rest)	Skin Temperature (End Ex.)	Δ°t	Thermal Gradient (Rest)	Thermal Gradient (End Ex.)
Forehead	33.6	36.1	2.5	-2.3	-4.8
Forearm	32.5	35.4	2.9	-1.2	-4.1
Upperarm	32.8	34.5	1.7	-1.5	-3.2
Back	32.9	34.8	1.9	-1.6	-3.5
Chest	32.8	35.4	2.6	-1.5	-4.1
Abdomen	32.7	34.5	1.8	-1.4	-3.2
Thigh	30.7	33.9	3.2	0.6	-2.6
Calf	29.1	33.2	4.1	2.2	-1.9

Heat Storage

Heat storage at rest, during prolonged wheelchair exercise and recovery in cool and warm conditions is shown in Figure 4. During both exercise and recovery in cool conditions, heat storage for the group was not elevated from rest at any time point (0.99 ±1.58 $J.g^{-1}$ and 0.00 ±1.18 $J.g^{-1}$ at the end of exercise and 30 minutes of recovery, respectively; P>0.05). At rest in the environmental chamber, prior to exercise in warm conditions, heat storage of 1.10 ±0.17 $J.g^{-1}$ was observed, increasing to 5.44 ±1.8 $J.g^{-1}$ at the end of exercise (P<0.05). After 30 minutes of recovery from exercise in warm conditions, heat storage decreased to 3.49 ±1.05 $J.g^{-1}$, but was still elevated above resting levels (P<0.05). Heat storage was greatest throughout exercise and recovery in warm when compared to cool conditions at every time point (P<0.05).

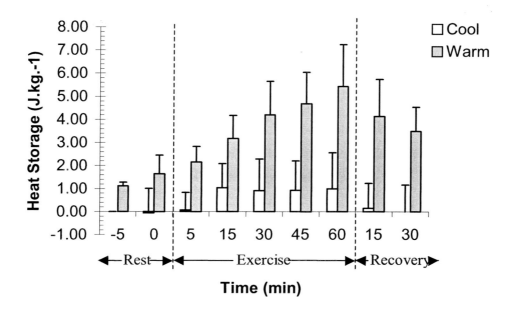

Figure 4. Heat storage for the athletes with a spinal cord injury at rest, during prolonged wheelchair exercise and recovery in cool (21.5 ±1.3°C; 54.2 ±6.3% relative humidity) and warm (31.3 ±0.4°C; 42.3 ±6.3% relative humidity) conditions.

Fluid Balance

No differences were observed for changes in plasma volume (-6.07 ±4.39% and -5.66 ±4.29%), fluid intake (428 ±349 ml and 361 ±291 ml) or total weight losses (-0.9 ±0.6 and -0.7 ±0.5 kg) during exercise in the cool and warm conditions, respectively.

Discussion

Physiological Responses

The physiological responses during cool conditions were similar and consistent with previous reports of athletes with a spinal cord injury during prolonged wheelchair exercise in cool conditions (Price and Campbell, 1999b). However, when compared to prolonged arm crank exercise the blood lactate response was lower than previous reports of both spinal cord injured and able-bodied subjects during exercise of a similar intensity and duration in cool conditions (Pimental et al., 1984; Price and Campbell, 1997, 2002). This has previously been reported to be due to differences in propulsion technique between the two modes of exercise (Price and Campbell, 1999b). The similar BLa responses during both environmental conditions reported in this chapter are consistent with the work of Dawson *et al.* (1994) and may represent the relatively low intensity and steady state aerobic exercise employed.

Aural Temperature During Exercise

The increase in aural temperature observed for the group was similar to observations of able-bodied athletes during prolonged arm crank exercise in cool and warm conditions (Price and Campbell, 2002). Values were also similar to aural and rectal temperature increases during short duration wheelchair exercise in similar conditions (~33°C; Armstrong *et al.*, 1995). The thermal strain of the athletes observed in this chapter was therefore similar to previous studies. It should be noted that aural temperature did not plateau during exercise in warm conditions suggesting that an imbalance existed between heat gain and heat loss during exercise. All athletes though completed the exercise duration demonstrating that the trained paraplegic athletes studied were able to tolerate increases in body temperature in the conditions examined. Interestingly, the able-bodied athletes cited for comparison (Price and Campbell, 2002), although exercising at similar relative exercise intensities to the present study, were exercising at greater absolute exercise intensities. This may suggest that although absolute heat production for the wheelchair athletes was lower, the reduced heat loss of this group resulted in similar core temperature responses to the able-bodied. Consequently, not only should the role of absolute and relative exercise intensities in this population be examined further but also conditions of greater exercise duration, higher intensities of exercise and greater thermal stress.

Aural Temperature During Recovery from Exercise

The decrease in aural temperature for the SCI subjects during the initial 10 minutes of recovery from exercise in the cool environment was similar to that observed by Gass *et al.* (1988) in low level paraplegics. Furthermore, at the end of the recovery period, aural temperature was similar to values observed at rest. This would suggest that the heat stored during exercise in cool conditions was effectively dissipated from the body within that time period. However, at the end of recovery from exercise in warm conditions, aural temperature for the group was 0.6°C greater than at rest. This is slightly higher than the 0.4°C elevation in aural temperature observed for able-bodied athletes at the end of recovery from prolonged arm crank exercise in similar conditions (Price and Campbell, 2002). Considering that arm crank exercise elicits greater heat storage when compared to wheelchair exercise (Price and Campbell, 1999b) this may represent a greater retention of heat within the body of the SCI during recovery from exercise in warm conditions. The greater thermal strain in warm conditions is also consistent with the elevated heart rates observed during the initial stages of recovery from exercise, a response that has been observed previously when compared to able-bodied athletes during recovery from exercise in cool conditions (Price and Campbell, 1999a).

Upper Body Skin Temperatures

During exercise in cool conditions skin temperatures for the paraplegic athletes, with the exception of the upper arm, remained unchanged from resting values. This suggests a balance between the heat production and heat loss mechanisms. During exercise in warm conditions, greater increases in skin temperature were observed when compared to exercise in the cool reflecting the presence of an external heat load. Furthermore, the increases in upper body skin temperatures for the group during exercise in the warm condition were similar to those observed for AB athletes (Price and Campbell, 2002). The similarity of upper body skin temperatures to those of able-bodied, upper body trained athletes suggests that the SCI group studied demonstrate comparable heat dissipation from the sensate upper body during exercise in both cool and warm conditions. However, as specific sweat rates were not measured during this study, whether differences exist between sweating responses of able-bodied and SCI subjects or indeed between subjects with spina bifida and traumatic SCI as employed within the present study is not known.

During exercise in cool conditions, a decrease in upper arm skin temperature was observed. It has previously been suggested that this may be due to local convective air currents as a result of arm movements during wheelchair propulsion (Price and Campbell, 1999b). During exercise in warm conditions upper arm skin temperature was maintained at a similar level to values observed at rest whereas other skin temperatures gradually increased. This may indicate that when compared to other skin sites, local cooling of the upper arm was effective. However, as aural temperature gradually increased throughout the exercise period, any regional cooling effect was unable to prevent increases in heat storage and body temperature in warm conditions.

Lower Body Skin Temperatures

During exercise in warm conditions increases in thigh and calf skin temperatures were greater for all athletes when compared to upper body sites. With both the absence of an increased local metabolic rate during exercise for the lower limb and the reduced sweating capacity due to spinal cord injury, such gains in heat are most likely to be passive in origin and not effectively dissipated. This would result in the retention of heat within the lower body and the subsequently greater skin temperatures. Interestingly, in warm conditions thigh skin temperature tended to be elevated earlier (although not statistically) during exercise than calf skin temperature possibly due to arterial blood flowing through the thigh segment prior to reaching the leg. A greater amount of heat would be available for transfer to the insensate tissues of the thigh resulting in less heat being transferred to the calf and a more delayed increase in calf skin temperature. Increases in calf skin temperature may therefore predominantly occur as a result of passive heat gain when compared to the thigh.

Lower body skin temperatures also remained elevated for all athletes throughout the recovery period in warm conditions when compared to the gradual decrease observed during recovery from exercise in cool conditions. Therefore the retention of heat within the lower body of the spinally injured during recovery from exercise in cool conditions is accentuated during exercise in warm conditions. Nevertheless, the retention of heat within the lower body during recovery from exercise in warm conditions did not prevent a significant decrease in aural temperature. The presence of sweating over the upper body may offset the retention of core body heat. It must be noted though that aural temperature did not completely return to pre-exercise levels after 30 minutes of recovery. This may have implications for treatment of heat injury in this population and warrants further study.

During recovery in warm conditions lower body skin temperatures and aural temperature remained elevated above resting values when compared to a return to pre-exercise values during the cool trial. In addition, heart rate was elevated during the initial five minutes of recovery during the warm trial. The former indicates greater thermal strain whereas the latter indicates greater physiological strain during recovery from exercise in warm conditions. The elevated heart rate may pertain to a decreased stroke volume from dehydration or a greater volume of blood redistributed to the skin for heat loss. As plasma volume changes were similar in both trials then it is unlikely that any reduced stroke volume would be due to dehydration alone. Further studies examining blood flow responses are required to elucidate the cause of this greater physiological strain. In the absence of such data we can only conclude that athletes with a spinal cord injury, although tolerating increases in body temperature during exercise, are under both greater physiological and thermal strain during recovery from exercise in warm conditions when compared to cool conditions.

Sweat Rates

Similar sweat rates and plasma volume changes were observed for the paraplegic athletes in both cool and warm conditions suggesting that maximal sweat rates were achieved during both trials. When compared to able-bodied individuals, at a given exercise intensity, a linear increase in sweat rate with ambient temperature is observed (Galloway and Maughan, 1997; Green et al., 2004). For example, previous studies examining able bodied subjects undertaking arm crank ergometry of between ~50 and 60% $\dot{V}O_2$peak have reported whole body sweat rates (based on body mass losses) of approximately 0.31 l.hour^{-1} at 15°C (Dawson et al., 1994), 0.8 l.hour^{-1} at 21°C, 1.3 l.hour^{-1} at 31°C (Price and Campbell, 2002) and 1.55 l.hour^{-1} at 38°C (Price and Mather, 2004). Thus, as environmental temperature increases so does the sweat output. However, due to the reduction of sweating capacity below the level of lesion in spinal cord injury, whole body sweat rates cannot increase to the same values as for the able-bodied. Therefore, although sweat rates for low level paraplegics and able-bodied individuals matched for training status are reported to be similar during exercise in cool conditions (Price and Campbell, 1997, 1999) this does not appear to be the case for warm conditions where the demand for increased evaporative cooling is increased.

From the results of previous studies, the low level paraplegics sweat rates' are approximately 0.5 l.hour^{-1} lower than for able-bodied individuals of similar training status exercising under similar environmental conditions (Price and Campbell, 2002). Interestingly, the evaporative cooling potential of the 0.8 l.hr^{-1} sweat rate observed (~464 Kcal) is greater than the total energy expenditure for the paraplegics during the 60 minute exercise period (~327 Kcal) and, if sweat rates were 100% efficient, would theoretically be more than adequate to dissipate the gains in heat from exercise per se. When compared to a similarly matched able-bodied population, in similar exercise and environmental conditions (Price and

Campbell, 2002), energy expenditure equated to ~588 Kcal with potential evaporative cooling of 755 Kcal. These values for potential evaporative cooling represent approximately 142% and 128% of the energy expenditure for paraplegics and able-bodied individuals respectively. When the differences in efficiency of arm crank and wheelchair ergometry are considered (~20% vs. ~10%, respectively; Price and Campbell, 1996b; Brown et al., 1990) the potential evaporative cooling for paraplegics and able-bodied subjects are similar (157% and 160%, respectively). It therefore appears that sweat rates for both groups are sufficient to balance heat production during exercise but, in the light of continual increases in aural temperature during exercise in warm conditions, are clearly not large enough to dissipate additional gains in body temperature from the environment. It must be noted though that the spinal cord injured subjects in the present study were trained and may have a greater thermal tolerance than spinal cord injured individuals that are untrained. Consequently, the gradual rise in core temperature observed in the present study for the athletes may be greatly accentuated in an untrained population, producing a potentially greater risk of heat injury.

Fluid Replacement

It is known that *ad libitum* drinking during exercise results in involuntary dehydration (Sawka, 1992). This chapter observed *ad libitum* fluid replacements representing 48 and 52% of fluid losses for the cool and warm conditions respectively. These values are lower than for able-bodied athletes during arm crank ergometry in cool and warm conditions (66 and 80%, respectively; Price and Campbell, 2002), female runners during 30 km time trials in 12, 17 and 25°C (63, 68, 73%) (Cheuvront and Haymes, 2001) but similar to 90 min treadmill walking in the heat (~42%, Armstrong et al., 1997). Values for voluntary fluid intake therefore appear to be within the lower range of what would be expected. However, more importantly, changes in body weight predominantly due to sweating were less than the 2% of body weight usually associated with decreased performance (Cheuvront et al., 2003). Although performance was not addressed in the present study, this aspect would be a useful progression in the study of thermoregulation and thermal strain in the spinal cord injured.

Heat Exchange in Cool and Warm Conditions

During exercise, the reduced sweating capacity of the area below the level of lesion results in increased skin temperatures (Fitzgerald et al., 1990) with previous authors noting the possibility of this region demonstrating dry exchange (Fitzgerald et al., 1990; Price and Campbell, 2003). For heat loss to occur via dry heat exchange skin temperature being must be greater than that of the environment and ideally for efficient heat flow there should also be a thermal gradient between the body core and skin. Consideration of local thermal gradients for each skin site measured demonstrates that at rest and post exercise in a cool environment, all skin sites measured would have allowed heat exchange from the skin surface to the environment. The cooler lower body of the paraplegic athletes (Price and Campbell, 1997) however, would produce a smaller thermal gradient and enable less heat exchange when compared to regions above the lesion, nevertheless, dry heat exchange would still be possible.

When initially entering the environmental chamber prior to warm-up, all skin sites demonstrated a greatly reduced thermal gradient with the environment. The thigh and calf showed a reversal of the gradient indicating heat gain. Heat storage may therefore have occurred in the lower body of the athletes at this stage. At the end of exercise in warm conditions, heat stored within the body had produced a thermal state where all skin surfaces, including the lower body, were warmer than the environment, and would allow dry heat loss to occur. The speed and effectiveness of heat flow from dry heat exchange and its importance in this population for heat balance has yet to be quantified.

At rest in cool conditions the difference in skin temperature between the abdomen, thigh and calf was much greater than after exercise in warm conditions. It is possible that skin temperatures below the level of lesion becoming similar may be an easily recognisable indicator of the amount of heat storage that has occurred. However, it must be noted that there is a large inter-individual variation in skin temperatures and their responses within this population, particularly below the level of spinal cord lesion. Furthermore, if lower body skin temperatures reach similar values, it is clear that a large amount of heat storage would have occurred, possibly pushing core temperature towards the likelihood of heat injury. Such a response is likely to occur a lot sooner in untrained or sedentary spinal cord injured individuals.

In summary, this study examined the thermoregulatory responses of athletes with a spinal cord injury during prolonged wheelchair exercise in cool and warm conditions. The athletes were able to tolerate gradual but increasing body temperatures during prolonged exercise in warm conditions, which may reflect their trained status and thermal tolerance. However, retention of heat within the lower body was observed suggesting a large amount of heat storage appeared to be peripheral in origin and resulting in greater thermal and physiological strain post exercise in warm conditions. Consequently, the area below the level of spinal cord lesion was a potent site for heat storage both during and post exercise in warm conditions. Studies involving subjects with high level spinal cord transection are required to examine these responses further.

References

Armstrong LE; Maresh CM; Gabaree CV; Hoffman JR; Kavouras SA; Kenefick RW; Castellani JW; Ahlquist LE. Thermal and circulatory responses during exercise: effects of hypohydration, dehydration and water intake. *Journ Appl Physiol*, 1997, 82, 2028-2035.

Armstrong LE; Riebe D; Kenefick RW; Castellani JW; Senk JM; Foley MF. Local cooling in wheelchair athletes during exercise-heat stress, *Med Sci Sports Exerc*, 1995 27, 211-216.

Armstrong LE; Crago AE; Adams R; Senk JM; Maresh CM. Use of the infra-red temperature scanner during triage of hyperthermic runners. *Sports Med Train Rehab*, 1994, 5, 243-245.

Brown DD; Knowlton RG; Hamill J; Schneider TL; Hetzler RK. Physiological and biomechanical differences between wheelchair-dependent and able-bodied subjects during wheelchair ergometry. *Eur J Appl Physiol Occup Physiol*, 1990, 60, 179-82.

Benzinger TH; Taylor GW. Cranial measurements of internal temperature in man. In Hardy, J.R., editor. *Temperature: Its Measurement and Control in Science and Industry. 3, Biology and Medicine.* New York, Reinhold, 1963; 111-120

Cheuvront SN; Carter R 3rd; Sawka MN. Fluid balance and endurance exercise performance. *Curr Sports Med Rep*, 2003, 2, 202-8.

Cheuvront SN; Haymes EM. Ad libitum fluid intakes and thermoregulatory responses of female distance runners in three environments. *J Sports Sci.* 2001, 19, 845-54.

Dawson, B; Bridle, F; Lockwood, R.J; Thermoregulation of paraplegic and able bodied men during prolonged exercise in warm and cool climates. *Paraplegia*, 1994, 32, 860-870.

Dill, DB; Costill, DL; Calculation of percentage changes in volumes of blood, plasma and red cells in dehydration. *Journal of Applied Physiology*, 1974, 37, 247-248.

Durnin, JGVA; Wormersley, J. Body fat assessment from total body density and its estimation from skinfold thickness: Measurements on 481 men and women aged 16-71 years. *British Journ Nut*, 1974, 32, 77-97

Fitzgerald PI; Sedlock DA; Knowlton RG. Circulatory and thermal adjustments to prolonged exercise in paraplegic women. *Med Sci Sports Exerc.* 1990 22, 629-35.

Galloway SDR; Maughan, RJ. Effects of ambient temperature on the capacity to perform prolonged cycle exercise in man. *Med Sci Sports Exerc*, 1997, 29, 1240-1249.

Gass, GC; Camp, EM; Nadel, ER; Gwinn, TH; Engel, P. Rectal and rectal vs. oesophageal temperature in paraplegic men during prolonged exercise. *Journ of Appl Physiol*, 1988, 64, 2265-2271

Goss, FL; Herbert, WG; Kelso, TB. A comparison of mean skin temperatures during prolonged cycle exercise. *Res Quart Exerc Sport*, 1989, 60, 292-296

Green JM; Pritchett RC; Tucker DC; Crews TR; McLester JR. Sweat lactate response during cycling at 30 degrees C and 18 degrees C WBGT. *J Sports Sci,* 2004, 22, 321-7.

Havenith, G; Luttikholt, VGM; Vrijkolte, TGM. The relative influence of body characteristics of humid heat stress response. *Euro Journ Appl Physiol*, 1995, 70, 270-279

Hopman, MTE; Oeseburg, B; Binkhorst, RA. Cardiovascular responses in persons with paraplegia to prolonged arm exercise and thermal stress. *Med Sci Sports Exerc*, 1993, 25, 577-583.

Hopman, MTE. Circulatory responses during arm exercise in individuals with paraplegia. *Int Journ Sports Med*, 1994, 15, 156-131

Petrofsky, JS. Thermoregulatory stress during rest and exercise in heat in patients with a spinal cord injury. *Euro Journ Appl Physiol*, 1992, 64, 503-507

Pimental, NA; Sawka, MN; Billings, DS; Trad, LA. Physiological responses to prolonged upper body exercise. *Med Sci Sports Exerc*, 1984, 16, 360-365

Price, MJ; Campbell, IG. Effects of spinal cord lesion level upon thermoregulation during exercise in the heat. *Med Sci Sports Exerc*, 2003, 35, 1100 – 1107.

Price, MJ; Campbell, IG. Thermoregulatory responses of able-bodied, upper body trained athletes to prolonged arm crank exercise in cool and warm conditions. *J Sport Sci*, 2002, 20, 519-527.

Price, MJ; Campbell, IG. Thermoregulatory responses of able-bodied, paraplegic and a tetraplegic athlete at rest, during prolonged upper body exercise and during passive recovery. *Spinal Cord*, 1999a, 37, 772-779

Price, MJ; Campbell, IG. Thermoregulatory and physiological responses of wheelchair athletes to prolonged arm crank ergometry and wheelchair ergometry. *Int Journ Sports Med*, 1999b, 20, 457-463

Price, MJ; Campbell, IG. Thermoregulatory responses of paraplegic and able-bodied athletes at rest during exercise and into recovery. *Euro Journ Appl Physiol*, 1997, 76, 552-560.

Price MJ; Mather MI. The effects of two cooling strategies during prolonged arm crank exercise in hot conditions. *Aviation Space Environ Med*, 2004, 75, 220-226,

Ramanathan, NL. A new weighting system for mean surface temperature of the human body. *Journ Appl Physiol*, 1964, 19, 531-533

Randall, WC; Wurster RD; Lewin, RJ. Responses of patients with high spinal transection to high ambient temperatures. *Journ Appl Physiol*, 1966, 21, 985-993

Sato, KT; Kane, NL; Soos, G; Gisolfi, CV; Kondo, N; Sato, K. Re-examination of tympanic membrane temperature as a core temperature. *Journ Appl Physiol*, 1996, 80, 1233-1239

Sawka, MN. Physiological consequences of hypohydration: exercise performance and thermoregulation. *Med Sci Sports Exerc*, 1992, 24, 657-670.

Wicks, JR; Oldridge, NB; Cameron, BJ; Jones, NL. Arm crank and wheelchair ergometry in spinal cord injured athletes. *Med Sci Sports Exerc*, 1983, 15, 224-231

In: Focus on Exercise and Health Research
Editor: Thomas B. Selkirk, pp. 221-238

ISBN 1-59454-349-6
© 2006 Nova Science Publishers, Inc.

Chapter IX

Exercise Pathophysiology in Patients with Juvenile Dermatomyositis

Tim Takken[1]*, Elisabeth F. Elst[2] and Janjaap van der Net[1]
[1]Department of Pediatric Physical Therapy & Exercise Physiology, and [2]Department of Pediatric Immunology, Wilhelmina Children's Hospital, University Medical Center Utrecht, the Netherlands

Abstract

Juvenile Dermatomyositis (JDM) is one of the idiopathic inflammatory myopathies in childhood. In this disease the immune system targets the microvasculature of the skeletal muscle and skin, leading to myopathy and a typical skin rash.

During episodes of active disease patients experience a significant reduction in exercise tolerance which is not only related to loss in muscle mass. In this chapter we propose a model consisting of 5 pathways that could explain the reduced exercise tolerance in children with JDM. The five pathways are 1) the increased concentration of intramuscular cytokines, 2) the systemic inflammation process 3) the inflammation of the capillaries in the muscle 4) the result of hypo-activity and 5) the effect of steroid treatment on body mass gain and protein breakdown.

Introduction

Juvenile Dermatomyositis (JDM) forms together with Juvenile Polymyositis and Sporadic Inclusion Body Myositis the idiopathic inflammatory myopathies in childhood. Of

---

* Dr Tim Takken MSc PhD Clinical Exercise Physiologist; Department of Pediatric Physical Therapy & Exercise Physiology; Wilhelmina Children's Hospital; University Medical Center Utrecht; Room KB2.056.0, PO Box 85090, NL 3508 AB Utrecht; The Netherlands; email (office): t.takken@umcutrecht.nl; +31 30 2504030 (phone); +31 30 2505333 (fax)

these three not commonly found diseases, JDM is the most frequent observed disease, the latter two are very rare diseases in childhood.

In JDM, the immune system targets the microvasculature of the skeletal muscle and skin, leading to myopathy and a typical skin rash [1, 2]. The pathophysiology of JDM is still unknown. In general the age of onset has two peaks, between 5 and 9 years as well as between 11 and 14 years. In all age groups there is a female predominance [3]. Since the introduction of new therapies, the attention has shifted from mortality towards morbidity and functional ability.

Generally the symptoms of weakness, muscles tenderness and stiffness follow the skin manifestations [4].

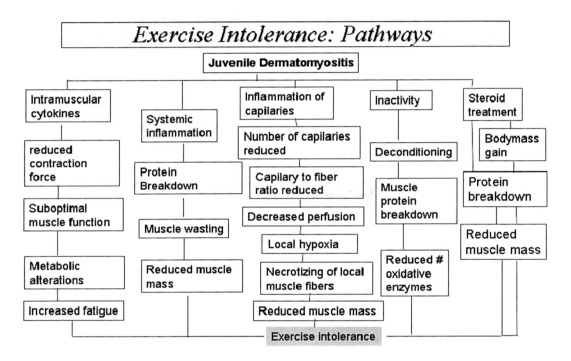

Figure 1. Pathways leading to exercise intolerance in JIIM patients.

The main pathological changes found in muscle biopsies are muscle fiber degeneration and necrosis with inflammatory infiltration in perivascular, perimysial and endomysial areas. Atrophied fibers, particularly in perifascicular areas, and fibers with an abnormal architecture may be found as well [5]. Since long the focus in clinical follow-up in JDM patients has been on muscle testing as muscle weakness was the most prominent clinical symptom [1, 6]. However, not only muscle strength is affected, other physiological properties such as exercise capacity as well [7, 8]. Other studies revealed disturbances in muscle metabolism of myositis patients [9-11]. This places the exercise capacity of diseased muscle in the focus of interest of clinicians [7, 8, 12, 13]. As a consequence, more physiological instruments, originally designed for the use in a healthy population, are being applied in a clinical population. In JDM patients, aerobic exercise tests have been used in the management and evaluation of their health status [7, 8]. These exercise tests were able to determine the aerobic exercise capacity (i.e. VO_{2peak}). Besides aerobic physical fitness, recent reports are suggesting the importance of anaerobic physical fitness (intensive exercise lasting < 2 minutes). This is not surprising, since the daily childhood activities consists of short-term bursts of intensive activities [14].

In this review, we propose 5 major pathways that could explain the exercise intolerance in JDM patients.

Exercise Intolerance in JDM: How Big is the Problem?

Broadly speaking, two general exercise forms can be distinguished, namely short-term intensive bouts of exercise, the so called anaerobic exercise capacity and the long-term endurance type of activity: the aerobic exercise capacity. The major energy (adenosine tri phosphate; ATP) production pathways in humans are displayed in Table 1. In the following paragraphs studies investigating exercise capacities in JDM patients will be reviewed.

Anaerobic Exercise Capacity

The Wingate Anaerobic exercise test (WAnT) is a 30 second all out cycle ergometry test, in which one must cycle against a rapidly progressive resistance. The test is found reliable and valid against other anaerobic indices such as invasively determined (by muscle biopsy) muscle metabolites and energy rich phosphates and muscle fiber type composition [15]. The WAnT has been used in healthy children [16], in patients with neuromuscular diseases [17] and in juvenile idiopathic arthritis [18, 19] to determine anaerobic exercise capacity. Recently we described the feasibility of the WAnT in JDM and Juvenile Polymyositis patients and found a decrease in their short-term anaerobic exercise capacity of approximately 30 percent compared to healthy controls (See Figure 2; 20). Hilario et al [21] found the greatest muscular atrophy in the gluteus maximus and the quadriceps muscle of patients with JDM, two muscles used in cycling exercise. In the light of these finding, the impaired anaerobic performance is not surprising. However, there was a broad scatter in performances in these patients ranging from – 80 percent to scores above reference values for healthy children.

Aerobic Exercise Capacity

We recently tested the feasibility of maximum exercise testing in fifteen patients (age 5-14 years) with JDM, and compared the obtained values with reference values for healthy children. Patients were tested using a motor driven treadmill and an apparatus for respiratory gas analysis, a so called metabolic cart, to volitional exhaustion conforming to the Bruce protocol [7].

In this study we found that all patients were able to perform the exercise test. Ten of the fifteen patients performed a maximal effort (heart rate > 180 beats/min or respiratory exchange ratio > 1.0). Five patients did not reach these criteria, since they experienced lag fatigue well before they were limited in their cardiovascular system.

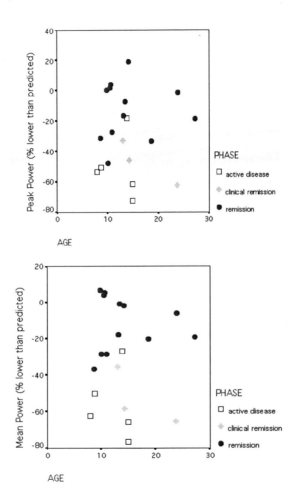

Figure 2. Percentage impairment in anaerobic capacity of JIIM patients in relation to age and disease phase. Values are expressed as a percentage difference compared to healthy subjects. A positive value indicated a value above predicted, a negative value indicate a lower value compared to healthy controls. The upper panel depicts the peak power, the lower panel depicts the mean power. From [20].

For the patients who had a maximal exercise performance, the mean VO_{2peak}, $VO_{2peak/kg}$ (related to body mass), and exercise time were respectively -1.82 (± 1.5), -2.83 (± 1.9), and -3.65 (± 1.9) standard deviations (SD-scores) lower compared to age and sex matched reference values ($p < 0.05$) (fig. 3). Expressed as percentage, patients with JDM had a 40% reduction in VO_{2peak}. The SD-scores for exercise time were significantly lower compared to SD-scores for absolute and relative VO_{2peak}, an indication of reduced muscular economy. The differences between VO_{2peak} and $VO_{2peak/kg}$ can be explained by a larger amount of non-metabolic active tissue (adipose tissue) in JDM patients (See also paragraph 5). These large reductions in exercise capacity have been confirmed by others in both adult dermato/polymyositis patients, as well as in patients with JDM. Wiesinger et al tested 8 patients with dermatomyositis and 3 patients with polymyositis and found a reduction of 47% in VO_{2peak} compared to healthy controls [12]. These data are comparable with the study of Hebert et al [13] in 11 polymyositis/dermatomysitis patients. They found a 54% reduction in VO_{2peak} in these patients compared to normal reference values. However, 3 of their patients performed the maximal exercise test within normal levels [13]. In children Hicks et al [7] tested 14 children and adolescents with JDM using a maximal bicycle exercise test. In this study they found a 37% reduction in VO_{2peak}. Moreover, VO_{2peak} correlated in this study significantly with disease damage indices such as physician global disease activity and damage and magnetic resonance imaging, suggesting the validity of the exercise testing measurements.

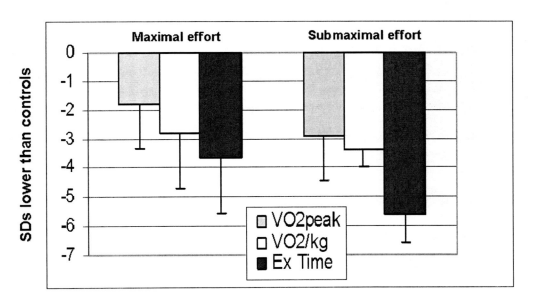

Figure 3. The exercise capacity in JDM patients during maximal treadmill exercise. The shaded bars represent the absolute maximal oxygen uptake, the white bars represent the maximal oxygen uptake per kg body mass, the dark bars represent the exercise time. All values indicate SD-scores. Redrawn after data from reference [7].

Economy

Park et al. [11] also suggest that JDM muscles have a lower economy (a larger energy cost per unit of work) when exercising at a sub-maximal exercise workload compared to healthy children. The discrepancy in Z-scores between the VO_{2peak} (absolute and relative) and

Z-scores for exercise time confirms this suggestion as running performance is influenced by muscular economy and VO_{2peak} [23]. This was recently confirmed in the study by Drinkard et al. [24], who found a reduced delta oxygen uptake/work rate slope in JDM patients compared to healthy controls. Our own data confirm this observation, as can be appreciated from Figure 4. Normal values for the delta oxygen uptake/workrate relationship are 8.4 to 10.3 ml/kg/min and might even be somewhat higher in elite athletes [25]. In this figure, 11 of 18 patients have a reduced delta oxygen uptake/work rate relationship. A reduced slope means that a larger part of the required energy production stems from anaerobic energy sources (anaerobic glycolysis). This is a disadvantage for the exercise capacity of the patient, since there are only limited stores of glucose and glycogen in the body. Moreover, the anaerobic glycolysis produces low amounts of energy from each glucose of glycogen molecule. Additionally, the anaerobic glycolysis forms metabolic waste products, such a lactic acid, which will increase lactate and H^+ concentrations in the blood what causes fatigue.

Table 1. Pathways for energy production in the muscle

Oxidative Phosphorylation:
$Glycogen_{(n)} + 6O_2 + 37Pi + 37 ADP \rightarrow glycogen_{(n-1)} + 6 CO_2 + 42 H_2O + 37 ATP$
$Glucose + 6 O_2 + 36 Pi + 36 ATP \rightarrow 6 CO_2 + 42 H_2O + 36 ATP$
$C_{16}H_{32}O_2$ (Fatty acids; palmitate) $+ 23 O_2 + 129 (ATP + Pi) \rightarrow 129 ATP + 16 CO_2 + 145 H_2O$
Glycolysis:
$Glycogen_{(n)} + 3 Pi + 3ATP \rightarrow glycogen_{(n-1)} + 2$ lactate $+ 2 H_2O + 2 ATP$
$Glucose + 2ATP + 2 NAD^+ + e^- + H^+ \rightarrow Pyruvate + NADH + H^+$
Creatine Kinase reaction
$ADP + PCr + H^+ \leftrightarrow ATP + Cr$
Adenylate kinase / AMP deaminase reactions
$2ADP \leftrightarrow ATP + AMP / AMP + H_2O \rightarrow NH_3 + IMP + 2 Pi$
ATP hydrolysis reaction
$ATP \rightarrow ADP + Pi +$ Energy

*Abbreviation*s: O_2: Oxygen, Pi: inorganic phosphate, ADP: adenosine triphosphate, CO_2: carbondioxide, H_2O: water, ATP: adenosinetriphosphate, PCr: creatine phosphaat, H^+: hydrogen, Cr: creatine, AMP: adenosinemonophosphate, NH_3: ammonia, IMP: inosinemonophosphate, NAD^+: Nicotinamide Adenine Dinucleotide, e-: electron. Table modified after reference [22].

The lower muscular economy and oxidative capacity might be a result of dysfunctional muscle mitochondria with a low cytochrome C-oxidase activity [26] and/or a changed magnesium status in the muscle [10].

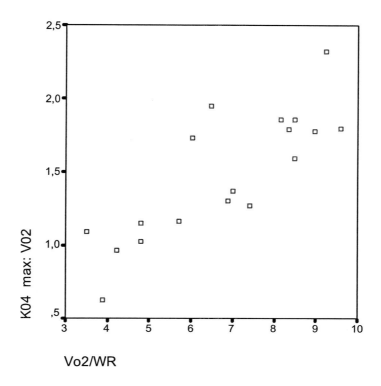

Figure 4. Relationship between maximal oxygen uptake and efficiency. (Takken et al, unpublished observations).

In conclusion, patients with JDM have a significantly impaired exercise capacity compared to healthy controls. These values are associated with disease activity and damage in the muscle.

Intramuscular Cytokines

An often observed phenomenon in inflammatory muscle diseases is that respiratory and skeletal muscles become weakened. During the early phase of the disease, muscle weakness may be severe without accompanying muscle atrophy, suggesting that other factors than loss of muscle mass are the cause of muscle weakness. Cytokines are likely to be potential mediators of this muscle weakness. Particularly tumor necrosis factor alpha (TNF-α) could play a main role in this observation. TNF-α can stimulate muscle wasting (see paragraph 2) but can also induce contractile dysfunction without overt catabolism.

In a recent study, Reid et al. [27] studied this process in murine diaphragm and limb muscle and found that TNF-α depressed tetanic force of the diaphragm and limb muscle to comparable degrees across a range of stimulus frequencies. Moreover, in isolated muscle fibers, TNF-α decreased tetanic force without altering tetanic calcium transients or resting calcium levels. From these observations two conclusions can be drawn, firstly TNF-α

compromises contractile function of muscle similarly, and secondly TNF-α decreases force by blunting the response of muscle myofilaments to calcium activation.

One of the other described observations in inflammatory diseases is a reduced muscle protein synthesis. This process might be also related to the higher cytokine levels, with again an important role for TNF-α [28]. The reduced myogenesis [29] results in a loss of muscle mass, since muscle breakdown is also increased under influence of again TNF-α, but also IL6 and IL-1β play a role in this process. This reduced muscle mass negatively influences muscle strength and exercise capacity [30].

Altered Muscle Metabolism

Patients with JIIM often experience strong exercise intolerance. Already in 1931 Steinitz & Steinfeld reported abnormal muscle creatine levels and glucose metabolism in muscle of a patient with dermatomyositis [31]. Since then, several authors reported abnormal levels of energy rich phosphates (adenosine triphosphate; ATP, phosphocreatine; PCr, inorganic phosphate; Pi) and metabolites (e.g. Magnesium) in patients with JIIM and IIM. These findings have been reported in both rest and during exercise as measured using 31-P magnetic resonance imaging and spectroscopy (MRS) [9-11]. Moreover, a defect in the purine -nucleotide cycle (adenosine monophosphate deaminase deficiency) in patients with IIM has been found [32].

Systemic Inflammation

Idiopathic Inflammatory Myopathies are known to be associated with elevated serum concentrations of inflammatory cytokines (e.g. IL-1β, TNF-α1. The crucial role of these cytokines in maintaining the balance between muscle protein synthesis and muscle protein degradation has been extensively studied in arthritic conditions by Roubenoff et al. [33]. This has lead to the notion of *rheumatoid cachexia*, a condition in which muscle protein degradation favors over muscle protein synthesis resulting in muscle wasting, impaired muscle strength and this is associated with increase of fat mass. The whole process is commonly referred to as 'cachexic obesity'. It is expected that the same *(similar)* cascade of events might influence muscle protein metabolism in IIM, *myopathic cachexia*, enhancing the effect of loss of muscle strength by the inflammatory damage to the muscle by the disease itself. The disease is thought to induce muscle necrosis following circulatory insufficiency resulting from vasculitis, leading to muscle wasting and reduction in muscle strength. Moreover, the inflammatory cytokines that are produced in that condition of vasculitis, themselves influence muscle protein metabolism as well. However, in both conditions, Rheumatoid Arthritis and IIM, the precise mechanism is not yet elucidated. Roubenoff proposes a model based on his work in animal studies with arthritic conditions [34]. An adapted version of that model hypothesizes the situation in IIM conditions, this model will be outlined in Fig 5.

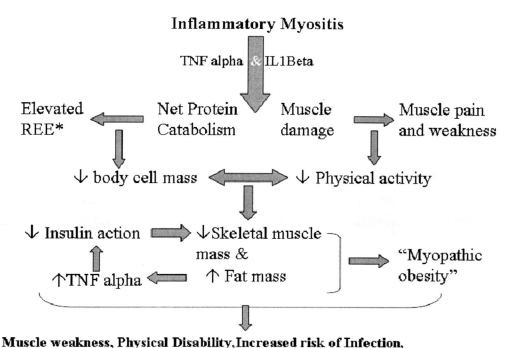

Figure 5. Summary of the metabolic consequences of inflammatory myopathies. The increased levels of inflammatory parameters leads to a loss of body cell mass, predominantly skeletal muscle mass, and reduced physical activity, which reinforce each other and lead to further losses of skeletal muscle mass and predispose to fat gain. *Resting energy expenditure (REE) is elevated in active inflammatoy diseases. Modified from Walsmith and Roubenoff [34].

The model 'explains' the role of the inflammatory cytokines. IL-1β and TNF-α acting synergistically to each other: A) a shift in protein metabolism towards a net catabolism is evident by a raised resting energy expenditure, B) furthermore these cytokines mediate muscle degradation, and cause muscle necrosis. This leads to a loss of body cell mass predominantly skeletal muscle mass, and reduced physical activity, which reinforce each other and lead to further losses of skeletal muscle mass and predispose fat gain. Fat gain increases circulating TNF-α. levels (produced by adipocytes) and predisposes to insulin resistance and further muscle loss. This reinforces the negative cycle of muscle loss and fat gain, and causes cachectic obesity. These metabolic alterations cause muscle weakness that may contribute to physical disability, as well as co-morbidity.

Clinically it is evident that muscle weakness and increased obesity are factors that progressively influence exercise tolerance in a negative way. Limited exercise tolerance is positively associated with loss of activities of daily living and reduced actiradius in daily life. These factors both contribute negatively to health-related quality of life.

Inflammation of Capillaries

The role of blood vessels in the pathogenesis of myositis was previously suggested based upon the decreased number of capillaries in the muscle tissue in recent-onset patients with dermatomyositis as well as the cytoplasmic inclusions in endothelial cells [35]. Moreover, these endothelial cells appeared thickened, ressembling the endothelial cells of high endothelium venules (HEV), which have a role in lymphocyte homing [36]. In the microvessels, arterioles and venules of patients with active myositis, there is an increased expression of certain proinflammatory cytokines such as Il-1α, adhesion molecules such as intercellular adhesion molecule 1 (ICAM-1) and vascular cell adhesion molecule 1 (VCAM-1) and class I major histocompatibility complex (MHC) [37]. Increased expression of these molecules was particularly evident in capillaries and small vessels in biopsy specimens from symptomatic muscles, both when these specimens contained inflammatory infiltrates and when such infiltrates where absent. This suggests that the decreased muscle function is more related to the expression of these molecules than to the mere presence of inflammatory cells in the affected muscles. This is an indication that the microvessels have a central role in the pathogenesis of inflammatory myositis.

Recent clinical research suggests that the abnormalities observed in some muscle biopsies are secondary to an impaired blood supply [38]. Hypoxia can upregulate both IL-1 and TGF-β, the cytokines most often detected in muscle tissues of patients with myositis [39, 40]. Hypoxia could be the result of a reduced number of capillaries reported in myositis biopsies, but it could also be generated in chronically inflamed tissue, as has been demonstrated in the synovial tissue of patients with rheumatoid arthritis [41].

The theory of an impaired blood supply is supported by the finding that in inflamed muscles hypoxia induces increased expression of angiogenic factors. Their impact however is insufficient to repair disease-associated reduction of the capillary network [34].

Several other studies have suggested that hypoxia of muscle fibres may have a role in the pathogenesis of JDM and therefore improving circulation to the muscles would be important. Circulation to the muscles is increased by exercise and therefore damage may be decreased if adequate blood and oxygen is supplied to the muscles. This may also have an impact upon the effects of TNFα, which are primarily pro-inflammatory and TNFα in increased amounts may increase the damage to muscles, but with improved circulation this effect may be reduced.

We found some excessive sweating in some of our JDM patients during exercise testing, although they were exercising at low workloads (Takken, unpublished observations). Recently it was found that the sweating response might be potentiated by muscle hypoxia [42].

Effects of Hypoactivity on Exercise Tolerance

There are several additional explanations for the decreased exercise tolerance of the patients with JDM. Sedentary subjects have fewer capillaries in their muscles per cross-sectional area compared to subjects with an active life-style [43, 44]. Also, the activity of the oxidative enzymes is reduced and will result in a decreased capacity of the skeletal muscle to extract oxygen from the blood [45]. Moreover, disease or inactivity induced skeletal muscle atrophy reduces the total amount of oxygen which can be consumed by the muscles[46].

Bed rest will also impair exercise capacity. Already in 1968 Saltin et al [44 described the detrimental effects of 3 weeks bedrest on exercise capacity in health young adults. In their widely cited Dallas Bedrest and Training Study, they described not only peripheral effects (in skeletal muscle) but also centrally (heart). The cardiac stroke volume during exercise was reduced after this period of bedrest. This lower stroke volume resulted in a reduced cardiac output. A recent follow-up of the original study participants, 30 years later showed that the reduction in exercise capacity after 3 weeks of bedrest was larger than the effects of 30 years of aging [47, 48]!

These inactivity-induced effects will lead to an impaired oxygen transport and extraction in the exercising muscle, higher mixed-venous oxygen content, and finally a reduced maximal oxygen uptake and exercise capacity.

Training

The reduced oxidative capacity of the muscles, which is probably caused by the low cytochrome oxydase levels, this is a key enzyme in the mitochondria of the skeletal muscles and regulates oxidative processes to produce ATP, might be improved by fitness training. A recent study showed that cytochrome oxydase levels could be improved in healthy adults using a fitness training program [49]. This indicates that fitness training might enhance the exercise capacity of JDM patients. Promising results have been found in physical training studies in adult dermatomyositis and polymyositis patients. Clinical trials from different laboratories have evaluated the effects of resistance training disease [50, 51] and endurance training [52, 53] in an adult dermato/polymyositis patients both with an active disease and in a clinically stable inactive condition. Arnadottir et al [54, 55] found in a pilot study that a 12-week period of home training was safe for patients with inclusion body myositis (another form of inflammatory myositis).

One of these studies performed muscle biopsies before and after a training program and observed an increase in percentage of type I muscle fibers and an increase in cross-sectional area of type II muscle fibers in polymyositis/dermatomyositis patients after a dynamic strength training program [56].

In children with IIM there is no exercise training program evaluated. However, Maillard found no increase in inflammation after performing moderate intensity exercises in JDM patients as evaluated using MRI derrived T2 relaxation times [55]. This study in children also shows that a moderate exercise program is safe to perform in children with myositis and that exercise does not increase the levels of inflammation within the muscles.

Disease activity (inflammatory parameters) and medication (e.g. the effects of cyclosporin A [28] and prednisone [29]) could diminish the trainability of patients with JDM. However, it is known from the literature that steroid-induced muscular atrophy (See paragraph 5), can be reversed by physical training [57, 58]. These findings need to be further investigated in the IIM/JDM patient population.

Nutritional Supplements

In a supplementation study with a group of patients with various neuromuscular disorders including adult dermatomyositis and polymyositis patients, a significant improvement in muscle strength in these patients was observed [59].

It needs to be further investigated if supplementation of creatine monohydrate in patients with JIIM could reduce the impairment in anaerobic exercise capacity [60].

Steroid Treatment

General Considerations

Glucocorticoids (GC) are among the most potent anti-inflammatory agents that can be used in the treatment of rheumatic diseases. However, the short term benefits are frequently outweighed by the long term side effects, particularly in children [61].

GC alter the regulation of many cellular processes, including enzyme synthesis and activity, membrane permeability, transport processes, hormone and receptor synthesis and function and production of structural elements. They also have major effects on carbohydrate, protein and fat metabolism. The former participate primarily in the adaptive response to stress and inflammation, the latter are necessary for maintaining homeostasis. Unfortunately, the antiinflammatory effects of GC cannot be separated from the metabolic effects because all the cells of the body use the same glucocorticoid receptor (GCR).

The typical cushingoid appearance, with centripetal obesity, acne, hirsutism, moon facies, buffalo hump and striae of the skin may already occur with low doses of GC. Other side effects include growth suppression, osteoporosis, cataract, hypertension and psychologic disturbances.

Two distinct types of steroid myopathy have been described with systemic GC therapy. The chronic (or classic) form is usually an insidious disease process, which causes weakness mainly to the proximal muscles of the upper and lower limbs and neck flexors. There is a wide interpatient variability in the time course of symptom onset. Inactivity sensitizes skeletal muscle to the catabolic effects of steroids [62]. Another study with a rat model showed that steroid myopathy could be prevented by even mild exercise [63]. Isokinetic muscle testing of hip flexor strength appears to be the most sensitive and objective test of proximal muscle weakness. Levels of enzymes of muscle origin such as creatine phosphokinase (CPK) and aldolase almost never are elevated, except for elevated urinary creatine excretion. Biopsy of affected muscle reveals non-specific atrophy of the type IIb fast-twitch glycolytic fibers. There are many reports showing preventive effects of either growth hormone or insulin-like growth factor I on steroid myopathy [64]. In an experimental model, steroid therapy interfered with insulin-like growth factor I signaling, leading to increased myocyte apoptosis [65]. The acute form of steroid myopathy is less common, is associated with rhabdomyolysis and occurs abruptly while the patient is receiving high-dose corticosteroids. Affected patients often have markedly elevated levels of CPK and diffuse necrosis of skeletal muscle on biopsy specimens. In both forms, recovery begins after GC tapering or withdrawal, but more than 6 months may be required for complete resolution of muscle weakness.

Specific Effects on Energy Expenditure

Increased Body Mass

A higher body mass is often the result of side effects of the GC resulting in a cushingoid appearance; this might account not only for the effects on psychosocial functioning, but an increased body mass (overweight) might restrict patients in the performance of activities of daily living.

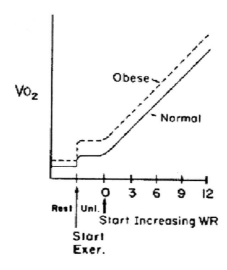

Figure 6. The effects of obesity on energy expenditure during a graded exercise test. Obese subjects have an increased energy expenditure (as measured by oxygen uptake; VO_2). Adapted from [25].

Figure 6 shows the increased energy expenditure during cycling, a non weight bearing activity. During unloaded cycling as well as during loaded cycling, the oxygen uptake is higher in obese subjects. This is caused by the increased weight of the legs, which costs extra energy to raise the legs during cycling. During weight bearing exercise this extra energy expenditure is even higher. The subject has to carry and extra load (body mass) and the leg swing of heavier legs also increases energy expenditure.

Decreased Muscle Mass

Muscle atrophy is a common problem in this population group due to the catabolic effects of GC. Muscle atrophy implies a smaller muscle mass to consume oxygen during exercise. In addition, the metabolic function of muscle fibers can be altered. Impaired aerobic metabolism (due to decreased mitochondrial volume and/or mitochondrial myopathy) or reduced capillarisation can occur after immunosuppressive therapy [66]. Muscle atrophy and altered muscle function are further aggravated by sedentary habits due to the catabolic effects that sedentarism and prolonged bedrest induce on skeletal muscle tissue [67]. As a result, muscle atrophy and early fatigue during low-to-moderate physical tasks become self-perpetuating conditions.

Conclusion

JDM is one of the inflammatory myopathies in childhood. Due to the disease process and consequences of the disease and treatment there are 5 pathways which contribute to the reduced exercise tolerance in these patients. The identification of these pathways make them a possible target for intervention therapies. Possible therapies include anti-TNF-α agents, Vascular Endothelial Growth Factor (VEGF) therapy, exercise and nutritional supplements. Exercise seems to have a possible important role in the treatment of JDM, since it might possibly upregulate VEGF expression and this enhancing angiogenesis in the muscle. Moreover, it reduced the inactivity related deconditioning and could prevent some of the deleterious effects of steroids (body mass gain and protein breakdown). However, no trials have been performed so far evaluating the effects of exercise in JDM patients. It is important to study the safety and effectiveness of exercise for treating JDM patients in a controlled trial before the shift from a bedrest-regime towards a more active treatment strategy can be made.

References

[1] Pachman LM (1995) Juvenile dermatomyositis. Pathophysiology and disease expression. *Pediatr Clin North Am* 42:1071-98.

[2] Wedderburn LR, Li CK (2004) Paediatric idiopathic inflammatory muscle disease. *Best Pract Res Clin Rheumatol* 18:345-58.

[3] Bowyer SL, Blane CE, Sullivan DB, Cassidy JT (1983) Childhood dermatomyositis: factors predicting functional outcome and development of dystrophic calcification. *J Pediatr* 103:882-8.

[4] Engel AG, Hohlfeld R, Banker BQ. Inflammatory myopathies. In: Basic and Clinical Myology. New-York: *McGraw-Hill;* 1994. p. 1335-1383.

[5] Jones DA, Round JM (1993) Skeletal muscle in health and disease. A textbook of muscle physiology Manchester University Press, Manchester

[6] Resnick JS, Mammel M, Mundale MO, Kottke FJ (1981) Muscular strength as an index of response to therapy in childhood dermatomyositis. *Arch Phys Med Rehabil* 62:12-9.

[7] Takken T, Spermon N, Helders PJ, Prakken AB, Van Der Net J (2003) Aerobic exercise capacity in patients with juvenile dermatomyositis. *J Rheumatol* 30:1075-80.

[8] Hicks JE, Drinkard B, Summers RM, Rider LG (2002) Decreased aerobic capacity in children with juvenile dermatomyositis. *Arthritis Rheum* 47:118-23.

[9] Newman ED, Kurland RJ (1992) P-31 magnetic resonance spectroscopy in polymyositis and dermatomyositis. *Arthritis and Rheumatism* 35:199-203.

[10] Niermann KJ, Olsen NJ, Park JH (2002) Magnesium abnormalities of skeletal muscle in dermatomyositis and juvenile dermatomyositis. *Arthritis Rheum* 46:475-88.

[11] Park JH, Niermann KJ, Ryder NM, Nelson AE, Das A, Lawton AR, et al. (2000) Muscle abnormalities in juvenile dermatomyositis patients: P-31 magnetic resonance spectroscopy studies. *Arthritis Rheum* 43:2359-67.

[12] Wiesinger GF, Quittan M, Nuhr M, Volc-Platzer B, Ebenbichler G, Zehetgruber M, et al. (2000) Aerobic capacity in adult dermatomyositis/polymyositis patients and healthy controls. *Arch Phys Med Rehabil* 81:1-5.

[13] Hebert CA, Byrnes TJ, Baethge BA, Wolf RE, Kinasewitz GT (1990) Exercise limitation in patients with polymyositis. *Chest* 98:352-7.

[14] Bailey RC, Olson J, Pepper SL, Porszasz J, Barstow TJ, Cooper DM (1995) The level and tempo of children's physical activities: an observational study. *Med Sci Sports Exerc* 27:1033-41.

[15] Inbar O, Bar-Or O, Skinner JS (1996) The wingate anaerobic test Human Kinetics, Champaign, Ill.

[16] Bar-Or O (1987) The Wingate anaerobic test. An update on methodology, reliability and validity. *Sports Med* 4:381-94.

[17] Tirosh E, Bar-Or O, Rosenbaum P (1990) New muscle power test in neuromuscular disease. Feasibility and reliability. *Am J Dis Child* 144:1083-7.

[18] Takken T, Van der Net J, Helders PJ (2003) Relationship between functional ability and physical fitness in juvenile idiopathic arthritis (JIA) patients. *Scand J Rheumatol* 32:174-178.

[19] Malleson PN, Bennett SM, MacKinnon M, Jespersen DK, Coutts KD, Turner SP, et al. (1996) Physical fitness and its relationship to other indices of health status in children with chronic arthritis. *J Rheumatol* 23:1059-65.

[20] Takken T, van der Net J, Helders PJM (2005) Anaerobic Exercise Capacity in Juvenile-onset Idiopathic Inflammatory Myositis (JIIM) Patients. *Arthritis and Rheumatism* 53:173-177.

[21] Hilario MO, Yamashita H, Lutti D, Len C, Terreri MT, Lederman H (2000) Juvenile idiopathic inflammatory myopathies: the value of magnetic resonance imaging in the detection of muscle involvement. *Sao Paulo Med J* 118:35-40.

[22] Lewis SF, Haller RG (1991) Physiologic measurement of exercise and fatigue with special reference to chronic fatigue syndrome. *Rev Infect Dis 13 Suppl* 1:S98-108.

[23] Bassett DRJ, Howley ET (2000) Limiting factors for maximum oxygen uptake and determinats of endurance performance. Medicine and Science in Sports and Exercise 32:70-84.

[24] Drinkard BE, Hicks J, Danoff J, Rider LG (2003) Fitness as a determinant of the oxygen uptake/work rate slope in healthy children and children with inflammatory myopathy. *Can J Appl Physiol* 28:888-97.

[25] Wasserman K, Hansen JE, Sue DY, Casaburi R, Whipp BJ (1999) Principles of Exercise testing and Interpretation. 3th Edition ed Lippincott, Williams & Wilkins, Baltimore, MD, USA

[26] Woo M, Chung SJ, Nonaka I (1988) Perifascicular atrophic fibers in childhood dermatomyositis with particular reference to mitochondrial changes. *J Neurol Sci* 88:133-43.

[27] Reid MB, Lannergren J, Westerblad H (2002) Respiratory and limb muscle weakness induced by tumor necrosis factor-alpha: involvement of muscle myofilaments. *Am J Respir Crit Care Med* 166:479-84.
[28] Tisdale MJ (2004) Cancer cachexia. *Langenbecks Arch Surg*.
[29] Langen RC, Schols AM, Kelders MC, Van Der Velden JL, Wouters EF, Janssen-Heininger YM (2002) Tumor necrosis factor-alpha inhibits myogenesis through redox-dependent and -independent pathways. *Am J Physiol Cell Physiol* 283:C714-21.
[30] Giordano A, Calvani M, Petillo O, Carteni M, Melone MR, Peluso G (2003) Skeletal muscle metabolism in physiology and in cancer disease. *J Cell Biochem* 90:170-86.
[31] Steinitz H, Steinfeld F (1931) Untersuchungen zum Kreatinstoffwechsel bei Dermatomyositis. *Zeitschrift fuer die Gesamte Experimentelle Medizin* 79:319-328.
[32] Sabina RL, Sulaiman AR, Wortman RL (1991) Molecular analysis of acquired myoadenulate deaminase deficiency in polymyositis (Idiopathic Inflammatory Myopathy). *Advances In Experimental Medicine And Biology* 309b:203-205.
[33] Roubenoff R, Roubenoff RA, Cannon JG, Kehayias JJ, Zhuang H, Dawson-Hughes B, et al. (1994) Rheumatoid cachexia: cytokine-driven hypermetabolism accompanying reduced body cell mass in chronic inflammation. *J Clin Invest* 93:2379-86.
[34] Walsmith J, Roubenoff R (2002) Cachexia in rheumatoid arthritis. *Int J Cardiol* 85:89-99.
[35] Kissel JT, Mendell JR, Rammohan KW (1986) Microvascular deposition of complement membrane attack complex in dermatomyositis. *N Engl J Med* 314:329-34.
[36] Girard JP, Springer TA (1995) High endothelial venules (HEVs): specialized endothelium for lymphocyte migration. *Immunol Today* 16:449-57.
[37] Englund P, Nennesmo I, Klareskog L, Lundberg IE (2002) Interleukin-1alpha expression in capillaries and major histocompatibility complex class I expression in type II muscle fibers from polymyositis and dermatomyositis patients: important pathogenic features independent of inflammatory cell clusters in muscle tissue. *Arthritis Rheum* 46:1044-55.
[38] Cea G, Bendahan D, Manners D, Hilton-Jones D, Lodi R, Styles P, et al. (2002) Reduced oxidative phosphorylation and proton efflux suggest reduced capillary blood supply in skeletal muscle of patients with dermatomyositis and polymyositis: a quantitative (31)P-magnetic resonance spectroscopy and MRI study. *Brain* 125:1635-1645.
[39] Falanga V, Qian SW, Danielpour D, Katz MH, Roberts AB, Sporn MB (1991) Hypoxia upregulates the synthesis of TGF-beta 1 by human dermal fibroblasts. *J Invest Dermatol* 97:634-7.
[40] Shreeniwas R, Koga S, Karakurum M, Pinsky D, Kaiser E, Brett J, et al. (1992) Hypoxia-mediated induction of endothelial cell interleukin-1 alpha. An autocrine mechanism promoting expression of leukocyte adhesion molecules on the vessel surface. *J Clin Invest* 90:2333-9.
[41] Paleolog EM (2002) Angiogenesis in rheumatoid arthritis. *Arthritis Res* 4 Suppl 3:S81-90.
[42] Eiken O, Mekjavic IB (2004) Ischaemia in working muscles potentiates the exercise-induced sweating response in man. *Acta Physiol Scand* 181:305-11.

[43] Wagner PD (1988) An integrated view of the determinants of maximum oxygen uptake. *Advances In Experimental Medicine And Biology* 227:245-56.

[44] Saltin B, Blomqvist G, Mitchell JH, Johnson RL, Jr., Wildenthal K, Chapman CB (1968) Response to exercise after bed rest and after training. *Circulation* 38:VII1-78.

[45] Holloszy JO, Coyle EF (1984) Adaptations of skeletal muscle to endurance exercise and their metabolic consequences. *J Appl Physiol* 56:831-8.

[46] Bar-Or O (1986) Pathophysiological factors which limit the exercise capacity of the sick child. *Med Sci Sports Exerc* 18:276-82.

[47] McGuire DK, Levine BD, Williamson JW, Snell PG, Blomqvist CG, Saltin B, et al. (2001) A 30-year follow-up of the Dallas Bedrest and Training Study: II. Effect of age on cardiovascular adaptation to exercise training. *Circulation* 104:1358-66.

[48] McGuire DK, Levine BD, Williamson JW, Snell PG, Blomqvist CG, Saltin B, et al. (2001) A 30-year follow-up of the Dallas Bedrest and Training Study: I. Effect of age on the cardiovascular response to exercise. *Circulation* 104:1350-7.

[49] Carter SL, Rennie CD, Hamilton SJ, Tarnopolsky MA (2001) Changes in skeletal muscle in males and females following endurance training. *Can J Physiol Pharmacol* 79:386-92.

[50] Alexanderson H, Stenstrom CH, Jenner G, Lundberg I (2000) The safety of a resistive home exercise program in patients with recent onset active polymyositis or dermatomyositis. *Scand J Rheumatol* 29:295-301.

[51] Alexanderson H, Stenstrom CH, Lundberg I (1999) Safety of a home exercise programme in patients with polymyositis and dermatomyositis: a pilot study. *Rheumatology* (Oxford) 38:608-11.

[52] Wiesinger GF, Quittan M, Aringer M, Seeber A, Volc-Platzer B, Smolen J, et al. (1998) Improvement of physical fitness and muscle strength in polymyositis/dermatomyositis patients by a training programme. *Br J Rheumatol* 37:196-200.

[53] Wiesinger GF, Quittan M, Graninger M, Seeber A, Ebenbichler G, Sturm B, et al. (1998) Benefit of 6 months long-term physical training in polymyositis/dermatomyositis patients. *Br J Rheumatol* 37:1338-42.

[54] Arnardottir S, Alexanderson H, Lundberg IE, Borg K (2002) Sporadic inclusion body myositis: pilot study on the effects of a home exercise program on muscle function, histopathology and inflammatory reaction. *J Rehabil Med* 35:31-35.

[55] Maillard S. Quantitative Assessment of the Effects of Exercise on Muscles in Children with Dermatomyositis [MSC]. London: City University; 2002.

[56] Esbjornsson-Liljedahl M, Dasmalchi M, Alexanderson H, Stahlberg M, Lundberg IE. Changed muscle morphology in myositis patients following a home exercise program. In: Klarlund Petersen B, Febbraio M, Fleshner M, editors. 6th International Society of Exercise Immunology Symposium; 2003; Copenhagen, Danmark; 2003. p. 47.

[57] Horber FF, Scheidegger JR, Grunig BE, Frey FJ (1985) Evidence that prednisone-induced myopathy is reversed by physical training. *J Clin Endocrinol Metab* 61:83-8.

[58] Hickson RC, Marone JR (1993) Exercise and inhibition of glucocorticoid-induced muscle atrophy. *Exerc Sport Sci Rev* 21:135-67.

[59] Tarnopolsky MA, Martin J (1999) Creatine monohydrate increases strength in patients with neuromuscular disease. *Neurology* 52:854-857.

[60] Tarnopolsky MA, Beal MF (2001) Potential for creatine and other therapies targetting cellular energy dysfunction in neurological disorders. *Ann Neurol* 49:561-574.

[61] Spahn JD, Kamada AK (1995) Special considerations in the use of glucocorticoids in children. *Pediatr Rev* 16:266-72.

[62] Ferrando AA, Stuart CA, Sheffield-Moore M, Wolfe RR (1999) Inactivity amplifies the catabolic response of skeletal muscle to cortisol. *J Clin Endocrinol Metab* 84:3515-21.

[63] Nakago K, Senda M, Touno M, Takahara Y, Inoue H (1999) Influence of exercise on muscle fibers in rats with steroid myopathy. *Acta Med Okayama* 53:265-70.

[64] Kanda F, Okuda S, Matsushita T, Takatani K, Kimura KI, Chihara K (2001) Steroid myopathy: pathogenesis and effects of growth hormone and insulin-like growth factor-I administration. *Horm Res 56 Suppl* 1:24-8.

[65] Singleton JR, Baker BL, Thorburn A (2000) Dexamethasone inhibits insulin-like growth factor signaling and potentiates myoblast apoptosis. *Endocrinology* 141:2945-50.

[66] Hickson RC, Marone RJ (1993) Exercise and inhibition of glucocorticoid-induced muscle atropy. *Exercise and Sport Science Reviews* 21:135-167.

[67] Lucia A, Earnest C, Perez M (2003) Cancer-related fatigue: can exercise physiology assist oncologists? *Lancet Oncol* 4:616-25.

Chapter X

Being From "Away" ... Focus on Exercise, Nutrition, and Health Research among Immigrant Older Adults

Shanthi Jacob Johnson[1,2*]

[1]School of Nutrition and Dietetics, Acadia University, Canada &
[2]Canadian Centre for Activity & Aging, University of Western Ontario

Abstract

In recent decades, both human life expectancy and general health among older adults have improved in industrialized nations. This trend is largely attributed to technological advancements and improved health practices that have been facilitated by research on biological and environmental determinants of health. While research can be a valuable tool in health promotion efforts, there are some segments of the population for which health concerns have not been adequately addressed, such as immigrants. Immigrants differ from non-immigrants and from other immigrant groups on many dimensions that have been associated with health outcomes, including cultural, socioeconomic, and linguistic characteristics. Immigrants also represent an increasing proportion of the population in Western nations, thus potentially influencing overall health data and necessitating their inclusion in modern health research. Health practices and outcomes among older immigrant adults are particularly important because health issues are likely to be more salient in old age, but this group is especially likely to be underrepresented in research. Health data among older immigrants is explored, highlighting trends in lifestyle choices, prevalence of health problems and service utilization. Methodological concerns

---

[*] C. Shanthi Jacob Johnson, PhD, PDt (corresponding author); Associate Professor; School of Nutrition and Dietetics; Acadia University; Wolfville, Nova Scotia B4P 2R6; Telephone: (902) 585 – 1204; Fax: (902) 585 – 1095; Email: shanthi.johnson@acadiau.ca

that influence current data are discussed as well as recommendations to increase cultural sensitivity in future research endeavors with this population subset.

Key words: Immigrant population, health, research, methodological considerations

Human populations have long been characterized by their diversity and dynamic nature. In recent decades, shifts in population demographics have been particularly prominent, especially in industrialized nations. Globalization efforts and advancements in technology have been associated with increased human migration, leading to unprecedented proportions of immigrant groups in countries such as Canada, the United States, the United Kingdom, and Australia. At the same time, increased understanding of human biology and health determinants have contributed to ever-increasing life expectancies in these nations. As a result, not only are immigrants making an increased presence overall, but the proportion of older immigrants is growing.

Older individuals, regardless of nativity, often differ from the younger members of a given population. This disparity is particularly salient in the field of health, as increased age is associated with physical and mental declines that influence levels of health and well-being and subsequently affect service utilization among older adults. In order to understand the health needs of older adults, researchers have developed theoretical frameworks of aging and make efforts to recruit elderly participants in health research projects. Seniors have presented themselves as a particularly challenging research demographic, however, because older adults exhibit a greater degree of within-group variability than their younger counterparts (Sallis, 2003). For example, the onset and rate of physical or mental decline is different from person to person, such that individuals that are 80 years of age may have larger health disparities than younger adults. Older persons are therefore not adequately classified under a single category that defines senior status as being at or above a set age because conclusions and generalizations based solely upon chronological age may not be indicative of real occurrences. While some researchers have proposed age categories such as "young old" and "old old" to accommodate for differences within the senior group, there is no consistent standard for the ages encapsulated by each level. In some models, aging is considered to begin at 50 and others do not include individuals less than 65 years of age.

Health research on seniors is further complicated by factors such as ethnicity and culture. As of 2001, over 18% of the Canadian population was comprised of foreign-born individuals, a proportion that had risen over 2% in the previous decade and is expected to continually rise in years to come (Statistics Canada, 2004). In addition, the number of seniors in Canada is expanding at twice the rate as that of the general population (Canada Mortgage and Housing Corporation, 2003). From these trends, it can be surmised that the proportion of foreign-born seniors is experiencing simultaneous growth. Immigrants are a very diverse subset of the population, differing from both non-immigrants and other immigrant groups in cultural, socioeconomic, and biological characteristics, all of which are associated with health outcomes. As a result, immigrant seniors amplify the heterogeneity of seniors in general, thus warranting increased attention from health researchers. Exploring health determinants that are particularly relevant to immigrant older adults would help create a valid knowledge base from which to implement programs and services that can address a broad spectrum of older persons. At present, there is a dearth of research on the health practices of immigrant seniors, and studies that have been conducted are often plagued by methodological concerns that confound the findings. However, awareness of demographic trends and the healthcare implications of increased immigrant senior populations have spurred research interest, creating many research opportunities in this field.

The Healthy Immigrant Effect

One of the most consistent findings among immigrant health studies in Canada is that recent immigrants have a health advantage over native-born Canadians, a phenomenon that is known as the healthy immigrant effect. However, as time in Canada increases, that health advantage disappears and immigrants' health levels converge with the levels of native-born Canadians, typically reaching similar levels within a decade (McDonald & Kennedy, 2004). The only noted exceptions are for infectious and parasitic diseases which may be treated or cured over time in Canada (DesMeules et al., 2004; Hyman, 2004). The healthy immigrant effect has been noted across all segments of the immigrant population, both in children and adults, regardless of gender (Ali, McDermott, & Gravel, 2004; Hyman, 2003).

There are many proposed explanations for the relatively better health of new immigrants, particularly citing immigration policies as a contributing factor. In Canada, non-refugee immigrants are admitted into the country only after undergoing a medical examination that is designed to prevent those with serious health problems from entering the country. Therefore, all immigrants who are granted admission have been deemed to have a satisfactory level of physical and mental health, which may exceed that of the general Canadian population. While the enforcement of such legislation can ensure that new immigrants have an acceptable level of health, it is unable to ensure that health levels will be maintained over time (Laroche, 2000). A prominent explanation of the apparent decline in immigrant health over the first decade in Canada is the process of acculturation, or adopting the behavioral patterns of the host culture. Immigrants may change their health behaviors and adopt habits such as smoking, drinking alcohol, or eating high fat diets which are all associated with negative health outcomes (Cairney & Østbye, 1999; Hyman, 2003; Johnson & Garcia, 2003). Among seniors, however, these behaviours may not be able to fully account for the noted convergence of health outcomes because although they do increase over time, they remain at a significantly lower level than those of native-born individuals (Ali, McDermott et al., 2004; Singh & Siahpush, 2002).

Other proposed explanations for the healthy immigrant effect suggest that immigrants who are healthier are more likely to participate in research projects while the ill or institutionalized are excluded from analysis and are therefore underrepresented (Hyman, 2004). While this explanation is able to account for some of the variability between new immigrants and native-born Canadians, it is unable to explain the gradual decline in immigrant health. One theory that does account for this decline suggests that immigrants may be subjected to specific health disadvantages after arriving in a new country, such as facing language barriers and discrimination (Dunn & Dyck, 2000). In one study of ageism, it was found that 91% of Canadian respondents and 84% of American respondents reported being subjected to at least one incident of ageism and many of these incidents occurred more than once (Palmore, 2004). Such barriers may lead to increased stress which can manifest itself in worsened physical and health outcomes over time. It has also been suggested by some that there is not a real difference in health outcomes among immigrants and native-born citizens and that the consistent finding of such data is merely the result of service utilization. New immigrants may face barriers to treatment, resulting in avoidance of medical services and subsequent under-diagnosis of medical conditions (Fisher, Bowman, & Thomas, 2003; Yu, Huang, & Singh, 2004). Emergency services and walk-in clinics tend to be popular service choices among new immigrants, but over time, as immigrants become more familiar with the medical system in the host country, they adopt regular medical services (Leduc & Proulx, 2004). This shift is associated with increased preventative treatment and doctor visits, which may correspond with more comprehensive care and more diagnoses.

The healthy immigrant among older immigrants has also been noted, but this population subset is unique in that it consists of two main demographic streams. The first is characterized by immigrants who migrated in early adulthood and are growing old in the host country while the second is characterized by immigrants who migrated as seniors, most often to join adult children in the host country (Boyd, 1991). Immigrants in the former group spend many years in the host country and tend to display acculturated living patterns that are congruent to native-born Canadians (Wilmoth, 2001). Immigrants from the latter group represent a very healthy group of older individuals, as those who suffer from severe health problems are frequently deterred by government policies. Although immigrants who migrate in later life are likely to be less acculturated than immigrants who migrated in early adulthood, they do show levels of adjustment that approach that are similar to the long-established group (Bagley, 1993). While age at immigration can influence the extent to which immigrants acculturate to the host environment, even immigrants who migrate late in life are apt to exhibit behavioral and attitudinal changes that may be associated with convergent health outcomes over time. Naturally, as individuals age they may be more likely to report health problems, thus making age a confounding variable of the healthy immigrant effect. However, even for studies that controlled for the aging of respondents, the healthy immigrant effect was still reported, indicating that other factors are responsible for the effect (Newbold & Danforth, 2003).

The pervasive nature of the healthy immigrant effect warrants additional attention and research. The numerous explanations that have been proposed to account for this effect indicate the multidimensional and complex nature of immigrant health and the lack of a universal immigrant health model to explain trends in health outcomes.

Health Practices of Immigrant Older Adults

A great deal of health research has focused on the determinants of health, or the various factors that can influence health outcomes. Health determinants and the interactions between them is the concern of the field of population health (Kindig & Stoddart, 2003). Health Canada (2003) proposed a Population Health Model in which income and social status, social support networks, education and literacy, employment and working conditions, social and physical environments, personal health practices, healthy child development, biology and genetic endowment, health services, gender, and culture were all indicated as health determinants. While all of these determinants may contribute to health outcomes, the socially based determinants including income, education, work, social support, health practices and health service utilization have been found to be particularly relevant for immigrants (Hyman, 2004). This is true for older immigrants, who face stressors both from growing older and from living in a culture that may be quite different than their own country's (Bagley, 1993). As a result, social determinants of health are highly relevant to health behaviors and outcomes.

One of the primary social determinants of health for older immigrants revolves around living circumstances. In Canada, as well as many other Westernized nations, there has been a shift in recent years regarding the country of origin for most immigrants. In the past, Canada would receive many immigrants from other Westernized countries such as the UK and the US, and these countries share many of the cultural values that are established in Canada. However, most immigrants today come from Asian countries in which cultural values may be quite different from those pervasive in North America. Western countries place a great deal of emphasis on individuality, stressing the importance of competition and self achievement over a sense of community. In many other nations of the world, including Asian nations, society is much more collectivist and the family and community are much more valued and relied upon. Perhaps as a result of this collectivist culture, many immigrants who come to Canada as seniors opt to live with their adult children, and are far more likely to reside with family than native-born individuals (Boyd, 1991). Although living arrangements may outwardly appear to have an indirect relationship to health, they influence the well being of older adults through the establishment of social support networks (Wilmouth, 2001). Among Chinese immigrants in Canada, for example, recent immigrants demonstrate extremely high levels of cultural retention, indicating that cultural values are maintained in the host country. Among these individuals, when there is a lack of social support, as indicated by the absence of the extended family, levels of hopelessness and depression were high (Bagley, 1993). However, among immigrants who have lived in Canada for longer periods of time, having immigrated as children or younger adults, the likelihood of living with family is very low and is not associated with any known health risks (Boyd, 1991). These results would appear to corroborate the acculturation hypothesis in which immigrants adopt the attitudes and beliefs of their host nation as a factor of their residency duration. Recent immigrants are less acculturated and therefore attempt to establish living environments that are conducive to their traditional cultural values, while well-established immigrants are likely to live in a similar fashion to the mainstream host society. If individuals are unable to live in an environment that supports their cultural values, they may experience emotional distress resulting in negative health outcomes.

Immigrant lifestyle choices are another predominant factor that can influence health outcomes, particularly choices regarding diet and fitness level. Negative health behaviors are positively associated with years since migration, and senior immigrants may be particularly at risk for health problems. In an examination of healthy eating and activity patterns among older immigrants in Ontario, nearly three-quarters of the respondents were identified as having moderate to high nutritional risk (Garcia & Johnson, 2003). Barriers that prevented adequate nutrition included language barriers, inability to cook, lack of ethnic food, lack of nutritional skills such as label reading, tooth and mouth problems, chronic conditions, polypharmacy, dining alone and financial constraints (Johnson & Garcia, 2003). Acculturation to Westernized food patterns may also be affiliated and results in an increased tendency to consume high fat convenience foods, eat large portions and stray from traditional dietary patterns such as a vegetarian or dairy-free diet (Carlsson & Johnson, 2004; Varghese & Moore-Orr, 2002). Individuals at risk are not consuming the recommended vitamins and nutrients that their bodies need in order to maintain health and longevity, thus predisposing them to a plethora of medical conditions. In order to improve eating habits among older immigrants, nutrition education may be beneficial. By providing healthy food alternatives that are easy to prepare and culturally appropriate, as well as teaching relevant food purchasing, preparation and safety skills to older immigrants, they may be able to boost their consumption of healthy foods and offset any potential health risks of having a poor diet.

Like nutritional concerns, fitness participation has been a problematic health area for older immigrants. Like many areas of research concerning immigrants, there is scant knowledge about physical activity or about the cultural and social influences that determine participation (or lack thereof) in fitness endeavors. Some studies report that immigrants engage in high rates of physical activity for working or running errands, but seldom report engaging in deliberate activity, thus possibly underestimating their overall fitness levels (Kandula, Kersey, & Lurie, 2004). Carlsson and Johnson (2004), however, found the exact opposite, with increased reports of deliberate exercise and decreased reports of physical activity for work or running errands decreasing. The latter also found that when asked to compare activity patterns before and after immigration, 64% of older immigrants indicate a change in activity level, with 31% reporting increased activity and 23% reporting a decrease since immigration. Although these results indicate a positive trend in the data, it was found that only 65% of respondents reported regular physical activity although 81% of respondents were not hampered by physical barriers that prevented exercise. Conflicting results may be the product of varying interpretations of fitness held by older immigrants. Levels of physical activity are commonly measured through self reports which are vulnerable to varying fitness perceptions and may not be culturally meaningful to all individuals. In order to account for reporting errors, objective measures can be used in order to map actual activity level and surveys can be reserved to assess other factors such as barriers that prevent exercise. The barriers that senior immigrants face regarding exercise include poor weather, lack of energy, medical conditions or illness, and lack of social support (Carlsson & Johnson, 2004; Garcia & Johnson, 2003). Immigrants who have lived in Canada for longer than ten years have been found to have higher levels of health motivation, thus indicating that the acculturation process may be helpful in reducing fitness barriers (Carlsson & Johnson, 2004). Educational interventions aimed at promoting exercise and physical activity among recent immigrants may therefore be particularly useful at encouraging involvement in activity and leading a healthier lifestyle.

The last factor that influences healthy lifestyle among older immigrants is the utilization of regular preventive measures and visits to health professionals. As previously discussed, recent immigrants are likely to make use of emergency services and walk-in clinics but increased time in the host country leads to the adoption of regular services. Although this would generally be associated with increased preventive measures, other variables are related to screening behaviours. For example, among multicultural women who are candidates for breast cancer screening, doctor recommendations and availability of insurance have been found to have the biggest impact on testing behaviours. Indications that many respondents had insurance as well as prompting from their physicians are promising, but there were also deterrents such as embarrassment or stress about mammograms (Magai, Consedine, Conway, Neugut, & Culver, 2004). Conceptualization barriers may be addressed using interventions that target the cognitions and emotions that immigrants may have concerning medical testing in order to reduce their apprehensions and improve screening rates.

Health utilization barriers may extend beyond cognitive factors and be found in physical, economical, and social facets of life. Barriers that prevent health service utilization include lack of transportation and lack of English language proficiency with which to communicate with health professionals (Pang, Jordan-Marsh, Silverstein, & Cody, 2003). Barriers may also result from lack of understanding of various healthcare approaches. Western medical practitioners and researchers often take an egocentric approach in which it is assumed that the most biological and scientifically proven treatments are the only way to effectively treat medical ailments. However, many immigrants, particularly those from Asian countries, are apt to use folk medicines, either as their sole form of treatment or in conjunction with Western medicine. If health care providers in Canada and other Western nations are not able to provide care that acknowledges folk remedies, immigrant patients may feel as though their cultural values are being undermined and may therefore seek treatment elsewhere. Confusing insurance policies and long waiting periods at clinics are also deterrents from help-seeking behaviours (Pang et al.). Many senior immigrants employ their own line of defense when faced with medical issues, using medical doctors and health staff as a last resort for very serious health concerns. Lesser health considerations are either tended to by themselves or by recruiting the assistance of family and friends if necessary.

The lifestyle choices made my individuals are closely related to their health outcomes. Culturally appropriate living arrangements, healthy dietary choices and exercise are all related to improved health and well-being, as is preventive health screening. However, older immigrants often face many barriers to health treatment due to their cultural differences from mainstream ideals and lack of adequate appropriate resources. These barriers not only deter older immigrants from engaging in proactive activities to improve their health outcomes, they can also negatively influence research that studies older immigrants.

Research Challenges and Opportunities

Researchers have the responsibility of presenting population health data in order to create a knowledge base from which policy makers and health care providers alike can implement programs and services that are best able to cater to the needs of the entire population. Decisions made by representatives within health regions require quality data (Paluck, Wiliamson, Milligan, & Frankish, 2001). Immigrant populations represent many unique methodological challenges to researchers, and senior immigrants are particularly challenging to adequately study (Johnson & Vissandjee, 2004).

One of the most prominent methodological issues is in collecting a suitable sample. Although the proportion of aging immigrants is continually rising in Canada and other nations, their absolute number is small, making it quite challenging to recruit a sufficient sample size from which conclusions or generalizations can be drawn. Further, immigrants that are from especially marginalized groups, including the institutionalized or aboriginal groups are often excluded from research due to having a sample size too insufficient to support any data analysis (e.g. Wilmoth, 2001). The small immigrant population from which to draw participants prohibits random selection, and necessitates the use of convenience sampling in many cases (e.g. Carlsson & Johnson, 2004). A convenience sample may differ from the immigrant population at large, due to volunteer bias. For example, in the Carlsson and Johnson study, 96% of respondents had completed high school or university and such a high level of education may act as a confounding variable to the data collected.

Research studies are further influenced by definitions of constructs under study, both in relation to the sample and the phenomenon to be studied. Many research projects use oversimplified conceptualizations of terms such as "culture" and "ethnicity" such that several ethnic groups are collapsed together in order to provide a significantly large sample size (Elliott & Gillie, 1998). The definition of terms used throughout the course of the research is also very important and perceptual differences can skew the results. Even terms that are very common in research may not be fully understood by respondents, including terms like ethnicity and race (Gaines & McDonald, 1999). Even the term healthy has many possible conceptualizations that are tempered by the social and cultural characteristics of respondents (Silverman, Smola, & Musa, 2000; Torres, 2003). Societal beliefs can even lead some people to deny a diagnosis due to social stigma, which can be troublesome when examining mental health issues. For example, some individuals may refuse to participate in studies of mental illness such as dementia due to the societal stigma of mental health problems and they may even deny that a problem exists in order to deny the burden of the disorder (Hinton, Guo, Hillygus, & Levkoff, 2000).

A final research consideration when examining the health of immigrant seniors is to select an appropriate research measurement. Older immigrants may not be able to accurately complete long and difficult surveys, so it is essential to use and develop tools that will pinpoint the desired issues while also being user-friendly. At present, a great deal of immigrant data is extracted from large national databases that were designed to accommodate the mainstream population, not to cater to the various cultural and social interactions experiences by immigrants. As a result, large surveys may not be able to capture the many cultural nuances that exist among various immigrant groups and they may be inappropriate both culturally and linguistically (Elder, 2003).

Despite methodological concerns, there are many research opportunities that exist within the field of older immigrant health. In order to conduct appropriate research, it is first essential for researchers to comprehend the diversity and complexity both of the concept of health and of the population to be studied. Barriers must be expected, comprehended, and systematically dissolved in order to gather valid and valuable data (Quandt, McDonald, Bell, & Arcury, 1999). These barriers can be dissolved by using culturally sensitive terminology and language and, when possible, conducting longitudinal studies to track changes in older immigrant health data. There are also many opportunities to explore information from a population health approach, in which several determinants of health and their interaction are explored. Few studies have examined multiple health behaviours, such as diet selection and exercise participation (Garcia & Johnson, 2003; Johnson & Garcia, 2003), thus indicating a research gap that could be bridged through increased study. Comprehensive and methodologically sound research could be very beneficial to immigrant older adults in improving their quality of life. Staff and board members from Canadian health regions indicated that research plays more than a moderate role in their decision making process, necessitating the best quality immigrant research possible.

Conclusion

Immigrants are a highly diverse population, and one that is continuing to increase in proportion in Western nations. Advancements in the human longevity and the simultaneous increase in the presence of immigrants in the West have resulted in an increase in older immigrants in Canada and other industrialized nations. Immigrants are a very diverse group, on factors such as cultural and social characteristics, and there variations are even more pronounced among older immigrants. As a result, older immigrants represent a unique population subgroup that requires the attention of researchers and policy-makers.

As the body ages it is likely to have some functional declines, both mentally and physically that result in decreased health. Despite this trend, there has been very little health research that has been conducted specifically on aging immigrants, creating a research gap that could result in a lack of knowledge and appropriate services to address their needs.

Present studies that have examined the health of older immigrants are often subject to criticism due to methodological shortcomings related to the sample, operational definitions, and measures used. Although such criticisms are valid, present studies have been useful in that they provide us with a basis from which to improve future studies and gather more accurate and robust data. The increasing diversity of immigrant groups and particularly older immigrants encourages further health research.

References

Ali, J. S., McDermott, S., & Gravel, R. G. (2004). Recent research on immigrant health from Statistics Canada's population surveys. *Canadian Journal of Public Health, 95*(3), I9-I13

Boyd, M. (1991). Immigration and living arrangements: Elderly women in Canada. *International Migration Review, 25*(1), 4-27.

Cairney, J., & Østbye, T. (1999). Time since immigration and excess body weight. *Canadian Journal of Public Health, 90*(2), 120-124.

Canada Mortgage and Housing Corporation. (2003). *Immigrant, Aboriginal, and Senior Populations Expand.* Retrieved August 17, 2004 from http://www.cmhc-schl.gc.ca/en/cahoob/desoec/desoec_03.cfm

Carlsson, L. & Johnson, C. S. J. (2004). Osteoporosis health beliefs and practices among Korean immigrants in Nova Scotia. *Journal of Immigrant Health, 6*(2), 93-100.

DesMeules, M., Gold, J., Kazanjian, A., Manuel, D., Payne, J., Vissandjée, B., et al. (2004). New approaches to immigrant health assessment. *Canadian Journal of Public Health, 95*(3), I22-I26.

Dunn, J. R., & Dyck, I. (2000). Social determinants of health in Canada's immigrant population: results from the National Population Health Survey. *Social Science and Medicine, 51*, 1573-1593.

Elder, J. P. (2003). Reaching out to America's immigrants: Community health advisors and health communication. *American Journal of Health Behavior, 27*(Suppl. 3), 196-203.

Elliott, S. J., & Gillie, J. (1998). Moving experiences: A qualitative analysis of health and migration. *Health & Place, 4*(4), 327-339.

Fisher, J. A., Bowman, M., & Thomas, T. (2003). Issues for south Asian Indian patients surrounding sexuality, fertility, and childbirth in the US health care system. *Journal of the American Board of Family Practice, 16*, 151-155.

Gaines, A. D., & McDonald, P. E. (1999). Aging and immigration: Who are the elderly? *Journal of Immigrant Health, 1*(2), 99-113.

Garcia, A. C., & Johnson, C. S. (2003). Development of educational modules for the promotion of healthy eating and physical activity among immigrant older adults. *Journal of Nutrition for the Elderly, 22*(3), 79-96.

Health Canada (2003, June 16). *Population Health: What Determines Health?* Retrieved July 5, 2004, from http://www.hc-sc.gc.ca/hppb/phdd/determinants/index.html

Hinton, L., Guo, Z., Hillygus, J., & Levkoff, S. (2000). Working with culture: A qualitative analysis of barriers to the recruitment of Chinese-American family caregivers for dementia research. *Journal of Cross-Cultural Gerontology, 15*, 119-137.

Hyman, I. (2004). Setting the stage: Reviewing current knowledge on the health of Canadian Immigrants: What is the evidence and where are the gaps? *Canadian Journal of Public Health, 95*(3), I4-I8.

Hyman, I. (2003). Canada's 'Healthy Immigrant' puzzle- A research report. *Women & Environments International Magazine, 60/61*, 31-33.

Johnson, C. S., & Garcia, A. C. (2003). Dietary and activity profiles of selected immigrant older adults in Canada. *Journal of Nutrition for the Elderly, 23*(1), 23-39.

Johnson, C. S., & Vissandjee, B. (2004). Health research involving Immigrant Populations: Opportunities and Challenges. Submitted for Considerations.

Kandula, N. R., Kersey, M., & Lurie, N. (2004). Assuring the health of immigrants: What the leading health indicators tell us. *Annual Review of Public Health, 25*, 357-376.

Kindig, D, & Stoddart, G. (2003). What is population health? *American Journal of Public Health, 93*(3), 380-383.

Laroche, M. (2000). Health status and health services utilization of Canada's immigrant and non-immigrant populations. *Canadian Public Policy, 26*(1), 51-75.

Leduc, N., & Proulx, M. (2004). Patterns of health services utilization by recent immigrants. *Journal of Immigrant Health, 6*(1), 15-27.

Magai, C., Consedine, N., Conway, F., Neugut, A., & Culver, C. (2004). Diversity matters: Unique populations of women and breast cancer screening. *Cancer, 100*(11), 2300-2307.

McDonald, J. T., & Kennedy, S. (2004). Insights into the 'healthy immigrant effect': Health status and health service use of immigrants to Canada. *Social Science & Medicine, 59*(8), 1613-1627.

Palmore, E. B. (2004). Research note: Ageism in Canada and the United States. *Journal of Cross-Cultural Gerontology, 19*, 41-46.

Paluck, E. C., Williamson, D. L., Milligan, C. D., & Frankish, C. J. (2001). The use of population health and health promotion research by health regions in Canada. *Canadian Journal of Public Health, 92*(1), 19-23.

Pang, E. C., Jordan-Marsh, M., Silverstein, M., & Cody, M. (2003). Health-seeking behaviors of elderly Chinese Americans: Shifts in expectations. *The Gerontologist, 43*(6), 864-874.

Quandt, S. A., McDonald, J., Bell, R. A., & Arcury, T. A. (1999). Aging research in multi-ethnic rural communities: Gaining entrée through community involvement. *Journal of Cross-Cultural Gerontology, 14*, 113-130.

Sallis, J. (2003). New thinking on older adults' physical activity. *American Journal of Preventive Medicine, 25*(3Sii), 110-111.

Silverman, M., Smola, S., & Musa, D. (2000). The meaning of healthy and not healthy: Older African Americans and Whites with chronic illness. *Journal of Cross-Cultural Gerontology, 15*, 139-156.

Singh, G. K., & Siahpush, M. (2002). Ethnic-immigrant differentials in health behaviors, mobidity, and cause-specific mortality in the United States: An analysis of two national data bases. *Human Biology, 74*(1), 83-109.

Statistics Canada (2004, April 25). *Proportion of Foreign-born Population, Proinces and Terrritories (2001 Census)*. Retrieved August 14, 2004 from http://www.statcan.ca/english/Pgdb/demo46a.htm

Torres, S. (2003). A preliminary empirical test of a culturally-relevant theoretical framework for the study of successful aging. *Journal of Cross-Cultural Gerontology, 18*, 79-100.

Varghese, S. & Moore-Orr, R. (2002). Dietary acculturation and health-related issues of Indian immigrant families in Newfoundland. *Canadian Journal of Dietetic Practice and Research, 63*(2), 72-79.

Wilmoth, J. M. (2001). Living arrangements among older immigrants in the United States. *The Gerontologist, 41*(2), 228-238.

Yu, S. M., Huang, Z. J., & Singh, G. K. (2004). Health status and health services utilization among US Chinese, Asian Indian, Filipino, and other Aisna/Pacific Islander children. *Pediatrics, 113*(1), 101-107.

Chapter XI

Pregnancy and Exercise: Should Healthy Pregnant Women Actively Train?

Jouko Pirhonen[1,*], *Elisabeth Rettedal*[1], *Tom Hartgill*[1] *and Pelle Lindqvist*[2]

[1]University of Oslo, Oslo, Norway
[2]University of Lund, Malmö, Sweden

Abstract

Background

The aim of this review article is to examine the evidence in the literature with regard to the safety of exercise in pregnancy.

Material and Methods

A literature search revealed fourteen randomised controlled trials which were systematically reviewed. The outcome measures looked at were both short and long term consequences of training in healthy pregnant women.

---

[*] Responsible author: Jouko Pirhonen, MD, PhD; Department of Obstetrics and Gynaecology, Ullevaal University Hospital, University of Oslo, N-0407 Oslo, Norway. Tel: +47-22118911; Email: tiina_jouko_pirhonen@hotmail.com; Jouko.pirhonen@medisin.uio.no

Results

The methodology of all included studies was qualitatively evaluated, though few were graded as good. The majority were small and had variable compliance from the volunteers. There was a lack of standardisation of the training schedules: the frequency ranged from 3 - 5 times per week, training intensities varied from age related maximal heart rates of 50 - 75% and exercise periods ranged from 20 – 60 minutes in length. Overall however, the exercise could be classified as moderate.

The literature revealed neither the fetus nor the mother derived harm from moderate exercise in pregnancy. Pregnant women who exercised in the above manner delivered normal healthy infants. With increasing intensity of exercise it appears the children are born with a lower percentage of body fat and thereby a lower birth weight, though still within normal range. This form of training does not appear to increase the incidence of preterm birth or caesarean section. The low number of studies and small patient numbers make it difficult to draw any conclusions with regard to teratogenic effects of hyperthermia. The exclusion of women who developed obstetric complications means it is not possible to draw any conclusions as regards exercise and the risk of placental abruption or bleeding.

Conclusion

Moderate exercise seems to have positive effects on pregnancy by way of improved physical well being. Moderate exercise also appears to increase psychological well being – the women feel better. Children born to mothers who exercised regularly showed no significant difference to those born to sedentary mothers in either a positive or a negative way. There was no apparent positive or negative effect on the infant at birth. From currently available data it appears that regular exercise of moderate intensity is both safe and commendable in pregnancy.

Further research in this area is required to assess whether physical activity can increase the risks of obstetric complications or cause significant effects from hyperthermia, particularly where exercise intensity is greater than as described here.

Introduction

Whether women can train or not during pregnancy is debated amongst healthcare professionals and lay folk, many studies have been carried out but results are not consistent. Only a few studies are large and of good quality, there are only two metanalysis [1, 2] which concluded with further research being required in this area.

There are few studies on exercise in pregnancy in Norway. Nordhagen found in one study, 70% of pregnant Norwegian women were physically active in at least two of three trimesters [3]. For information regarding physical activity in pregnancy women seek advice from their Primary Healthcare Centres, General Practitioners or the internet. It is important therefore for healthcare workers to have access to accurate information on what type and intensity of exercise is acceptable in pregnancy for mother and child. Currently there is no consensus of opinion on whether or not pregnant women can train or to what intensity they can exercise which reflects a general lack of knowledge.

Pregnancy is a major physiological stress on a woman; physical activity produces some of the same physiological changes. The main concern related to exercise and pregnancy is of potential harm caused to the fetus. Harmful effects on the fetus may be caused by hyperthermia which is a known teratogen, hypoxia due to reduce blood flow to the uterus, fetal growth restriction and trauma. Potential negative effects on the pregnant woman are increased risk of obstetric complications such as bleeding, preterm labour and an increased risk of caesarean section. However, one would also expect physical activity during pregnancy to be beneficial, particularly for the women, for example reducing the risk of depression and gestational diabetes. On a smaller scale physical activity may improve self esteem and thereby their work capacity and could reduce complications during labour.

There are many women who stop training when they become pregnant, though exercise had been a positive experience and one can only speculate as to the reasons for stopping. It is likely this is due to a relative uncertainty with regard to safety for both mother and baby; whether there are any positive gains is also important.

In this article we have undertaken a qualitative, systematic review of randomised controlled trials concerning exercise and pregnancy. The aim of this review is to investigate whether or not there is evidence in the literature on the safety of exercise in pregnancy and secondly whether aerobic exercise should be recommended to pregnant women.

Explanation of Terms

Healthy Pregnancy: A pregnancy without known obstetric or medical complications (for which physical activity would increase the risks to the fetus or pregnant woman).

Exercise: In the context of this review means aerobic physical activity with a minimum heart rate increase of 50% of the age related maximum.

Literature Search

The literature search was done in 2002-2003. Search terms used were "pregnancy + exercise + consequences/effects" in the Medline/Pubmed database and the Cochrane Library. Reference lists and related literature were used, authors were not contacted and only published data was used. The results of the literature search gave 14 randomised controlled trials concerned with exercise and pregnancy.

The Type of Publication

The main criterion for inclusion of a study was randomisation. When investigating whether a factor has an effect (positive or negative) the most important question is whether subjects were allocated randomly to the intervention or control group. Randomisation is the only technique which without bias gives comparable groups. In studies with sufficient participants randomisation ensures balance of known and unknown confounding or prognostic factors [4]. Chalmers [5] showed that not blinding which category participants were allocated to often lead to uneven distribution of prognostic factors, which may have a greater effect on the study than the intervention itself [6]. The literature search revealed many studies on exercise and pregnancy though only in a minority was randomisation performed. In most studies women who were already physically active were selected to the intervention group, then the control group selected based on known prognostic factors without taking into account the many unknown prognostic factors.

The second inclusion criterion was a physical activity level leading to a rise in the heart rate at a minimum of 50% of the age related heart rate. Many of the potentially harmful effects of exercise, particularly to the fetus, would be expected to occur when a significant proportion of the maternal blood flow was diverted to skeletal muscle, away from the uterus and fetus. Sufficient energy expenditure is also required to raise maternal body temperature to a level that may be harmful to the fetus.

The third criterion was a healthy pregnant woman, with no known obstetric or medical complications prior to inclusion in the study.

The fourth criterion was parameters measured looked at the effects of exercise on the pregnant woman or the fetus.

There were no limits as to the size, date or language of the studies though only English language studies were found. In areas where the selected publications could not reach conclusions, the literature was reviewed to show where current research stands today. This is meant as a perspective for readers and not a definitive answer.

Examination of Methodology for Included Studies

Studies were scored in relation to the randomisation procedure and information on participant drop out. The scoring method used was developed by Jadad et al [7], with scoring from 0-3 where 3 is the highest score. Thereafter the methodological quality of the included studies were assessed using the "12 questions to help assess a randomised controlled study" developed by the Critical Appraisal Skills Programme (CASP, Oxford). The CASP system categorises the studies as "very good, good, average or poor." The studies with their CASP scores are presented in Table 1.

Overall none of the studies were of "very good" quality, of the 14 studies included only 5 were of "good" quality with the rest being of "average" quality. When applying Jadad's criteria: 3 studies scored 3 points, 8 scored 2 points and 3 scored 1 point. The process of randomisation used is important in assessing if the procedure itself was adequately performed; an important part of the randomisation process is concealed random allocation, whereby those who are carrying out the study do not know which group a participant is in, this principle (blinding) should also be extended to those who are analysing the results. Lee [15] specified that he used a randomisation table; Clapp [10, 11] used anonymous envelopes without further clarification in both studies. None of the other studies specified how the randomisation was performed or whether any form of blinding was used.

Table 1. Included studies – method assessment

Study	Year published	Method	Scoring (Jadad) QA
Bell, Palma [8]	2000	Randomised, only 52% of the women agreed to randomisation. All the women included in the study wished to train 5 times/week or more. With allowances for dropouts. Poor compliance 61 women randomised, 33 continued to train 5 times/week, 28 reduced it to 3 times/week.	Jadad:2 QA: average
Carpenter, Sady, Sady Haydon, Thompson, Coustan [9]	1990	Randomised, further details not given. No info. with regards to dropouts or compliance. EG – 7, CG - 7	Jadad:1 QA: Average
Clapp, Kim, Burciu, Lopez [10]	2000	Randomised by use of anonymised envelopes. Participants included pre-pregnancy. Originally 50, 4 dropouts – 2 from EG non-compliant, 1 premature birth in each group. Compliance excellent EG – 22, CG – 24,	Jadad:3 QA: good
Clapp, Kim, Burciu, Schmidt, Petry, Lopez [11]	2002	Randomised by use of anonymised envelopes. Participants included in the study pre-pregnancy. Originally 80, 5 dropouts – 2 non-compliance, 2 premature births, 1 IUGR and bleeding. Unclear which groups these belonged to. Dropouts excluded from analysis. Compliance excellent. 3 training groups: Hi-Lo – 26, Mod-Mod – 24, Lo – Hi – 25	Jadad:3 QA: good
Collings, Curet, Mullin [12]	1982	The first 5 self-selected which group, the remaining 15 were randomised. Dropouts not taken into account. EG – 12, CG – 8	Jadad:1 QA: average
Erkkola [13]	1976	Randomised, not explained further. Originally 83, 7 did not want to participate, 14 drop outs, 3 moved in both groups, 1 spontaneous abort in EG, 1 threatened abortion in both groups, 2 premature deliveries in CG, 1 in EG, 1 termination in EG, 1 unknown dropout. EG – 31, CG – 31. Primigravidae.	Jadad:2 QA: average
Kulpa, White, Visscher [14]	1986	Randomised, not explained further. Originally 141, 56 dropouts- spontaneous abortion (n=8), non-compliance (n=2) those who stopped (n=20) were eliminated from study. Serious obstetric complications analysed separately(n=26, 10 from EG and16 from CG). Studied over 2,5 years. EG – 17 primigravidae, 21 multigravidae CG – 20 primigravidae, 27 multigravidae	Jadad:2 QA: average

Table 1. Included studies – method assessment (Continued)

Study	Year1 published	Method	Scoring (Jadad) QA
Lee [15]	1996	Randomised by randomisation table Originally 370, 19 dropouts Variable compliance;15,4% did not participate, 27,4% minimum participation. 1/week for 1-5 weeks, 34,3% 1 /week for 6-15 weeks, 22,9% 1/week for minimum16 weeks EG – 176, CG – 177.	Jadad:3 QA: good
Marquez-Sterling, Kaplan, Halberstein, Signorlie, Perry [16]	1997	Randomised, not explained further Originally 20, 5 dropouts– 1 in EG moved, 2 in CG due to work, 2 in CG lost contact EG – 9 primigravidae, CG – 6 primigravidae	Jadad:2 QA: average
Pijpers, Wladimiroff, McGhie [17]	1984	Randomised, , not explained further Primigravidae. No dropouts. EG – 14, CG – 14	Jadad:2 QA: good
Prevedel, Calderon, Abadde, Borges, Rudge [18]	2001	Randomised, not explained further No information on dropouts or compliance EG – 22, CG – 19.	Jadad:1 QA: average
Sibley, Ruhling, Cameron-Foster, Christensen, Bolen [19]	1981	Randomised., not explained further No dropouts and good compliance EG – 7, CG – 6	Jadad:2 QA: average
South-Paul, Rajagopal, Tenholder [20]	1988	Randomized, not explained further Originally 23, 6 dropouts – 3 (2 from EG) due to work, 1 had twins(EG), 1 appendicitis (EG), 1 placenta previa (EG). EG – 10, CG – 7, primi- og multigravidae.	Jadad:2 QA: good
Varassi, Bazzano, Edwards [21]	1988	Randomised, not explained further Originally 36. Multips. 4 excluded from CG for other medical intervention, 2 excluded from EG unwilling to train. EG – 13, CG – 17	Jadad:2 QA: average

EG- Exercise Group, CG- Control Group, QA- Qualitative Assessment.
Hi-Lo: reducing from 60-20min exercise in week 24, Mod-Mod: exercised 40 min throughout pregnancy, Lo-Hi: increased from 20-60 min in week 24.

Several of the studies included details of participants withdrawing from the studies, though only Lee [15] included these in the analysis. If one wishes to have robust data it is best to include the participants who withdrew in their group, when analysing the data. Such "intention to treat" analysis strengthens the results [4]. This type of study allows one to analyse these results even though they were not a parameter originally planned for investigation. The complications which the participants develop may be a result of exercise and thus need to be included in order to advise women on exercise in pregnancy.

The limited randomised studies available indicate this is a difficult area to investigate, in Bell's study [8] only 51% of participants wanted to be randomised, the remainder did not want to risk limiting their physical activity. Lee's study [15] was the only large study with 351 participants. Bell [8], Clapp [10], Erkkola [12] and Kulpa [14] were studies with over 60 participants. The other studies were small, making it difficult to infer anything from the results, unless there is a large and / or statistically significant difference.

In order to establish an effect from an intervention it is necessary to minimise other variables, a good starting point is to study the groups at the beginning in order to assess their baseline physical fitness and ensure equality between the groups. Only a few of the studies compared the groups at the start of the study. It is important that the groups are otherwise treated similarly [4], however this is difficult to achieve in this type of study. By treating the groups with a similar follow-up and ensuring blinding of the investigators it is possible to reduce bias, though several studies actually had more frequent monitoring of the intervention group.

Instructions (or lack of) given to the control groups are also of importance; knowing or limiting the extent of physical activity undertaken during the study period allows some control over the study. In 4 studies the women were asked to continue their normal daily activity [10, 11, 12 and 15] and Kulpa [14] allowed them to train a maximum of once a week. Some of the studies gave diaries for participants to fill in with physical activity and other variables such as diet to record.

In most studies the training regime was organised and undertaken with an instructor making it easier to ensure participants followed the programme. Four studies [8, 10, 11 and 13] allowed participants to do their own training regime, documenting the exercises in a diary. Intuitively, one would expect organised training regimes to give better compliance, though Lee's study [15] demonstrated poor compliance despite organised training. A few studies gave information on compliance varying from very good to poor, though many studies did not give information on compliance. Where compliance with an exercise regime is poor it makes interpreting the results difficult: if participants have not completed the regime the results may be misinterpreted.

Literature Review as a Method

In a systematic review, one aims to use all available information from around the world on a subject. This entails searching all relevant databases, reference lists and contacting authors with regard to unpublished data [4]. In this article we have searched for all randomised controlled studies on the subject, though cannot exclude that others may exist in other databases or unpublished. Authors were not contacted directly, which could have increased the quality of this study certainly with regard to precise questions surrounding methods and results of the included studies but also of unpublished data. Within exercise and pregnancy there are many studies though few were randomised controlled. Other criteria for selection in the literature could have been used such as number of participants, however we wanted to look at the effect of exercise during pregnancy so only chose randomised controlled studies where the groups were comparable.

The author's assessment of the included studies is important, there is an advantage in several people have looked at the articles critically. In this study only the principle author has reviewed the articles using a scoring system developed by Jadad et al [7] and the checklist developed by CASP. Few studies were of "good" quality though none were assessed as "poor" quality. An exclusion criterion that could be used were on those studies which excluded participants who developed obstetric complications but this would have left only one study. There were large variations in method quality and number of participants, those studies assessed as "good" were given greater weight.

The studies under examination should be homogenous in a systematic review [4], the studies included in this review examined the same phenomenon: physical activity in pregnancy, but they did not measure the same parameters and end points varied between studies making a meta-analysis difficult. In addition most of the studies were small and not of "very good" methodology so statistic analysis of the studies is not advisable. A meta-analysis would have improved the quality of the review as the results would be objective rather than subjective as in a qualitative review. In order to objectify the review as much as possible scoring systems such as those of Jadad [7] and CASP were used.

Empirical Results of Included Studies

Table 1 shows an alphabetical list of the 14 studies included, the type of exercise performed varied from walking, jogging, rowing, cycling, swimming, aerobics and cross country skiing. All the infants born were healthy at birth; preterm birth and caesarean section were the only obstetric complications used as an outcome measures. Lee [15] was the only investigator who did not exclude participants from the analysis when obstetric complications arose, the six other studies [8, 10, 11, 12, 13 and 16] which had recorded obstetric complication subsequently removed them from their analysis.

The training regimes in the different studies varied. Pijpers looked only at short term effects of 2 sessions lasting 5 minutes [17]. The other studies had exercise programmes over longer time periods. Two studies investigated the consequences of different exercise intensities [8, 11] on participants who were all in physical training programmes at recruitment. Bell [8] started with a regime of 5 times per week, reducing to 3 times per week at 25 weeks in 28 0f 61 participants. Clapp [11] had 3 groups: Lo-Hi increased from 20 to 60 minutes in week 24, Mod-Mod exercised for 40 min throughout pregnancy and Hi-Low reduced from 60 to 20 minutes in week 24. All three groups exercised 5 times per week.

The remaining 11 studies looked at sedate women who were randomly allocated to the exercise group or control group. Exercise intensity, length of training times and number of training sessions per week varied: Intensity varied from 50% to 80% of maximal age related heart rate, some studies gave heart rates for the participants to achieve varying from 120 to 156 beats per minute. Sibley [19] chose individual intensities for each participant without giving further explanation. Two studies [9, 15] did not give information on the intensity of the exercise regimes. Length of regimes varied from 20 to 60 minutes, three studies [14, 18 and 20] did not give this information. In the majority of studies the participants trained 3 times per week, Clapp's [10] study trained 3 to 5 times per week, whereas Kulpa's [14] study did not state how often participants trained.

The studies also varied in relation to when the intervention started and stopped in the pregnancy. Bell [8], Clapp [10, 11], Erkkola [12] and Kulpa [14] started in the first trimester, the others in the second trimester. Most continued to delivery though Carpenter [9], Erkkola [13], Prevedel [18], Sibley [19] and South-Paul [20] terminated their studies in the third trimester.

Table 2 shows the results of different outcome measures. Results for individual studies in relation to a given outcome measure reads directly from the same line as the study is placed. All studies used the student's t-test for statistical analysis; P values for statistical significance were mostly $P < 0.05$ though some were as low as $P < 0.001$.

Only three studies had preterm labour as an outcome measure, but four other studies recorded how many delivered preterm though excluding them from the analysis. None of these studies [8, 10, 11, 12, 13, 15 and 16] showed a statistically significant difference in the number of preterm births. Frequency of caesarean section was an outcome measure in three studies [12, 15, 16], but no statistically significant difference was found. Half of the studies [10, 11, 12, 14, 15, 16 and 19] looked at the Apgar scores which were all over 8 for all the children at birth.

Seven studies also looked at birth weight; all the children weighed over 3kg. Clapp [10] found in fact children born to mothers who exercised weighed significantly more, though the other six studies found no significant difference. Bell [8] who compared two exercising groups found those women who continued to train 5 times per week gave birth to bigger children but the difference was not significant. Clapp [11] comparing three training regimes found again significant differences: women in the Lo-Hi group (increasing from 20 -60 minutes at week 24] gave birth to children with significantly lower birth weight. In both of Clapp's studies [10, 11] he also compared the ponderal index, in the control group study there was no difference but in the study with 3 training regimes the ponderal index was significantly lower in the Lo-Hi and Mod-Mod groups.

Pijpers [17] looked at only short term effects of exercise including fetal heart rate five minutes after exercise; the heart rate was between 120-160 beats per minute. Two other studies [12, 19] compared fetal heart rates, Colling's [12] found a significant increase during exercise though within normal range (120-160) and five minutes after exercise. Sibley [19] found two of the seven participants in the exercise group had fetal heart rates over 160 beats per minute during training, though all were within normal (120-160) range five minutes after exercise again.

Two studies comparing an exercise group with a control group looked at the placental volume. Clapp [10] found the placentas in the exercise group had significantly larger volume, more villi and less non functional tissue. In his study with 3 training regimes [11] Clapp also found significant increase in growth rate in those who reduced training at 24 weeks (Hi-Lo group). Colling's study [12] showed a larger placental volume in the exercise group, though this was not statistically significant.

Table 2. Outcome measures – results

Outcome	Studies	Participants	Results
Premature birth (PB)	Bell	Dropout	1 PB in each of the groups
	Clapp (2000)	Dropout	1 PB in each of the groups
	Clapp (2002)	Dropout	2 PB in each of the groups
	Collings	20	No s.s difference
	Erkkola	Dropout	1 PB in EG, 2 PB in CG
	Lee	351	No s.s difference
	Marquez-Sterling	15	No s.s difference
Caesarean Section	Collings	EG 12/20	2 caesarean sections in CG, 0 in EG, no s.s difference
	Lee	EG 176/351	No s.s difference
	Marquez-Sterling	EG 9/20	1/3 caesareans in each of the groups
Apgar score (AS) 1 and 5 min. after birth	Clapp (2000)	46	AS 8 or over in all, no s.s difference
	Clapp (2002)	75	AS 8 or over in all, no s.s difference
	Collings	20	AS 8 or over 5 min. postpartum, No s.s difference
	Kulpa	85	No s.s difference
	Lee	351	No s.s difference
	Marquez-Sterling	15	No s.s difference
	Sibley	13	AS 9 or over 5 min. postpartum, no s.s difference AS 8 or over, no s.s difference
Birth weight (average weight per group, in grams)	Bell	61	Increased birth weight in those that trained 5 times/week not s.s
	Clapp (2000)	46	EG – 3750, CG – 3490, s.s difference
	Clapp (2002)	75	Lo-Hi – 3370, s.s. lower (Mod-Mod 3430, Hi-Lo 3820)
	Collings	20	EG – 3600, CG – 3350, No s.s difference. (figures not given)
	Kulpa	85	EG – 3286, CG – 3325, no s.s difference
	Lee	351	EG – 3515, CG – 3722, no s.s difference
	Marquez-Sterling	15	
Ponderal Index	Clapp (2000)	46	No s.s difference
	Clapp (2002)	75	Lo-Hi og Mod-Mod groups s.s lower.
Fetal heart rate (FHR) during og 5 min. after training	Collings	20	FHR 120-160 bpm during and 5 min. after training
	Pijpers	28	FHR 120-160 bpm 5 min. after training
	Sibley	13	FHR over 160bpm in 2 cases during training, otherwise 137-160 bpm during and 5 min. after training
Placenta Volume and growth rate	Clapp (2000)	46	Placental volume s.s increased in EG, less non-functional tissue
	Clapp (2002)	75	Placentas growth rate s.s. increased in the Hi-Lo group
	Collings	20	Placental volume increased in EG, not s.s.

Table 2. Outcome measures – results (Continued)

Outcome	Studies	Participants	Results
Physical form Objectively measured at beginning and end	Carpenter Collings Erkkola Kulpa Marquez-Sterling Prevedel Sibley South-Paul	14 20 62 85 15 41 13 17	Pulse oximetry s.s increased in EG, but not MVO2, SV, HR MVO2 s.s. increased in TG from 2nd to 3rd trimester PWC s.s. increased in EG in weeks 26 and 38. MVO2 s.s increased in TG TG s.s improved fitness TG s.s increased training capacity, reduction in CG MVO2 s.s. increased in EG EG maintained their fitness, reduced in CG, not s.s Increased fitness in EG, not s.s.
Blood Pressure	Erkkola Lee Sibley	62 351 13	Increased diastolic pressure in CG from 10th to 38th week, not s.s. Somewhat lower diastolic pressure in EG, not s.s.
Weight gain during pregnancy (in kg)	Collings Clapp (2000) Clapp (2002) Kulpa Marquez-Sterling Prevedel	20 46 75 85 15 41	EG - 15,8, CG - 14, No s.s difference EG - 15,7, CG - 16,3, No s.s difference The Lo-Hi group put on less weight s.s less (12 vs. 14,6 og15,5) Multigravida in CG put on s.s more EG - 16,2, CG - 15,7, No s.s difference EG - 14,5, CG - 12,5, No s.s difference
Duration of second stage	Collings Kulpa Lee	20 85 351	No s.s difference Primips in EG s.s shorter duration No s.s difference
Pain during birth	Lee Varassi	351 20	No s.s difference EG expressed s.s. less pain experienced during birth
Experience of physical and psychological well-being	Lee Marquez-Sterling Sibley	351 15 13	S.s higher in EG S.s higher in EG S.s higher in EG
Post-natal depression	Lee	351	No s.s difference
Post-partum incontinence	Lee	351	No s.s difference

[1] SS: statistical significance, MVO2: maximal oxygen uptake, PWC: physical work capacity, BPM: beats per minute, HR: heart rate, SV: stroke volume, O2puls: pulse oximetry

Eight studies investigated whether participants in the exercise groups got the improvement in their physical condition. Several parameters were used to measure physical fitness such as work capacity, estimated maximal oxygen uptake and aerobic capacity. In order to collectively review the results, the term objectively measured physical fitness is used. In Sibley's study [19] the exercise group maintained their fitness levels, whereas in the control group it fell, the results were not significant. Results from Collings [12], Erkkola [13] and Prevedel [18] demonstrated a significant rise in maximal oxygen uptake in the exercise groups; Carpenter [9], Kulpa [14], Marquez-Sterling [16] and South-Paul [20] also showed improvement in physical fitness in the training groups.

Blood pressure was measured at different stages of the pregnancy and was an outcome measure in three of the studies. Erkkolas [13] study showed an increase in diastolic pressures from 10th to 38th week of gestation in the control group, whereas Sibley [19] found lower diastolic pressures in the exercise group (not statistically significant). Lee [15] found no differences between their groups.

Weight gain during the pregnancy was an outcome measure in six studies, the five studies comparing exercise with control group found only small changes [10, 12, 14, 16 and 18]. Kulpa [14] found multigravida in the control group increased their weight significantly more than in the other three groups. In his study with three exercise regimes [11] there was a significantly lower increase in the group which increased their training regime (Lo – Hi group).

Kulpa [14] and Lee [15] examined the duration of the second stage of labour. Lee found no difference between the exercise and control groups; though by distinguishing between primigravida and multigravida, Kulpa found significantly shorter second stages in the primigravidae as compared to the control group. Personally experienced pain (as measured by pain score questionnaires) during labour was an outcome measure in two studies; Varassi [21] found women in the exercising group experienced less pain whereas Lee [15] saw no difference between the groups. The way in which exercise effected the women's physical and psychological well being was an outcome measure in three studies: all three found a significant increase in the parameters measured [15, 16 and 19].

Discussion

Extensive physiological changes occur in pregnancy, for a majority of which, hormones appear to be a prerequisite. Major cardiovascular changes occur which affect the ability to exercise; Cardiac output increases in the first trimester, reaching its nadir (a 30-50% increase) in the second trimester. This increase is due to a fall in total peripheral vascular resistance and concomitant increase in stroke volume and heart rate. The diastolic blood pressure falls by 5-10 mmHg through the second trimester and the systolic pressure either falls slightly or shows no change. The blood pressure then rises again towards term eventually reaching pre-pregnancy levels. Blood volume gradually increases by 40-50% through the first and second trimester, though the increase is greater in plasma volume than erythrocytes leading to the physiological anaemia of pregnancy [22]. Blood flow distribution is also significantly altered, increasing flow to the visceral organs ensuring good flow to the uterus and thereby securing blood flow to the feto-placental unit [23]. Respiration is also altered in pregnancy: tidal volume increases 50% and maximal oxygen uptake increases by 10-20%. This increased ventilation reduces the arterial carbon dioxide tension (paCO2) inducing a mild maternal alkalosis which in turn facilitates gas exchange across the placenta so hindering fetal acidosis [23]. The hormonal changes can cause mechanical alterations by relaxation of ligaments which in turn lead to greater joint instability [24]. Basal metabolic rate and heat production increase also in pregnancy; pregnant women require circa 300kcal extra per day and the fetal body temperature is approximately 1°C higher than maternal [25] allowing heat transfer from fetus to mother [26].

Physical activity gives similar changes to a woman's physiology as a pregnancy. The changes that occur are increased heart rate, a fall in peripheral resistance and unlike pregnancy a raised blood pressure (greater systolic change than diastolic); these changes lead to an increase in cardiac output [27]. With increasing work intensity core body temperature may also rise, though this is not scientifically proven in humans. A 20 minute exercise regime at 70% intensity can theoretically increase core body temperature by 1.5°C [28]. Physical activity leads to a redistribution of the blood supply moving it from visceral organs and skin, to the exercising skeletal muscle, as intensity increases so does the redistribution [23]. Respiratory changes are increased respiratory rate and tidal volume [27]; physical activity also raises the basal metabolic rate as the exercising muscle requires energy. Over time regular aerobic training will increase oxygen uptake, raise stroke volume, lower the resting pulse rate and may help lower blood pressure [29].

In the studies included in this review, the exercise groups trained aerobically 3 – 5 times per week for 20 – 60 minutes with a work intensity of between 50 – 75% of maximal age related heart rate. The extent to which the participants reached the desired training effect was looked at in eight of the studies [9, 12, 13, 14, 16, 18, 19 and 20]. The majority found the exercising group gained a significant improvement in physical fitness. A few found the women merely maintained fitness whereas the control groups fell in fitness; this may be due to the effects being masked by the changes of pregnancy.

Theoretical risks to the fetus from the combination of the physiological changes of aerobic exercise and pregnancy are fetal hypoxia, growth restriction, hyperthermia and trauma. The redistribution of blood flow during training can be great enough to cause a reduction in blood flow to the placenta thereby inducing fetal hypoxia. Active skeletal muscle may be able to alter the energy substrate accessibility to such a degree as to cause fetal growth restriction. Hyperthermia is a known teratogen leading to increased risk of neural tube defects [30]. Fetal trauma is of particular risk in contact sports where there is a risk of a blow to the uterus. Trauma was not investigated by the included studies and will therefore not be discussed further in this review.

Fetal oxygen deprivation is difficult to measure in utero and carries a risk of preterm labour, though indirectly the fetal heart rate and its variability can be used. Those studies which did assess fetal heart rate patterns [11, 17 and 18] demonstrated normal parameters 5 minutes after training. In only one study did the fetal heart rate rise above 160 beats per minute during the training regime in two of seven participants otherwise fetal heart rate recordings were unremarkable.

Physical exercise tends to direct blood flow away from the visceral organs, including the placenta, thus a possible cause of reduced transport of oxygen and nutrients to the fetus. Three studies investigated the placental volume [10, 11 and 12] of which two compared with a control group [10, 12], both studies showed larger placental volume in the exercise group though only one was statistically significant. Clapp [10] demonstrated a larger proportion of functional and villous tissue in the placentas of exercising groups. The third study [11] looking at three training regimes demonstrated a significant increase in placental growth rate in the reducing exercise (Hi-Lo) group. These results suggest the placenta adapts to regular exercise by increasing its volume and quantity of functional tissue, thereby compensating for the reduction in blood flow during exercise.

Birth weight is an indicator of fetal growth restriction [22] and among the five studies [10, 12, 14, 15 and 16] with a control group comparison only one study showed the exercise group delivered significantly larger babies [10]. The other studies had no significant differences in birth weight, in fact all studies where birth weight was recorded, these were within the normal ranges. Significantly smaller babies were born in the group where exercise was increased (Lo-Hi, 11), these children had significantly less body fat, and ponderal index suggested symmetrical growth thus not growth restricted. Maternal weight gain in pregnancy is a poor, non-specific measure of pregnancy wellbeing [22], those studies measuring this parameter [10, 12, 14, 16 and 18] found small differences all within the normal range. Clapp's study [11] found those who increased their training regime (Lo-Hi group) showed a significant lack of weight gain. Overall the results indicate moderate training has little effect on the babies' birth weight but that increasing exercise intensity can lead to a reduction in birth weight principally through reduced body fat.

Birth weight is an important predictor of fetal morbidity, if physical exercise led to an increased risk of preterm birth, perinatal complications would also be expected to rise. None of the studies found an increase in preterm deliveries and all who measured, had Apgar scores of 8 or over. The Apgar score indicates fetal vitality and scores of 8 – 10 of 10 suggests normal vital functions at birth. The results were consistent through all the studies included in this review.

Maternal body temperature was not measured during exercise; however a teratogenic effect might become apparent through an increase in children born with anatomical abnormalities to women in the exercise groups. Approximately 3% of all babies born have this type of abnormality [22], therefore a large cohort is required in order to test this hypothesis. No babies in these studies were born with abnormalities. A recently published longitudinal study [31] investigating core body temperature in an exercising group where work intensity was 85% of age related maximum showed a fall in maternal core body temperature, which may assist in protecting the fetus from hyperthermia.

Healthcare workers are most concerned with possible harmful effects of physical activity on the pregnant woman and their unborn child. Obstetric complications such as abruptio placenta, gestational diabetes, pre-eclampsia, preterm delivery, increasing the incidence of caesarean section or direct injury to ligaments and joints of the women caused by the changes in connective tissue and altered posture which occurs in pregnancy. Injuries were not reported in any of the studies and cannot be commented on further in this review. The obstetric complications which occurred during the pregnancy, in many of the studies lead to the exclusion of that person, whereas complications arising in labour were an outcome measure. Those studies [8, 10, 11, 12, 13, 15 and 16] which used preterm labour and caesarean section as outcome measures found no differences between exercising or control groups. Some complications, such as first trimester spontaneous miscarriage could not be assessed as most studies started in the second trimester.

Three studies [13, 15 and 19] followed blood pressure changes during the exercise periods, when compared to control groups the differences were small and insignificant. Had a positive effect of exercise (as might be expected) been apparent, this would have been interesting for those who develop pre-eclampsia. Regular aerobic exercise can lower blood pressure [29], though none of the reviewed studies demonstrated this effect.

The incidence of obesity and diabetes mellitus during pregnancy is increasing in westernised societies [22], even though in pregnancy fasting blood sugar levels tend to be lower [32]. An indirect and rough guide to whether exercise affects blood sugar regulation and thereby appetite would be changes in weight. The studies in which weight was an outcome measure [10, 12, 14, 16 and 18] showed normal weight gain in all groups, only the study [11] with three exercise regimes demonstrated a significantly smaller weight gain in those who increased their training (Lo-Hi). Other studies [33, 34] not included in this review of gestational diabetes have shown exercise, diet control and insulin use all have a similar effect on lowering blood sugar levels. Regular aerobic exercise gives lower, more stable blood sugar and can therefore form part of a treatment regime. There is no information on the incidence of gestational diabetes in the studies reviewed, and a large population (greater than all the 14 studies reviewed here put together) would need to be investigated to see a significant difference. Further investigation in this area is required.

The myth that women who maintain physical fitness have shorter, easier deliveries compared with their more sedate counterparts is popular, only one of the studies [14] investigating the length of the second stage of labour found a difference. The primigravida who exercised had a shorter second stage of labour; the two other studies [12, 15] found no difference. Two studies looked at pain scores during labour [15, 21], one found lower pain scores in those who exercised [21] whereas the other found no difference.

Regular exercise during pregnancy could also have other positive effects, for example less risk of depression. Many women experience postnatal depression. Exercise increases serotonin levels in the brain, which may have a protective effect against depression. Nordhagen [3] found lower levels of depressive symptoms in physically active pregnant women than in sedate women, in his retrospective study. Lee [15] found no difference in rates of postnatal depression between exercising and control groups.

Longstanding exercise regimes could also reduce the risks of incontinence after delivery; Lee's study [15] showed no differences between their groups though none of the studies employed pelvic floor training in their exercise regimes. Pelvic floor exercises have been shown to reduce the frequency of incontinence after delivery in other studies [35].

The most consistent positive outcome measure found in the studies was the personally experienced effect of exercise on physical and psychological wellbeing of the women. All the studies investigating this parameter demonstrated a significant improvement in the exercise group, though in medical terms this is not the most important, for the women to feel better was very important.

None of the studies in this review followed the children postpartum; there are retrospective studies looking at morphometry and neuropsychological development of children in mothers who actively trained in pregnancy [36, 37]. These children had similar if not higher scores on neuropsychological testing. The studies included in this review all delivered healthy children and it would be interesting to have follow up studies of their development. None of the studies in this review showed a direct positive effect on the fetus or child of physically active women.

References

[1] Lokey EA, Tran ZV, Wells CL, Myers BC, Tran AC Effects of physical exercise on pregnancy outcomes: a meta-analytic review. *Medicine and Science in Sports and Exercise* 1991; Vol. 23, No. 11; 1234-9.

[2] Kramer MS. Aerobic exercise for women during pregnancy (Cochrane review) In: *the Cochrane Library, Issue* 2, 2002.

[3] Nordhagen IH, Sundgot-Borgen J. Fysisk aktivitet hos gravide i relasjon til svangerskapsplager og depressive symptomer. *Tidsskrift for den Norske Lægeforening nr.* 5, 2002; 122: 470-4.

[4] Bjørndal A, Flottorp S, Klovning A. Medisinsk kunnskapshåndtering. *Gyldendal Akademisk* 2000.

[5] Chalmers TC, Celano P, Sacks HS, Smith H. Bias in treatment assignment in controlled clinical trials. *New England Journal of Medicine* 1983; 309:1358-61.

[6] Kuns R, Oxman AD. The unpredictability paradox: review of empirical comparisons of randomised and non-randomised clinical trials. *British Medical Journal* 1998; 317: 1185-90.

[7] Jadad AR, Moore RA, Carroll D, Jenkinson C, Reynolds JM, Gavaghan DJ, McQuay HJ. Assessing the quality of reports of randomised clinical trials: is blinding necessary? *Controlled Clinical Trials* 1996; 17: 1-12.

[8] Bell R, Palma S. Antenatal exercise and birth weight. *Australian and New Zeeland Journal of Obstetrics and Gynaecology* 2000; 40; 1: 70-73.

[9] Carpenter MW, Sady Sp, Sady MA, Haydon BB, Coustan DR, Thompson PD. effects of exercise training in midpregnancy: a randomised controlled trial. Annual meeting – society for gynaecologic investigation 1990; 497.

[10] Clapp JF, Kim H, Burciu B, Lopez B. Beginning regular exercise in early pregnancy: effect on fetoplacental growth. *American Journal of Obstetrics and Gynaecology* 2000; 183: 1484-8.

[11] Clapp JF, Kim H, Burciu B, Schmidt S, Petry K, Lopez B. Continuing regular exercise during pregnancy: effect of exercise volume on fetoplacental growth. *American Journal of Obstetrics and Gynaecology* 2002; 186: 142-7.

[12] Collings CA, Curet LB, Mullin JP. Maternal and fetal responses to a maternal aerobic exercise program. *American Journal of Obstetrics and Gynaecology* 1983; 145: 702-707.

[13] Erkkola R. The influence of physical training during pregnancy on physical work capacity and circulatory parameters. *Scandinavian Journal of Clinical Laboratory Investigations* 1976; 36: 747-54.

[14] Kulpa PJ, White BM, Visscher R. Aerobic exercise in pregnancy. *American Journal of Obstetrics and Gynaecology* 1987; 156: 1395-403.

[15] Lee G. Exercise in pregnancy. *Modern Midwife* 1996; 6: 28-33.
[16] Marquez-Sterling S, Perry AC, Kaplan TA, Halberstein A, Signorlie JF. Physical and psychological changes with vigorous exercise in sedentary primigravidae. *Medicine and Science in Sports and Exercise* 2000; 32 (1): 58-62.
[17] Pijpers L, Wladimiroff JW, Mcghie J. effect of short-term maternal exercise on maternal and fetal cardiovascular dynamics. *British Journal of Obstetrics and Gynaecology* 1984; 91: 1081-6.
[18] Prevedel TTS, Calderon IMP, Abadde JF, Borges VTM, Rudge MVC. Maternal effects of hydrotherapy in normal pregnant women. *Journal of Perinatal Medicine* 2001; 29 (Suppl 1, part 2): 665-6.
[19] Sibley L, Ruhling RO, Cameron-Foster J, Christensen C, Bolen T. Swimming and physical fitness during pregnancy. *Journal of Nurse Midwifery* 1981; 26, 3-12.
[20] South-Paul JE, Rajagopal KR, Tenholder MF. The effect of participation in a regular exercise program upon aerobic capacity during pregnancy. *Obstetrics and Gynaecology* 1989; 71; 175-9.
[21] Varassi G, Bazzano C, Edwards T. Effects of physical activity on maternal plasma beta-endorphin levels and perception of labour pain. *American Journal of Obstetrics and Gynaecology* 1988; 71: 175-9.
[22] Bergsjø P, Maltau JM, Molne K, Nesheim BI. Obstetrikk. *Gyldendal Akademisk* 2000, 3. utgave.
[23] Artal R. Exercise and pregnancy. *Clinics in Sports Medicine* 1992; 11; 2; 363-76.
[24] Calguneri M, Bird HA, Wright V. Changes in joint laxity occurring during pregnancy. *Ann Rhem Dis* 1982; 41; 126-8.
[25] Hytten FE, Chamberlain G. Clinical Physiology in Obstetrics. Oxford. *Blackwell,* 1980.
[26] ACOG Technical Bulletin Number 189. Exercise during pregnancy and the postpartum period. *International Journal of Gynaecology and Obstetrics* 1994; 45: 65-70.
[27] Berne RM, Levy MN. Principles of physiology. *Mosby* 2000, 3. edition.
[28] Artal R, Wiswell RA, Drinkwater BL. Exercise in pregnancy. Baltimore; *Williams and Wilkins* 1991, 2. edition.
[29] Halbert JA, Silagy CA, Finucane P, Withers RT, Hamdorf PA, Andrews GR. The effectiveness of exercise training in lowering blood pressure: a meta-analysis of randomised controlled trials of 4 weeks or longer. *Journal of Human Hypertension* 1997; 11 (10): 641-9.
[30] Edwards MJ. Hyperthermia as a teratogen: a review of experimental studies and their clinical significance. *Teratogenesis Carcinog Mutagen* 1986; 6: 563-82.
[31] Lindqvist PG, Marsal K, Merlo J, Pirhonen JP. Thermal response to submaximal exercise before, during and after pregnancy: a longitudinal study. *Journal of Maternal and Fetal Neonatal Medicine* 2003 Mar; 13 (3): 152-6.
[32] Clapp JF, Seaward BL, Sleamaker RH, Hiser L. Maternal physiologic adaptations to early human pregnancy. *American Journal of Obstetrics and Gynaecology* 1988; 159; 1456-60.
[33] Bung P, Artal R, Khodiguian N. Regular exercise therapy in disorders of carbohydrate metabolism in pregnancy – results of a prospective, randomised longitudinal study. *Journal of Perinatal Medicine* 1993 Mar; 53 (3): 188-93.

[34] Jovanovic-Peterson L, Durak Ep, Peterson CM. Randomised trial of diet versus diet plus cardiovascular conditioning on glucose levels in gestational diabetes. *American Journal of Obstetrics and Gynaecology* 1989; 161: 415-9.

[35] Harvey MA. Pelvic floor exercises during and after pregnancy: a systematic review of their role in preventing pelvic floor dysfunction. *Journal of Obstetrics and Gynaecology Canada* 2003 Jun; 25 (6): 487-98.

[36] Clapp JF, Simonian S, Lopez B, Appelby-wineberg S, Harcar-sevcik R. The one-year morphometric and neurodevelopmental outcome of the offspring of women who continued to exercise regularly throughout pregnancy. *American Journal of Obstetrics and Gynaecology* 1998; 178; 594-9.

[37] Clapp JF, Capeless El. Neonatal morphometrics after endurance exercise during pregnancy. *American Journal of Obstetrics and Gynaecology* 1990; 163: 1805-11.

Index

A

abdomen, 3, 206, 218
acetylcholine, 192
acid, 4, 40, 54, 64, 65, 81, 82, 83, 86, 95, 98, 100, 116, 117, 119, 123, 189
acidosis, 65, 87, 201, 262
acne, 232
ACTH, 132, 133, 134, 138, 139, 140, 141, 143, 144, 153, 154, 156, 161
activities of daily living, viii, 62, 66, 69, 83, 229, 233
adaptation, ix, 88, 91, 132, 138, 152, 155, 156, 157, 159, 160, 175, 178, 237
adenosine triphosphate, 226, 228
adipocyte, 100, 160
adipose, 95, 96, 99, 100, 101, 112, 114, 118, 120, 122, 123, 124, 128, 153, 224
adolescents, 225
adrenal gland, 16
adrenal insufficiency, 157
adrenaline, 39
adulthood, 242
aerobic exercise, viii, 14, 61, 64, 65, 66, 67, 70, 74, 76, 79, 84, 109, 113, 119, 133, 214, 222, 223, 253, 263, 265, 266
afferent nerve, 183
African Americans, 249
age, vii, xii, 1, 3, 26, 32, 68, 70, 72, 73, 74, 76, 84, 107, 126, 134, 166, 170, 205, 222, 223, 224, 237, 240, 242, 252, 253, 254, 258, 263, 264
agonist, 173, 174
albumin, 42
alcohol, 241
aldolase, 232
alkalosis, 262
allele, 122
amino acid, 40
amputation, 79
anaerobic, vii, 1, 3, 24, 136, 223, 224, 226, 232, 235
anal, 64, 266
angiogenesis, 234
angiography, 103
angioplasty, 66, 87
angiotensin converting enzyme, 70, 72, 74, 76
ankles, 187
anorectic, 135
anorexia nervosa, 135, 156, 158, 159
antagonism, 192, 201
anterior, 159
antibody (Ab), 14
antigen, 125
anti-inflammatory, 151, 232
anti-inflammatory agents, 232
antioxidant, 62, 63, 68, 72, 74, 83, 84, 86, 87, 88, 89, 90, 91
aorta, 16, 187
apoptosis, 232, 238
appearance, 95, 98, 117, 120, 232, 233
appendicitis, 256
appetite, 265
arginine, 122
arterioles, 230
artery, 41, 66, 70, 87, 103, 104, 124
arthritis, 223, 235
AS, 86, 260
ascorbic acid, 86, 91
asymptomatic, 98, 103, 121, 124
atherogenesis, 62, 104, 124, 126
atherosclerosis, viii, 15, 85, 88, 89, 90, 93, 94, 98, 103, 104, 105, 117, 118, 120, 121, 124, 125, 126

atherosclerotic plaque, 103, 104, 125
atrophy, 195, 223, 231, 232, 233
attenuated, 111, 113, 117, 133, 195, 201
Australia, 163, 240
autonomic nervous system (ANS), 56, 184

B

bacterial, 147
balloon angioplasty, 87
basal ganglia, 37, 38, 59
basal metabolic rate, 263
beta blockers, 72
bilateral, 168
binding, 42, 43, 50, 63, 96, 99, 101, 102, 104, 121, 122, 126, 148, 149, 157, 159, 160
biology, 56, 85, 240, 243
biopsy, 110, 230, 232
birth weight, xii, 252, 259, 260, 264, 266
bleeding, xii, 252, 253, 255
blood, vii, x, 1, 2, 3, 4, 6, 7, 9, 11, 12, 13, 14, 18, 39, 40, 41, 42, 43, 44, 49, 51, 53, 54, 55, 57, 59, 64, 66, 73, 84, 86, 89, 91, 94, 95, 101, 102, 120, 124, 126, 135, 138, 147, 153, 158, 159, 181, 182, 184, 185, 186, 187, 188, 189, 190, 191, 192, 193, 194, 195, 196, 197, 198, 200, 204, 206, 207, 213, 215, 216, 219, 226, 230, 231, 236, 253, 254, 262, 263, 265, 267
blood pressure, vii, x, 1, 2, 4, 6, 7, 11, 12, 13, 14, 18, 39, 55, 181, 182, 184, 185, 186, 187, 190, 191, 192, 193, 194, 195, 196, 197, 200, 262, 263, 265, 267
blood vessels, 184, 193, 230
blood-brain barrier (BBB), 55, 59
body composition, 117
body density, 219
body fat, xii, 76, 90, 152, 153, 154, 161, 252, 264
body mass, xi, xii, 6, 74, 111, 170, 204, 205, 216, 221, 224, 225, 233, 234
body mass index (BMI), 6, 74, 76, 79
body weight, 15, 68, 74, 79, 107, 122, 170, 217
bowel, vii
bradycardia, 192, 193
bradykinin, 188, 189
brainstem, 38, 40, 42, 43, 49
breakfast, 109, 113
breast cancer, vii, 245, 248
breathing, 63
bypass graft, 70

C

cachexia, 228, 236
calcification, 234
calcium, 6, 15, 16, 70, 72, 74, 76, 227
calcium channel blocker(s), 70, 72, 74, 76
Canada, 239, 240, 241, 242, 243, 244, 245, 246, 247, 248, 249, 268
cancer, vii, 236
capillary(ies), xi, 95, 101, 206, 207, 221, 230, 236
carbohydrate, 12, 15, 112, 120, 128, 129, 232, 267
carbohydrate metabolism, 12, 15, 267
carbohydrates, 101, 102, 111
cardiac, xi, 3, 66, 70, 71, 72, 73, 76, 78, 83, 101, 104, 117, 126, 130, 182, 183, 184, 187, 192, 193, 195, 196, 197, 199, 200, 201, 231, 263
cardiac muscle, 101
cardiac output, 182, 183, 184, 187, 192, 193, 195, 197, 200, 231, 263
cardiac reserve, 193, 195
cardiovascular disease, 2, 12, 124
cardiovascular function, 186
carotene, 62, 84
carotenoids, 73, 89
carotid arteries, 104
carrier, 65
cast, 48
catabolism, 69, 95, 97, 105, 122, 134, 227, 229
catalyst, 40
cataract, 232
catecholamines, viii, 17, 40, 41, 42, 43, 44, 46, 47, 48, 49, 50, 52, 54, 57, 58, 60, 149
caudal, 198
cell(s), 2, 4, 12, 13, 14, 15, 16, 22, 39, 40, 42, 54, 67, 84, 88, 89, 91, 95, 99, 100, 102, 119, 120, 124, 132, 139, 143, 147, 148, 155, 159, 160, 195, 201, 219, 229, 230, 232, 236
cell membranes, 2, 4, 12
central nervous system (CNS), 18, 22, 35, 38, 39, 42, 43, 44, 50, 51, 52, 53, 57, 141, 173
cephalic, 123
cerebellum, 40
cerebral blood flow, 36
childhood, xi, 221, 223, 234, 235
children, xi, xii, 69, 70, 221, 223, 225, 231, 232, 234, 235, 238, 241, 242, 243, 249, 252, 259, 264, 265
cholesterol, ix, 6, 9, 85, 93, 94, 96, 97, 98, 103, 104, 105, 106, 111, 118, 121, 124, 126, 128
chromatography, 6, 64, 86, 98, 104, 160

chronic fatigue syndrome, 235
chronic renal failure, 89
chylomicron(s), ix, 93, 94, 95, 96, 97, 98, 99, 100, 101, 104, 110, 114, 115, 117, 119, 120, 121, 123, 125, 127, 130
cigarette smoke, 72, 73
cigarette smokers, 72, 73
cigarette smoking, 73, 74
clinical trials, 83, 266
cluster of differentiation (CD), 86, 125, 127, 159, 237
coagulation, 125
cognition, viii, 17, 18, 19, 22, 24, 34, 35, 36, 37, 38, 39, 40, 41, 42, 43, 46, 47, 49, 50, 51, 52, 54, 59, 60
coma, 43
communities, 249
complement, 236
complications, xii, 3, 13, 252, 253, 254, 255, 257, 258, 264
concentration, ix, x, xi, 10, 11, 12, 13, 16, 42, 60, 87, 97, 99, 100, 103, 104, 105, 106, 107, 111, 114, 116, 117, 122, 124, 127, 132, 133, 137, 139, 153, 156, 181, 206, 207, 221
congestive heart failure, 3, 195, 199
connective tissue, 264
consumption, xi, 11, 65, 66, 73, 74, 84, 113, 204, 244
contamination, 41
control, x, 13, 15, 25, 28, 33, 36, 37, 42, 46, 48, 52, 53, 55, 59, 73, 74, 75, 76, 81, 82, 98, 100, 102, 103, 108, 109, 110, 111, 112, 113, 115, 116, 122, 124, 126, 133, 136, 148, 153, 154, 163, 165, 166, 167, 168, 171, 172, 173, 174, 176, 181, 183, 184, 185, 188, 190, 191, 196, 197, 198, 199, 200, 201, 204, 253, 257, 258, 259, 262, 263, 264, 265
controlled study(ies), 254, 257
controlled trial(s), xii, 234, 251, 253, 266, 267
coronary artery disease, viii, 61, 62, 88, 90, 98, 121, 124, 125, 126, 127, 130
coronary heart disease, ix, 3, 13, 90, 93, 94, 125, 127, 130, 153, 160
cortex, 36, 37, 38, 40, 44, 48, 49, 54, 55, 56, 59, 173, 184
corticosteroid(s), 157, 159, 160, 232
corticosteroid therapy, 157
corticotropin, 132, 156
cortisol, ix, 131, 132, 133, 134, 135, 136, 137, 138, 139, 140, 141, 142, 143, 144, 145, 146, 147, 148, 149, 151, 152, 153, 154, 155, 156, 157, 158, 160, 161, 174, 177, 238
creatine phosphokinase, 232
creatinine, 6, 9, 66, 87, 88
culture(s), 59, 145, 154, 240, 241, 243, 246, 248
cutaneous, 200
cycling, 23, 28, 46, 65, 111, 114, 182, 219, 223, 233, 258
cystic fibrosis, 69, 70
cytochrome, 226, 231
cytokine(s), xi, 81, 147, 152, 159, 221, 228, 229, 230, 236
cytoplasm, 96

D

death, 104, 126
degradation, 64, 90, 96, 97, 106, 228, 229
dehydration, 216, 217, 218, 219
dementia, 246, 248
dendritic cell (DC), 14, 15, 87, 158, 219
dephosphorylation, 99
depression, vii, ix, 132, 134, 135, 156, 243, 253, 261, 265
dermatomyositis, 225, 228, 230, 231, 232, 234, 235, 236, 237
desensitization, 139, 147
developed countries, 152
dexamethasone suppression test, 154
diabetes, 3, 15, 72, 76, 117, 130, 265
diabetic patients, 107, 116
diagnosis, 73, 160, 175, 242, 246
dialysis, 73, 74, 79, 80, 83, 88, 89
diaphragm, 227
diastolic blood pressure, 11, 262
diastolic pressure, 261, 262
diet, viii, 15, 62, 64, 74, 83, 111, 113, 120, 129, 243, 247, 257, 265, 268
dietary fat, 94, 95, 98, 117, 119, 121, 123, 124
differentiation, 153, 160
diffusion, 13, 42
digestion, 94, 119
dihydroxyphenylalanine, 55
dilated cardiomyopathy, 78, 201
disability, 229
discomfort, 33, 206
disease activity, 225, 227
distal, 185
diuretic, 70, 76

dopamine, viii, 17, 39, 40, 41, 42, 43, 44, 50, 51, 56, 57, 58, 59
dopamine precursor, 58
dorsal, 39, 187, 188, 190
dorsal horn, 190
duodenum, 94
dyslipidemia, 11, 72, 130

E

EEG, 40, 53
efficacy, 166, 170, 175, 176, 177, 178
elderly, 15, 89, 90, 158, 240, 248, 249
emotions, 18, 19, 34, 38, 39, 42, 50, 52, 245
encouragement, 164
endocrine, ix, 56, 132
endogenous, viii, ix, 12, 13, 16, 62, 83, 84, 107, 129, 131, 138, 141
endothelial cells, 91, 94, 102, 120, 230
endothelium, 67, 84, 101, 104, 106, 230, 236
endurance, ix, x, 11, 14, 54, 63, 66, 83, 106, 107, 108, 110, 112, 114, 126, 127, 128, 131, 132, 134, 135, 137, 138, 139, 140, 141, 143, 144, 145, 146, 147, 148, 149, 152, 153, 155, 156, 157, 158, 160, 163, 164, 171, 172, 173, 176, 177, 178, 219, 223, 231, 235, 237, 268
energy, ix, 43, 66, 87, 91, 93, 100, 108, 109, 110, 112, 113, 119, 123, 128, 131, 132, 135, 158, 201, 216, 223, 225, 226, 228, 229, 233, 238, 244, 254, 263
enzyme(s), 42, 73, 88, 95, 98, 114, 123, 148, 149, 231, 232
epinephrine, viii, 17, 39, 40, 41, 42, 43, 44, 46, 47, 49, 51, 58, 157
equilibrium, 38
erythrocyte(s), vii, 1, 2, 4, 5, 6, 7, 8, 9, 10, 11, 12, 13, 14, 15, 16, 73, 86, 89, 91, 262
ethanol, 68, 72, 73, 74
ethnicity, 74, 240, 246
evolution, 85, 86, 107
excess body weight, 247
excretion, 69, 135, 137, 149, 151, 156, 160, 232
exercise performance, 55, 219, 220, 224
exertion, 55, 57, 60, 66, 67, 69, 78, 195, 207
exogenous, viii, 62, 83, 115, 129, 160
extracellular, xi, 12, 145, 148, 182

F

facies, 232
factor i, 2, 16, 52, 72
fasciculation, 187
fasting, vii, ix, 2, 4, 6, 9, 10, 12, 93, 103, 104, 105, 106, 107, 110, 114, 116, 117, 118, 119, 121, 123, 125, 153, 265
fat, ix, 74, 76, 93, 94, 95, 100, 101, 102, 105, 107, 108, 109, 110, 111, 112, 113, 114, 115, 116, 117, 120, 124, 125, 127, 128, 130, 152, 153, 160, 219, 228, 229, 232, 241, 244, 264
fat soluble, 94
fatigue, 18, 23, 24, 53, 54, 55, 56, 58, 85, 149, 151, 169, 173, 224, 226, 234, 235, 238
fatty acid(s), 4, 5, 15, 42, 43, 64, 81, 82, 83, 90, 94, 95, 96, 98, 99, 100, 102, 110, 113, 114, 116, 117, 118, 122, 123, 124, 130
feedback, 43, 139, 142, 143, 154, 169, 183, 191
females, 166, 237
fertility, 248
fetal growth, 253, 263, 264
fetus, xii, 252, 253, 254, 263, 264, 266
fibers, x, 67, 181, 184, 185, 186, 187, 188, 189, 190, 191, 197, 199, 200, 222, 227, 231, 232, 233, 235, 236, 238
fibroblasts, 236
fibrosis, 69
fitness, x, 3, 14, 15, 23, 28, 32, 49, 54, 60, 71, 112, 164, 166, 175, 176, 223, 231, 235, 237, 243, 244, 257, 261, 263, 265, 267
flexor, 186, 232
fluorescence, 14
follow-up, 77, 79, 124, 149, 222, 231, 237, 257
food intake, 109, 113, 139, 143, 153, 154, 155
fruits, 62

G

gastric, 94, 117
gastrocnemius, 67, 185, 186
gastrointestinal, 117
gender, 73, 241, 243
gene, 67, 91, 95, 114, 119, 122, 128, 129, 132, 159, 240, 246
gene expression, 91, 114, 128, 129, 159
genotype, 125
Germany, 206
gestation, 262

gestational diabetes, 253, 264, 265, 268
glands, 139
glatiramer acetate (GA), 16, 85, 91, 156, 198, 199, 200
glucocorticoid(s), ix, 131, 132, 138, 149, 152, 153, 157, 158, 159, 160, 232, 237, 238
glucose, 6, 9, 12, 15, 43, 100, 123, 135, 153, 155, 161, 226, 228, 268
glucose regulation, 135
GLUT, 129
glutathione, 66, 84, 91
gluteus maximus, 223
glycerol, 123
glycogen, 42, 43, 226
glycolysis, 42, 190, 226
growth factor, 232, 238
growth hormone, 15, 157, 232, 238
guidelines, 63

H

hamstring, 79
heart disease, vii, 124
heart failure, 195, 196, 197, 199, 200, 201
heart rate, xi, xii, 3, 6, 11, 18, 24, 26, 27, 29, 30, 31, 32, 72, 138, 182, 186, 187, 191, 192, 193, 196, 200, 204, 206, 207, 214, 216, 224, 252, 253, 254, 258, 259, 260, 261, 262, 263
heat shock protein, 66
height, vii, 1, 4, 5, 7, 8, 9, 10, 12, 68, 70, 76
hematocrit, 4, 6, 9
hemiparesis, 175
hemisphere, 36
hemodialysis, 73, 75, 78, 82, 89
hemoglobin, 6, 9, 36
heparin, 114
hepatic, ix, 3, 81, 90, 93, 96, 97, 98, 99, 105, 106, 110, 115, 116, 119, 120, 121, 126, 127
hepatocyte(s), 96, 99
heredity, 127
heterogeneity, 97, 120, 240
high blood pressure, 15
high density lipoprotein, 6, 9, 126, 128
hippocampus, 38, 39
hirsutism, 232
homeostasis, 19, 24, 90, 182, 232
homogenous, 13, 153, 258
homovanillic acid, 41
homozygous, 99

hormone(s), 16, 39, 40, 99, 100, 132, 133, 136, 138, 148, 149, 156, 158, 159, 160, 232, 262
host, 241, 242, 243, 244
hydrolysis, 94, 95, 97, 99, 100, 101, 102, 104, 114, 116, 117, 118, 226
hyperemia, 198
hyperglycemia, 122
hyperinsulinemia, 12, 15, 99, 122
hyperlipidemia, 121
hypersensitivity, 153
hypertension, 2, 3, 8, 9, 11, 12, 14, 15, 16, 72, 88, 232
hyperthermia, xii, 252, 253, 263, 264
hypertriglyceridemia, 122, 125
hypertrophy, 144
hyperventilation, 187
hypoglycemia, 133, 139
hypotension, 182
hypothalamus, 39, 41, 42, 43, 44, 49, 50, 51, 132
hypothesis, 16, 19, 33, 38, 44, 49, 65, 66, 70, 71, 78, 81, 85, 106, 114, 134, 139, 143, 144, 147, 152, 160, 169, 173, 174, 195, 243, 264
hypoxia, 66, 230, 253, 263

I

identification, 234
idiopathic, xi, 221, 223, 234, 235
IL-6, 145, 146, 147, 154, 155, 159
immune response, 67
immune system, ix, xi, 131, 132, 221, 222
immunohistochemistry, 120
in situ hybridization, 120
in vitro, 12, 64, 85, 86, 89, 95, 96, 98, 120, 145, 147, 154, 155
in vivo, 42, 58, 59, 64, 95, 96, 98, 99, 100, 101, 102, 114, 115, 116, 120, 122, 123, 125, 126, 129, 160
indication, 4, 170, 172, 224, 230
infant(s), xii, 252, 258
infection, 85
inflamed, 230
inflammation, xi, 67, 85, 89, 90, 221, 231, 232, 236
inflammatory, viii, xi, 61, 62, 67, 147, 152, 221, 222, 227, 228, 229, 230, 231, 234, 235, 236, 237
inflammatory cells, 230
inflammatory disease, 228
inflammatory response, viii, 61, 62, 67, 147
ingestion, 109, 133
inhibitor, 16, 57, 70, 76

insulin, vii, 2, 6, 9, 10, 11, 12, 13, 15, 16, 98, 99, 100, 115, 122, 123, 129, 133, 139, 153, 155, 160, 161, 229, 232, 238, 265
insulin dependent diabetes, 12
insulin resistance, 11, 15, 153, 155, 229
insulin sensitivity, 12, 15, 122, 155
interactions, 51, 88, 139, 166, 198, 242, 246
intercellular, 230
intercellular adhesion molecule (ICAM), 230
interleukin (IL), 145, 146, 147, 154, 155, 159, 176, 177, 178, 228, 229, 230, 236
intestine, ix, 93, 94, 117, 119
intima, 103, 104, 124, 125
intracellular, 12, 13, 42, 99, 114, 145, 148, 149, 152
intravascular, x, 181
intravenous (IV), v, ix, xi, 93, 95, 96, 97, 110, 111, 115, 121, 182, 184, 185, 186, 187, 188, 189, 190, 191, 196, 198
ischemia, 65, 66, 67, 71, 73, 87, 192, 193, 197, 198, 199
ischemic, 66, 124, 198, 200

J

joints, 187, 188, 264
jugular, 41

K

ketone, 116
kidney, 149
kinetic, 157

L

labor, vii
lactate dehydrogenase, 87
lactic acid, 65, 67, 73, 75, 189, 226
laminectomy, 184
Langerhans cells (LC), 126, 157
left ventricle, 184
leptin, 158
lesion(s), 54, 98, 204, 205, 208, 216, 217, 218, 219
leukemia, 15
leukocytes, 67
lifestyle changes, 83
ligaments, 262, 264
line of defense, 245

lipase, 94, 95, 96, 99, 105, 106, 120, 122, 123, 124, 126, 127, 128, 129
lipemia, viii, 93, 103, 105, 106, 107, 109, 110, 112, 113, 114, 115, 116, 117, 118, 119, 121, 124, 125, 126, 127, 128, 129, 130
lipid(s), viii, ix, 4, 12, 42, 55, 61, 62, 63, 64, 65, 67, 68, 69, 70, 73, 75, 76, 77, 78, 79, 83, 85, 86, 87, 89, 90, 91, 93, 94, 95, 96, 97, 99, 100, 103, 104, 105, 110, 117, 118, 122, 123, 124, 125, 126, 128, 129
lipid peroxides, viii, 61, 64, 65, 76, 87, 91
lipolysis, 42, 97, 99, 104, 105, 106, 121, 122, 130
lipoproteins, viii, 86, 93, 94, 95, 96, 99, 103, 104, 118, 119, 120, 121, 122, 124, 125, 127, 128, 129, 130
liver, 86, 94, 96, 97, 99, 102, 105, 115, 116, 117, 118, 120, 121, 155
locus, 39, 99
longevity, 244, 247
low-density lipoprotein (LDL), ix, 62, 85, 89, 90, 93, 94, 95, 96, 97, 99, 103, 104, 106, 121, 122, 124, 127, 129, 130
lumen, 95, 96
lymph, 95
lymphocyte(s), 147, 159, 230, 236
lysine, 141, 159

M

macrophage, 90
magnesium, 84, 91, 226
magnetic resonance imaging (MRI), 225, 228, 231, 235, 236
magnetic resonance spectroscopy (MRS), 190, 228, 234, 235, 236
major histocompatibility complex (MHC), 230, 236
males, 102, 116, 147, 153, 166, 171, 237
mat, vii, 1, 25, 29, 73, 76, 103, 134, 145, 216, 224
matrix, 72
mean, vii, 1, 3, 6, 12, 24, 30, 48, 68, 69, 70, 71, 75, 76, 80, 81, 82, 106, 151, 166, 182, 185, 190, 199, 204, 205, 207, 208, 219, 220, 224
mean arterial pressure, 182, 190, 199
medulla, 41, 42, 43, 44, 49, 50, 51, 183, 190
memory, 25, 30, 35, 36, 37, 39, 44, 48, 53, 54, 57, 60
men, vii, ix, 3, 14, 68, 70, 83, 84, 87, 98, 99, 102, 103, 104, 105, 107, 117, 118, 121, 122, 124, 125, 126, 127, 128, 130, 132, 133, 134, 135, 136, 137, 138, 139, 140, 141, 143, 144, 145, 146, 147, 148,

149, 151, 152, 153, 155, 156, 157, 158, 159, 160, 176, 186, 187, 200, 219
menopause, 153
messenger RNA (mRNA), 91, 95, 100, 114, 132
meta-analysis, 122, 124, 164, 258, 267
metabolic disorder, 3, 105, 119, 155
metabolic syndrome, ix, 15, 132, 158
metabolism, viii, xi, 15, 41, 43, 51, 54, 56, 93, 94, 95, 98, 99, 103, 105, 107, 108, 109, 110, 111, 112, 113, 117, 118, 119, 120, 121, 122, 123, 124, 126, 127, 128, 129, 130, 148, 152, 153, 154, 160, 182, 186, 189, 190, 191, 195, 199, 201, 222, 228, 229, 232, 233, 236
metabolites, 40, 41, 47, 160, 189, 190, 192, 223, 228
methylation, 41
microcirculation, 13
migration, 236, 240, 243, 248
mineralocorticoid, 160
miscarriage, 264
mitochondria, 226, 231
mitral valve, 3
mode, 103, 204
modelling, 175
molecule, 62, 94, 96, 226
monoclonal antibody (mAb), 64
monolayer, 94
mood, 177, 178
morbidity, viii, 2, 61, 62, 153, 222, 229, 264
morphology, 237
mortality, viii, 2, 14, 61, 62, 65, 87, 153, 222, 249
multiple sclerosis (MS), 85, 91, 121, 266
muscle atrophy, 227, 231, 234, 237
muscle biopsy, 223
muscle mass, xi, 221, 227, 228, 229, 233
muscle strain, 190
muscle strength, 84, 178, 222, 228, 232, 237
music, 164, 172
myelin, 189
myocardial infarction, 72, 78, 90, 105, 122, 125, 126, 127
myocardium, 194, 195
myocyte, 232
myofibril, 67
myogenesis, 228, 236
myoglobin, 86
myopathy, xi, 221, 222, 232, 233, 235, 237, 238
myosin, 173
myositis, 222, 230, 231, 237

N

NADH, 66, 226
nausea, 43
necrosis, 222, 228, 229, 232, 236
nerve, 16, 22, 39, 182, 184, 185, 186, 187, 188, 189, 190, 198, 199, 201
nerve fibers, 184, 186, 187, 188, 189
neurogenic, 133
neuroimaging, 55, 60
neuromuscular diseases, 223
neurons, x, 39, 41, 50, 52, 132, 181
neurotransmitter(s), viii, 17, 35, 39, 40, 41, 42, 43, 47, 48, 50, 52, 53, 58
neurovascular, 199
neutrophils, 67
nitric oxide synthase, 84, 91
node, 192, 198
non-insulin dependent diabetes, 12
norepinephrine (NE), viii, 6, 9, 10, 16, 17, 39, 40, 41, 42, 43, 44, 46, 47, 49, 51, 54, 55, 157, 192
nucleic acid, 62
nucleotide, 228
nucleus, 39, 132, 190
nutrients, 62, 244, 263
nutrition, vi, 239, 244, 248

O

obesity, vii, ix, 74, 76, 89, 117, 122, 130, 132, 152, 153, 154, 155, 156, 158, 160, 161, 229, 232, 233, 265
obsessive-compulsive disorder, 56
occlusion, 66, 87, 184
old age, xii, 239
organ, 186
organism, ix, 39, 131, 132
osteoporosis, vii, 232
overweight, 76, 233
oxidation, 43, 67, 85, 89, 91, 106, 110, 113, 114, 116
oxidative damage, 81
oxidative stress, viii, 61, 62, 63, 65, 66, 67, 69, 70, 71, 73, 76, 79, 81, 83, 84, 85, 86, 87, 88, 89, 90, 91
oxygen, xi, 11, 13, 23, 65, 66, 67, 85, 88, 190, 200, 203, 205, 208, 225, 226, 227, 230, 231, 233, 235, 237, 261, 262, 263

P

pain, 88, 186, 188, 199, 261, 262, 265, 267
paralysis, 187
parasympathetic, 174, 183, 192, 197, 198, 199, 201
parasympathetic nervous system, 174
parenchymal cell, 101
parietal cortex, 36
pathogenesis, viii, ix, 14, 61, 62, 73, 93, 103, 154, 230, 238
pathogenic, 236
pathology, ix, 132, 153, 155
pathophysiology, 12, 222
pedal, 48
pelvic, 265, 268
percutaneous, 66
perfusion, 13, 195, 196, 200
perinatal, 264
peripheral nervous system, 40, 42
persuasion, 175
pH, 4, 51, 72, 190, 199, 201
phagocytosis, 67
phenotype, 99, 122, 127
phenylalanine, 40
phosphate(s), 73, 188, 223, 226, 228
phospholipids, 94, 95, 96, 105, 119
phosphorylation, 236
physical activity, xii, 30, 55, 59, 66, 81, 107, 112, 135, 177, 229, 244, 248, 249, 252, 253, 254, 257, 258, 263, 264, 267
physical training, 2, 12, 15, 57, 195, 231, 237, 258, 266
physiology, 53, 123, 138, 156, 234, 236, 238, 263, 267
physiopathology, 135
pituitary gland, 158
placebo, 57, 109, 112, 165, 167
placenta, 256, 262, 263, 264
placenta previa, 256
placental abruption, xii, 252
plasma, vii, viii, xi, 2, 4, 6, 9, 10, 11, 12, 13, 16, 17, 41, 42, 43, 44, 46, 47, 54, 55, 57, 58, 63, 64, 65, 66, 67, 69, 72, 76, 77, 83, 84, 86, 87, 88, 89, 90, 91, 93, 94, 95, 96, 97, 99, 101, 102, 103, 104, 105, 106, 107, 109, 110, 111, 113, 114, 115, 116, 117, 118, 119, 120, 121, 122, 124, 125, 126, 127, 128, 129, 131, 132, 133, 134, 135, 137, 138, 139, 142, 144, 145, 148, 152, 154, 156, 157, 159, 204, 206, 213, 216, 219, 262, 267
plasma levels, 67, 95, 125, 126, 159
plasma membrane, 4
plasma proteins, 148
plasticity, 145, 147, 152, 194, 196
platelet(s), 12, 64, 86, 90
polymorphism, 95, 99, 119
polymyositis, 225, 231, 232, 234, 235, 236, 237
polyunsaturated fatty acids, 64, 85, 86
pons, 40
population, xii, 55, 73, 106, 124, 149, 189, 204, 205, 214, 216, 218, 222, 231, 233, 239, 240, 241, 242, 245, 246, 247, 248, 249, 265
postnatal, 265
potassium, 6, 9, 188, 189
precursor cells, 160
prednisone, 231, 237
pregnancy, xii, 251, 252, 253, 254, 255, 256, 257, 258, 259, 261, 262, 263, 264, 265, 266, 267, 268
preterm delivery, 264
prevention, 2, 11, 13, 15, 91
primate, 54
probe, 138
prognostic, 254
progression, ix, 93, 103, 104, 125, 217
proliferation, 37, 81, 153
promoter, 95, 114, 119
protein, xii, 67, 85, 88, 94, 95, 96, 98, 101, 102, 114, 119, 121, 123, 127, 129, 134, 221, 228, 229, 232, 234
protein synthesis, 134, 228
proteins, 62, 63, 66, 100, 126, 159
proximal, 232
public health, viii, 61, 65, 76, 152
pulmonary, 87, 185
pulse, 261, 263
purine, 228

Q

quadriceps, 223
quality of life, 229, 247

R

RA, 14, 120, 159, 196, 198, 200, 219, 236, 266, 267
race, ix, 87, 114, 115, 131, 138, 204, 246
rash, xi, 221, 222
reactive oxygen, 62, 88
reagents, 6

receptor(s), x, 12, 16, 42, 70, 74, 76, 81, 96, 97, 98, 99, 106, 120, 121, 122, 129, 148, 153, 159, 181, 183, 184, 188, 189, 197, 199, 232
rectal, 206, 214, 219
rectal temperature, 206, 214
red blood cell(s), 64, 89
reflexes, xi, 169, 182, 184, 188, 198
regeneration, 67
regression, 6, 34, 45, 46, 103
regulators, 114
renin, 6, 9, 10
replication, 74, 75
respiration, 66
respiratory, x, 3, 15, 18, 39, 63, 64, 66, 67, 181, 182, 185, 187, 197, 199, 223, 224, 227, 263
respiratory failure, 63
respiratory rate, 18, 39, 263
response, viii, ix, 4, 32, 36, 37, 38, 39, 41, 47, 48, 50, 51, 54, 58, 60, 62, 67, 72, 73, 76, 77, 81, 82, 83, 84, 87, 103, 106, 107, 108, 110, 111, 112, 113, 114, 115, 116, 117, 127, 130, 132, 133, 134, 139, 141, 143, 145, 149, 153, 154, 155, 156, 157, 158, 159, 174, 177, 182, 184, 185, 186, 187, 188, 189, 190, 191, 192, 193, 194, 195, 196, 197, 198, 199, 200, 201, 207, 213, 214, 218, 219, 228, 230, 232, 234, 236, 237, 238, 267
reticulum, 95
rhabdomyolysis, 232
rheumatic diseases, 232
rheumatoid arthritis, 79, 230, 236
rhythm, 134, 157, 158
risk, vii, viii, xii, 11, 12, 61, 65, 73, 76, 81, 83, 85, 90, 104, 106, 117, 124, 125, 127, 151, 159, 217, 243, 252, 253, 257, 263, 264, 265
risk factor(s), 11, 106, 117, 124, 125, 159
RNA processing, 119
rodents, 123, 132

S

sadness, 38
saliva, 135, 142, 144, 145, 148, 149, 152, 154, 160, 174
satellite, 67
secrete, 115
secretion, ix, 40, 41, 42, 43, 44, 49, 50, 51, 94, 95, 96, 98, 99, 114, 115, 116, 118, 119, 123, 129, 132, 133, 134, 135, 137, 138, 139, 141, 143, 145, 147, 150, 152, 153, 154, 155, 156, 157, 158, 161

sedentary, xii, 14, 83, 84, 107, 109, 114, 127, 133, 134, 135, 137, 138, 139, 140, 141, 142, 143, 145, 147, 148, 149, 152, 156, 218, 233, 252, 267
selective serotonin reuptake inhibitor, 56
self-efficacy, 166, 175
sensitivity, ix, xii, 12, 132, 138, 139, 141, 143, 144, 145, 147, 148, 152, 153, 154, 155, 158, 159, 160, 240
septum, 39
serotonin, 39, 54, 56, 57, 58, 188, 265
serum, 6, 9, 64, 66, 73, 75, 83, 86, 87, 89, 95, 111, 125, 128, 133, 160, 174, 228
short-term memory, 28, 30, 53
side effects, 232, 233
simulation, 57
sinus, 176, 192, 198
sinus arrhythmia, 176
skeletal muscle(s), xi, 84, 85, 87, 88, 90, 96, 100, 101, 102, 113, 114, 123, 128, 129, 182, 184, 188, 195, 196, 197, 198, 199, 200, 201, 221, 222, 227, 229, 231, 232, 234, 236, 237, 238, 254, 263
skin, xi, 187, 188, 203, 204, 206, 207, 209, 210, 211, 212, 215, 216, 217, 218, 219, 221, 222, 232, 263
skinfolds, 205
small intestine, 94, 119
smoking, 72, 73, 241
smooth muscle cells, 104
SNS, 41, 43, 50, 51
soleus, 185, 186
solution, 4, 165, 170
somatic, 18, 178, 201
species, 62, 71, 88, 104, 105, 106, 126, 143
specificity, 64, 206
sphygmomanometer, 4
spina bifida, 215
spinal cord, xi, 182, 184, 185, 188, 190, 197, 203, 204, 205, 206, 208, 209, 210, 211, 213, 215, 216, 217, 218, 219, 220
spinal cord injury, xi, 203, 204, 205, 209, 210, 211, 213, 215, 216, 218, 219
spindle, xi, 182, 186, 197
splanchnic, 96, 118, 130, 193, 195
spontaneous abortion, 255
sports, 20, 21, 55, 57, 164, 166, 167, 175, 176, 205, 206, 263
standard deviation, 68, 70, 75, 80, 151, 224
steady state, xi, 24, 34, 49, 51, 203, 206, 214
stenosis, 78
steroid(s), xii, 159, 221, 231, 232, 234, 238
stigma, 246

stimulus, ix, 37, 60, 131, 133, 175, 227
strain, x, xi, 48, 135, 181, 189, 204, 214, 216, 217, 218
striae, 232
striatum, 40, 58
stroke, vii, xi, 182, 187, 192, 193, 195, 196, 197, 198, 216, 231, 261, 262, 263
stroke volume, xi, 182, 187, 192, 193, 195, 196, 197, 198, 216, 231, 261, 262, 263
structural gene, 99
structural protein, 94
style, 230
subcutaneous (SC), 100, 101, 102, 118, 119, 123, 126, 153
sweat, xi, 18, 39, 204, 215, 216
sympathetic nervous system, 16, 173, 174
symptom, 72, 73, 195, 222, 232
syndrome, 151, 160
synergistic, 112
synovial tissue, 230
systolic pressure, 185, 262

T

T cell, 147
T3, xi, 203, 204, 205, 208
T4, 205
tendon, x, 181, 185, 186, 187
teratogen, 253, 263, 267
testosterone, 134, 158
thalamus, 38, 39
thallium stress test, 72, 88
therapeutic targets, 124
thoracic, 95
threatened abortion, 255
threshold, vii, 1, 3, 15, 31, 44, 49, 54, 57, 58, 65, 106, 133, 158, 185, 190
tissue(s), x ix,, 41, 63, 64, 66, 69, 84, 85, 86, 94, 96, 100, 101, 102, 105, 114, 118, 119, 120, 123, 132, 136, 138, 145, 148, 149, 152, 153, 154, 155, 158, 159, 160, 181, 189, 207, 2 215, 24, 230, 234, 236, 259, 260, 263
tissue perfusion, 66
tobacco smoke, 62
tonic, 38
total cholesterol, 9
transection, 218, 220
transfer, 31, 32, 35, 37, 43, 47, 95, 105, 119, 125, 126, 127, 215, 263
transformation, 54

transforming growth factor (TGF), 125, 230, 236
translocation, 96, 123
trauma, 253, 263
treatment, xii, 2, 11, 15, 28, 45, 56, 216, 221, 232, 234, 242, 245, 265, 266
triceps, 174, 206
triglycerides, 119, 129
tryptophan, 40, 42, 53, 54
tumor, 227, 236
tumor necrosis factor (TNF), 159, 227, 228, 229, 230, 234, 236
tympanic membrane, 220
type 2 diabetes, 124, 127, 129
tyrosine, 40, 42, 43
tyrosine hydroxylase, 40, 42

U

ultrasound, 103
uniform, 42
unilateral, 170
unmasking, 159
unstable angina, 85
uric acid, 87
urine, 13, 148, 149
uterus, 253, 254, 262, 263

V

vascular, ix, xi, 91, 101, 120, 125, 131, 132, 182, 183, 184, 187, 191, 192, 193, 194, 198, 230, 262
vascular cell adhesion molecule (VCAM), 230
vasculitis, 228
vasoconstriction, 183, 192, 193, 195, 201
vasodilation, 182
vasopressin, 132, 141, 143, 156, 159
vegetables, 62
VEGF expression, 234
vein, 41, 95, 206
venipuncture, 4
venous, 41, 193, 206, 207, 231
ventilation, 185, 197, 201, 262
ventricle, 185
venules, 230, 236
very low density lipoprotein (VLDL), ix, 90, 93, 94, 96, 97, 98, 99, 104, 105, 107, 110, 114, 115, 116, 118, 120, 121, 122, 125, 126, 130
vesicles, 42
vessel(s), 78, 192, 230, 236

viral infection, 147
vital, 264
vitamin(s), 67, 68, 72, 73, 74, 83, 86, 87, 89, 90, 244
vitamin C, 84
vitamin E, 67, 83, 86, 87, 89, 90

W

walking, 2, 3, 12, 15, 32, 69, 108, 109, 110, 111, 112, 113, 128, 195, 217, 258
weakness, 222, 227, 229, 232, 236
weight gain, 264, 265
weight loss, 213
weight ratio, 170
women, vii, xii, 14, 68, 70, 83, 84, 88, 102, 103, 107, 117, 124, 127, 128, 130, 135, 137, 153, 154, 155, 156, 157, 158, 160, 161, 204, 219, 245, 247, 248, 251, 252, 253, 254, 255, 257, 258, 259, 262, 263, 264, 265, 266, 267, 268

Y

yeast, 62
young adults, 99, 107, 128, 231